THE
BRAIN BOOSTING DIET
FEED YOUR MEMORY

by NORENE GILLETZ
and EDWARD WEIN, PhD

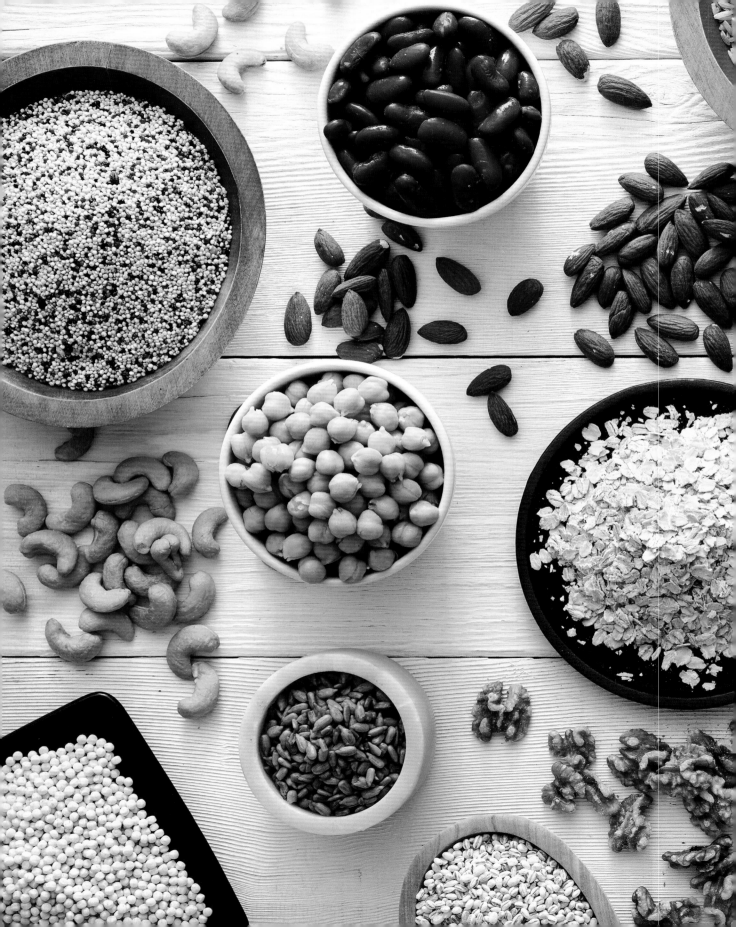

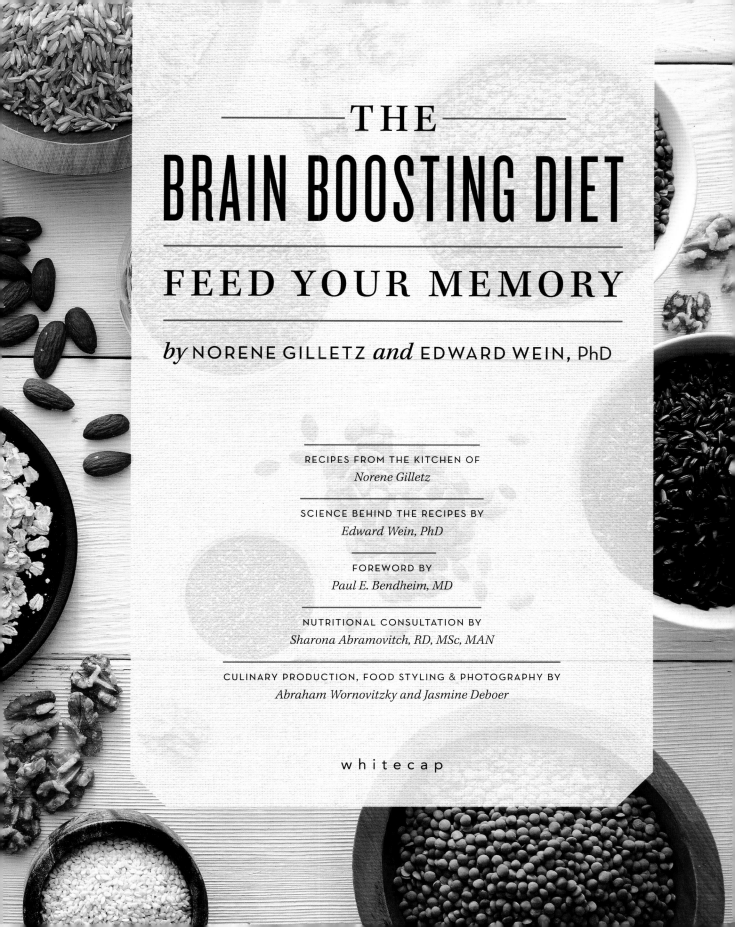

THE
BRAIN BOOSTING DIET
FEED YOUR MEMORY

by NORENE GILLETZ *and* EDWARD WEIN, PhD

RECIPES FROM THE KITCHEN OF
Norene Gilletz

SCIENCE BEHIND THE RECIPES BY
Edward Wein, PhD

FOREWORD BY
Paul E. Bendheim, MD

NUTRITIONAL CONSULTATION BY
Sharona Abramovitch, RD, MSc, MAN

CULINARY PRODUCTION, FOOD STYLING & PHOTOGRAPHY BY
Abraham Wornovitzky and Jasmine Deboer

whitecap

EDITOR AND PROOFREADER Patrick Geraghty
DESIGN Andrew Bagatella
CULINARY PRODUCTION, FOOD STYLING & PHOTOGRAPHY BY Abraham Wornovitzky and Jasmine Deboer

Library and Archives Canada Cataloguing in Publication

Title: The brain boosting diet : feed your memory / by Norene Gilletz and Edward Wein, PhD.
Names: Gilletz, Norene, author. | Wein, Edward, author.
Description: Includes bibliographical references and index.
Identifiers: Canadiana 2019018339X | ISBN 9781770503212 (softcover)
Subjects: LCSH: Memory disorders—Diet therapy. | LCSH: Memory—Nutritional aspects. |
    LCSH: Brain—
    Diseases—Nutritional aspects. | LCSH: Memory disorders—Prevention. | LCSH:
    Brain—Degeneration—
    Prevention. | LCGFT: Cookbooks.
Classification: LCC RC394.M46 G55 2019 | DDC 641.5/63—dc23

We acknowledge the financial support of the Government of Canada through the Canada Book Fund (CBF) for our publishing activities and the Province of British Columbia through the Book Publishing Tax Credit.

Nous reconnaissons l'appui financier du gouvernement du Canada et la province de la Colombie-Britannique par le Book Publishing Tax Credit.

7 6 5 4 3 2 1
Printed in South Korea through Four Colour Print Group, Louisville, Kentucky, USA

For our families and future generations.

A small contribution to help those

at risk of cognitive decline.

FOREWORD

Paul E. Bendheim, MD
Clinical Professor of Neurology
University of Arizona College of Medicine - Phoenix

Founder, BrainSavers® - *The Fitness Program to Remember*™
Author of *The Brain Training Revolution: A Proven Workout for Healthy Brain Aging*

Let food BE thy medicine and medicine your food
—Hippocrates

Who does not relish a tasty meal or invigorating midday snack? Who does not know the importance of healthy nutrition for virtually all aspects of health and healthful aging? On the other hand, who in North America is not bombarded with endless marketing advertisements about the "miraculous" benefits of this particular berry, beverage, or brain supplement? Given the constant, never-ending, and changing advice from so many so-called experts and marketing professionals, how is the concerned consumer to decide what to buy and how to consume it? How can we be certain that a certain ingredient, whole food, snack, or meal is health-promoting?

The role of diet and nutrition in preventing and mitigating many chronic diseases is being increasingly recognized as critically important for good health and a resilient brain. Although many specific foods and nutrients have been identified for their functional activities, the accumulating evidence is that it is the whole diet with all its varied components and their interactions that really makes the difference.

Nutritional science is formidably complex due to the number and interactions of all the foods and their constituent components. There are estimated to be up to 350,000 plant species on planet earth, of which at least 50,000 are edible. There are an estimated 3000 fish, 10,000 bird, and 5000 mammal species in total. Of course, we humans don't eat from all species, but you understand where I am going. Each natural, edible food has innumerable proteins, carbohydrates, fats (collectively the macronutrients), and minerals and vitamins (micronutrients). These macro- and micro nutrients have evolved and our bodies have co-evolved with them over millions of years to extract maximum nutritional and thus health benefits from natural foods (unadulterated foods that nature provides). Unraveling the composition and mechanisms of actions involved from digestion to organ destination, then to structural contributions and metabolic activities, of the nutrients in a single food is a herculean undertaking.

Fortunately, Dr. Ed Wein and Norene Gilletz have come to our aid. They have taken a grounded-in-science and practical approach in developing and presenting the *Brain Boosting Diet: Feed Your Memory*. In this book you will find a comprehensive yet understandable description of the dos and don'ts of eating well for your brain and, in fact, for your whole body. Michael Pollan wrote about the unfortunate path North Americans have taken in our movement away from "food" and into "nutritionism"—our obsession with extracting nutrients and repackaging them as processed, often unrecognizable edibles. Ed and Norene are making an invaluable contribution in teaching how to reverse this unfortunate and unhealthy trend by moving us back to real food, with the inclusion of 200 delicious and easy-to-prepare recipes.

Dr. Ed Wein, an experienced and deeply knowledgeable nutritional scientist, presents here a comprehensive treatise on multiple aspects of nutrition as it relates to the brain, and his section is packed full of the latest science regarding nutrition and the brain. Dr. Ed's contributions are replete with nutritional facts as currently understood and debated. For those readers who wish to understand the science behind the many recipes, the first part of this book will serve as an excellent resource. This is particularly true for those with a particular interest or question about the critical nutrients and foods required for maximizing memory and cognitive functions, and reducing the risk of Alzheimer's disease and other dementias.

Norene's recipes are creative and easy to follow, and you will savor the tasty and nutritional results. She employs ingredients that are easily obtainable and easy to prepare, and, importantly, the resulting dishes are simply delicious. There is nutritional science infrastructure in these recipes. In a delightful compendium to the recipes, "Dr. Ed" adds comments on the brain-health benefits of Norene's ingredients.

As I have written previously, "What is brain-healthy food? Food that you find in gardens, fields, orchards, rivers and seas. The less processed it is, the better it is for you." And as Dr. Jeff Victoroff wrote: "Eat right, exercise some. Break free of the chains of obesity, return to the virtues of our ancient dietary heritage, take the time to enjoy a good meal, and the time to enjoy the active life that meal makes possible. These are some of the most powerful things you can do to unleash the amazing potential of your brain." *The Brain Boosting Diet: Feed Your Memory* is an invaluable contribution to this movement back to natural, healthy nutritional practices.

Ed and Norene's book belongs on every health-conscious individual's kitchen cookbook shelf. Knowledge, health, taste, and enjoyment are here for your benefit. Savor them.

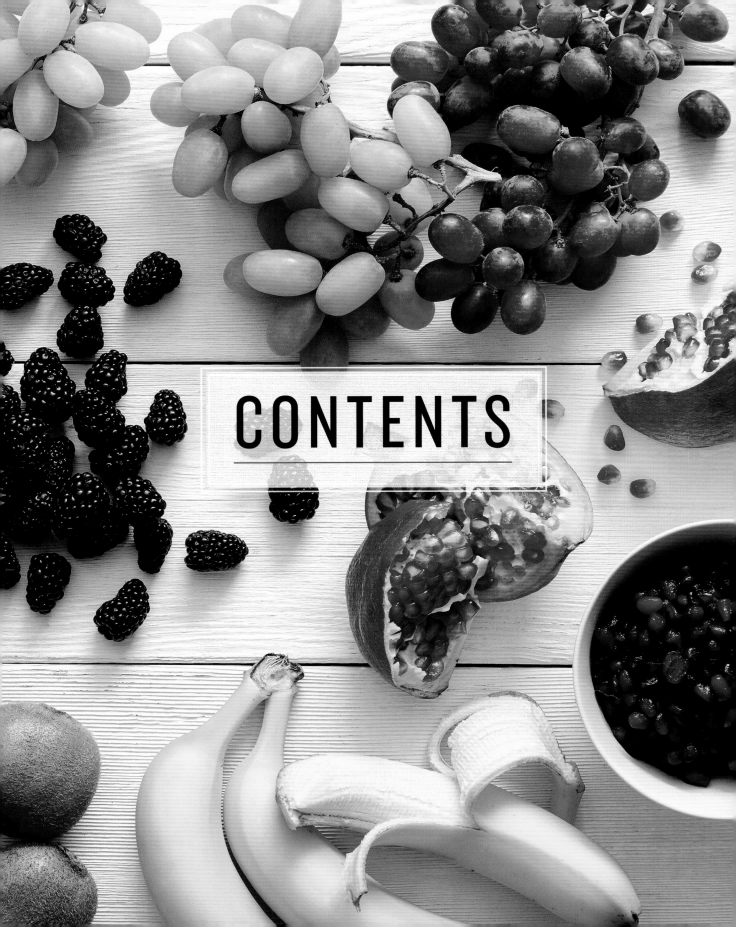

CONTENTS

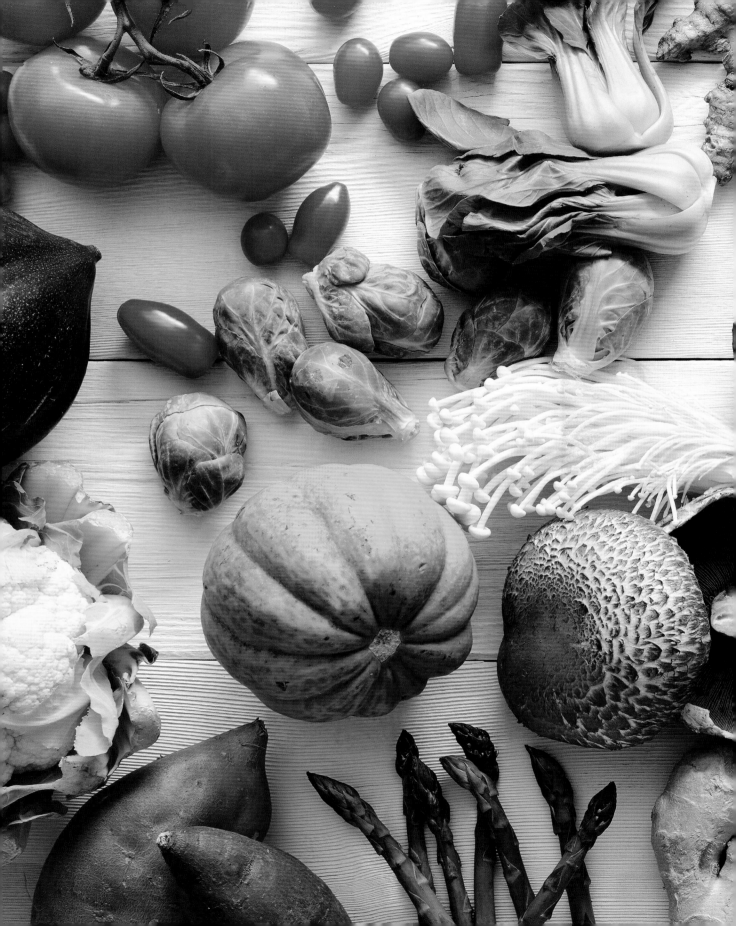

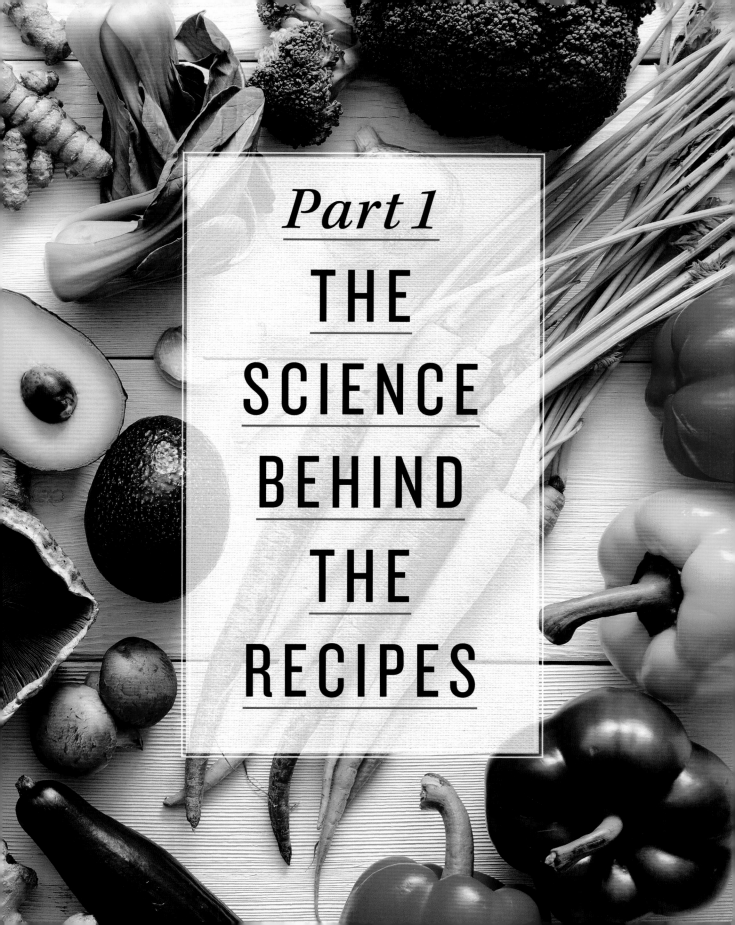

Part 1

THE SCIENCE BEHIND THE RECIPES

1. INTRODUCTION

WHAT IS THIS BOOK ABOUT?

Of all the things I've lost, I miss memory the most
—Mark Twain

In this quote, Mark Twain captures the key concern that people have with memory loss. Although some memory loss is a normal function of aging, too often it is a slippery slope leading to cognitive impairment, and ultimately to Alzheimer's disease (AD) and other dementias. Dementia and AD have many symptoms, but the most common, and the one most people focus on, is memory loss—and for good reason.

Memory is about who you are. It's about your experiences, your beliefs, your relationships, your education and knowledge, your communication with family and those around you. In short, it's about your very identity, because personal identity is defined by individual memory and personal identity determines who you are. So, it's understandable that people fear losing memory the most as they age. We fear losing our awareness of self.

The main purpose of this book is to show the reader how he or she can slow down and reduce the risk of memory loss and the more serious impacts of cognitive impairment, dementia, and AD through diet.

Other books have been published with various techniques for reducing the risk of memory loss, dementia, and AD, including brain exercises, physical exercises, social interaction, diet, and adequate sleep. All these interventions have a significant role to play in maintaining memory.

However, not a lot of books have been published solely on the role of nutrition and brain health, primarily because this is a relatively new field. The result is that nutrition is often an add-on when discussing lifestyle factors that affect the brain (e.g., physical exercise, mental exercise, and social interactions), especially in terms of preventing memory loss and reducing AD/dementia risk, and nutritional messages tend to get diluted, misdirected, or not fully addressed.

This comprehensive book's focus on nutrition and its impact on brain health is an easy-to-read resource for anyone wanting current scientific information in addition to nutritious recipes. We teach our readers ways to "get smart" about nutritional choices, and we suggest recipes to "cook smart" as well.

Our primary focus is on how to use diet and nutrition to help maintain memory and reduce the risk of AD/dementia through smarter food choices and healthier recipes. We discuss our current, generally poor-quality North

American diet and its three deadly sins, identify "good" and "bad" foods with simple scientific explanations, and compare the best current diet plans for brain health. We also go one step further, the end result of which is our own enhanced Brain Boosting Diet plan.

Readers will benefit from our practical "shopping cart," filled with brain-healthy ingredients arranged in order of their nutritional benefit, while our culinary advice ranges from simple, general guidelines on broad categories such as foods to eat and specific food groups and menu plans, to the 200 easy-to-follow recipes with hundreds of culinary and nutritional tips. We have included a section on recommended supplements, as well as appendices and references for those who want more information. Furthermore, because different readers have different needs, we offer alternatives within a brain-healthy diet plan for different dietary needs, whether you're vegan, have celiac disease, or planning a meal for Passover.

Finally, we have incorporated several bonuses for the reader, including supplementary historical, cultural, and scientific comments that accompany the main text. A unique aspect of our book is that we show the reader how to combine and prepare ingredients specifically for their maximum brain benefit—something we have not seen in other books.

Our recipes come complete with nutritional analyses as well as options for individual and small-family serving sizes. Throughout, we recommend using fresh and unprocessed foods whenever possible, and, when using packaged foods, we advise the reader on how to make smart nutritional choices and reduce excessive consumption of available carbohydrates, sugar, and salt.

THE ROLE OF FOOD IN PRESERVING MEMORY

Eat your food as your medicines. Otherwise you have to eat medicines as your food
—Anonymous

The use of food and food ingredients as medicine is a relatively recent phenomenon. Humans have evolved to ingest nutrients to maintain and grow a healthy body, and these nutrients are provided in the foods that we eat. Until the turn of the 20th century, however, the main emphasis was on obtaining sufficient calories, without much concern for nutritional content. There were isolated observations that some foods contained important elements for health—for instance, the discovery by the British in 1762 that citrus fruits on board their ships could prevent scurvy in the crew—but for the most part, people were concerned about where their next meal was coming from rather than its nutrient content. Under these circumstances, adequate nutrition and health could only be achieved through eating sufficient quantities of a variety of foods, a choice that was available for only a small part of the population.

Did You Know? Our human hunter-gatherer ancestors of 10,000 years ago had better nutrition than our farming ancestors until a couple of hundred years ago. This was because they ate a variety of foods they could find, rather than trying to subsist on one or a few farmed crops offering limited nutrition.

As the 20th century dawned with its many technological innovations, there was a greater emphasis put on identifying nutritional factors in foods that contributed to health, well-being, and growth. The term "vitamine" was coined in 1912 as an abbreviation of "vital amine," representing important factors in the diet, even though amines are not relevant to vitamins as we know them today. The first vitamin, thiamine, was isolated in 1913 and used to prevent beriberi (thiamine deficiency). An understanding of the role of minerals such as calcium, which is essential for the development and maintenance of healthy bones and teeth, also began to emerge.

Since those early beginnings, many more vitamins and minerals have been identified and their nutritional roles determined.

Did You Know? Of the thousands of substances involved in human metabolism, only about 50 need to be supplied by the diet. The other compounds can be derived through the metabolic processes of the body.

In addition, other essential nutrients were identified, such as essential fatty acids and essential amino acids. Together with a better understanding of the role of diet and health, technological innovations such as the development of the internal combustion engine and electricity resulted in greater efficiencies in the production of food and corresponding cost reductions. This allowed people to be more selective in their food choices both in taste and health.

The discovery of important nutrients in the diet led to a proactive approach by the US and Canadian governments to add key nutrients to commonly consumed foods, so as to improve the health of the population. It was found that large segments of the population were deficient in certain nutrients due to extensive food processing, food consumption patterns, and local situations. In order to prevent the deficiency diseases that would result, the government initiated programs to fortify commonly used foods.

Starting in 1924, iodine was added to salt to prevent goiter. In the 1930s, vitamin D was added to milk to prevent rickets. In 1940, a standard was enacted for enriched flour that specified the addition of iron (to prevent anemia) along with thiamine (to prevent beriberi), and riboflavin and niacin (to prevent pellagra).

Fortification has continued to improve over the years due to actions of both the federal government and other groups, such as the American Public Health Association, the Council on Food and Nutrition of the American Medical Association, the Food and Nutrition Board of the National Research Council, and the National Academy of Sciences. The most recent fortification legislation in 1996 required the addition of folic acid to foods such as grains and cereals to prevent neural tube defects in infants.

That was good progress, but keep in mind that all these actions were taken to ensure we have a nutritional profile in our diet that is sufficient for normal health and growth. What it didn't consider was the use of food and food ingredients beyond basic nutritional needs to prevent, treat, and mitigate disease. That started about 40 years ago, with research looking at food components that hurt the body, such as saturated fats, trans fats, and sugars, but also looking at food components such as antioxidants, Omega-3 fish oils, and anti-cancer agents that have helped stave off chronic disease and maintain normal body function.

In 1980, the US Department of Agriculture (USDA) and the Federal Department of Health and Human Services (HHS) started issuing a major document called Dietary Guidelines for Americans, visible at http://health.gov/dietaryguidelines/2015/.

Did You Know? The dietary guidelines were an attempt by the government to condense and focus all the confusing and multisource dietary advice being issued prior to the guidelines, and to give them a stamp of authority and credibility.

This document is reviewed and revised every five years to incorporate new scientific information. It provides science-based advice on how you can use your diet to promote health and reduce the risk of chronic disease.

It also forms the basis for the many dietary and health publications, as well as the recommendations of both governmental and non-governmental organizations.

Most of the guidelines for using diet to maintain health and reduce the risk of disease have focused on the usual-suspect diseases: heart disease, cancer, and diabetes. However, more recently, probably because of the aging population, there has been a lot of work done relating diet to prevention of memory loss and brain diseases such as Alzheimer's disease (AD) and other dementias. Very significant data have been developed on how diet and dietary components can reduce memory loss and the risk of dementia and AD, both by eliminating certain food components that harm, and by incorporating those food components that are beneficial. As will be seen later in this book, these changes can even slow down cognitive decline by 30–90%, depending on food choices and the age at which you start a brain-healthy diet.

Did You Know? Most diet-based studies on populations above 60 years of age show risk reductions with appropriate diets such as the MED or MIND diets, of about 30%-50%. One major study in Finland in 2014, however, had a 90% risk reduction, but the average age of the participants was considerably lower (50 years of age).

The key is to start early—the best time to prevent Alzheimer's and other dementias is before symptoms such as severe memory loss start to appear. Therein lies the thrust of this book—to show the reader how he or she can manipulate his or her diet at a level of their choice to minimize memory loss and the threat of dementia and AD.

2. MEMORY LOSS AND COGNITIVE DECLINE (AND WHAT YOU CAN DO ABOUT IT)

Not all people with memory loss have AD/dementia, but most people with AD/dementia will experience significant memory loss.

Dementia is a collection of brain disorders that results in a decline in reasoning ability and memory to the extent that it affects daily living. Alzheimer's disease (AD) is the most common form of dementia, representing 45–80% of all dementia, and memory loss is the most common symptom.

The incidence of AD is double what it was 20 years ago. Age is the most important factor—the older you are, the greater your likelihood of being diagnosed with AD. One in nine people aged 65 and older has Alzheimer's. For those who are 75 and over, approximately 40% suffer from AD. There is currently no known reversal or cure.

Did You Know? A report in 2014 found that in the period 2002-2012, 244 compounds were tested for AD with a 99.6% failure rate towards preventing, curing, or improving symptoms of the disease. Only one drug was approved in this time period.

According to the Alzheimer's Association, an estimated 5.7 million Americans are currently suffering from AD, out of which approximately 5.5 million are 65 and over. The total number of Americans with AD is expected to rise to 14 million by 2050. According to the Alzheimer's Association of Canada, there are approximately 564,000 Canadians living with AD and other forms of dementia, and this number is expected to increase to 937,000 by 2033. Worldwide, current estimates are that 44 million people, mostly over 60, are living with AD and other forms of dementia, and that by 2050 this figure is projected to increase to 131.5 million. The Alzheimer's Association (www.alz.org) estimates that more than 15 million caregivers have provided more than 18.1 billion hours of unpaid care for AD/dementia patients.

AD not only debilitates, it also kills. It is the sixth leading cause of death in the US and the fifth leading cause for people age 65 and older. The death rate from AD has increased by 71% from 2000 to 2015, compared to a significant reduction in mortality for other diseases (e.g., heart disease deaths, which have declined by 14% in the same period). The risk of developing AD is almost double for women.

Did You Know? Canadian data shows that 71% of AD patients are women—perhaps partially because they live longer than men.

As mentioned in the previous section, dementia is a collection of brain disorders of which AD is the most prevalent. A summary of the most common forms of dementia is shown in Table 1.

Table 1. Types of dementia.

Type of Dementia	Prevalence	Symptoms
Alzheimer's disease (AD)	45–80%	**Early symptoms** are short term memory lapses, apathy, and depression. **Later symptoms** include impaired communication and judgment, disorientation, confusion, and behavior changes. Swallowing, walking, and speaking impairment usually happen near the end.
Vascular dementia	10–15%	**Early symptoms** are impairment of executive functions such as planning, organizing, and decision-making, as well as mood changes such as depression and apathy. **Later symptoms** may include deficiencies in language, communication, and memory, as well as increased confusion and behavioral changes such as aggression and unacceptable social behavior.
Mixed dementia	10%	**Symptoms** can be a combination of the symptoms of the most common dementia forms, as several dementias may exist simultaneously.
Lewy body dementia	4–5%	**Early symptoms** are likely to include motion problems, hallucinations, and sleep disturbances. **Later symptoms** can include cognitive and memory impairment similar to AD.

Each of the dementias has somewhat different symptom patterns, as shown in Table 1, and these, along with imaging tests and biomarker analysis, enable classification of the dementias.

The first thing we notice about Table 1 is the large variation in prevalence of AD and vascular dementia. The reason for this is that, until relatively recently, clinical diagnosis of the various types of dementia depended on clinical presentation. This included a variety of symptoms such as memory impairment, executive thinking (mental ability to get things done) dysfunction, and language or visual problems.

Because clinical diagnosis is difficult to standardize across different geographical locations, and because dementia can simultaneously be a mixture of different types, we end up with a range of prevalence from different sources for the major dementia types. However, with modern technological techniques, diagnosis is getting better.[1]

Currently, doctors diagnose dementia with a combination of clinical presentation and imaging techniques such as PET and MRI. These identify the presence of biomarkers, such as beta amyloid, tau protein, and hippocampus volume, which can be used as diagnostic tools. In the near future, the use of these and other biomarkers will enable us to diagnose dementia even before clinical symptoms appear.[2]

The most common form of dementia by far is AD, followed by vascular dementia. For this reason, most treatment studies have been carried out on these two targets.

Each form of dementia has somewhat different symptom patterns, as shown in Table 1, and these, along with imaging tests and biomarker analysis, enable classification of the dementia.

For AD, the usual microscopic, pathological characteristics are a build-up of specialized proteins called beta amyloid (outside the brain neurons) and tau (inside the neurons), and there appears to be a correlation between the extent of this build-up and the severity of the AD. These protein clumps choke off the neurons and eventually kill them. As diagnostic techniques improve in identifying these and other markers of AD, doctors will be able to identify the disease at very early stages before symptoms appear, which bodes well for treating AD.

For vascular dementia, as the name implies, the causes are problems with the blood vessels in the brain. Any pathology of these blood vessels can lead to dementia because they result in a lack of blood to neurons, which then die. The pathology can include constriction of the vessels, which occurs in atherosclerosis, and stroke caused by blood clots, or by the rupturing and bleeding of arteries. AD and vascular dementia seem intricately linked and often times both pathologies exist together. Amazingly, a paper published in late 2016 found for the first time that patients with AD and heart disease actually had beta amyloid bodies in their heart tissue.[3] This could mean that AD results in heart disease or vice versa.

Lewy body dementia (LBD) is characterized by abnormal accumulation of a protein called alpha synuclein in neurons. It is thought that these clumps of protein result in dementia because they interfere with the production of neurotransmitters. Interestingly, the same Lewy bodies are also present in Parkinson's disease.

Did You Know? The difference between Parkinson's disease and dementia is that the Lewy bodies accumulate in different regions of the brain for each disease.

Many dementias are combinations of several types of dementia, making them more difficult to diagnose and characterize. In a 2016 study on Medicare and Medicaid patients in the US, it was found that 93% of all dementia diagnoses were for dementia not otherwise specified.[4] Lack of specific diagnosis can hinder treatment; it has been found that the type of mixed dementia a patient has will determine the rapidity with which cognition will decline. In a paper published in November 2016, it was found that the fastest progression of AD was when it was combined with Lewy body dementia, and the slowest progression was when it was combined with vascular dementia.[5]

LIFESTYLE RISK FACTORS FOR AD/DEMENTIA

Although we know that the most common forms of dementia are due to various pathologies in the brain, we also now know that lifestyle has a great impact on the probability of getting dementia. Two papers, published by *The Lancet Neurology* in 2011 and 2014, summarized the risks of various lifestyles for development of AD/dementia.[6,7] Some risk factors were not included. For example, the risk of having the genetic variant APOE4 was not included because it was not a lifestyle factor and cannot be controlled. As well, certain lifestyle risk factors, such as diet, use of statins, impact of social support, and others, were also not included due to a lack of data.

A summary of the key risk factors and how they increase the risk of getting AD/dementia is summarized in Table 2, based on combining the results of both of these key papers.

Table 2. Lifestyle risk factors for AD/dementia.

Risk Factor	Relative Increased Risk of Dementia (%)	Relative Increased Risk of AD (%)	Comments
Physical inactivity	39	82	Lower risk of dementia overall than of AD.
Depression	80	65	Risk is much higher for late-life depression than for midlife depression.
Smoking	16	59	Lower risk of dementia overall than of AD.
Midlife hypertension	61	n/a	In later life, hypotension either resulting naturally or from meds increases the risk of dementia overall.
Midlife obesity	60	59	In later life, being underweight is a greater risk factor.
Cognitive inactivity	40.0	59	
Diabetes	47	46	
Poor diet*	30–90	30–90	Based on a comparison of Mediterranean-type and non-Mediterranean-type diets.**

*Although diet was recognized as a significant risk factor in this paper,[6] it was not included at the time of publication due to a lack of data. We have now included this risk factor based on extensive recent studies and will define "poor diet" in the following sections of the book.

**The risk factor for diet varies quite widely based on the foods and population age used for Mediterranean-type diet studies and will be explored more fully in our chapter titled *Pulling it All Together: Menu Plans.*

Considering all the risk factors above and their prevalence in the population, it was determined that more than 50% of all forms of dementia could be avoided or delayed if all lifestyle risk factors were eliminated. The main risk factors are summarized below:

POOR DIET is probably the one biggest determinant of whether an individual will develop AD/dementia due to lifestyle factors. Not only is poor diet a risk factor in itself, but it can also lead to other risk factors. For example, obesity is directly related to a poor diet in that excess empty calories from snacks or junk food are usually to blame as the cause of obesity. Diabetes can also be related to a poor diet in the form of metabolic syndrome or prediabetes, which are often precursors to diabetes and can develop as a result of obesity, excess sugar, or available carbohydrate intake. Finally, it is well known that hypertension can be controlled through diet, by controlling weight, and by increasing vegetable consumption (the DASH Diet, which has many aspects in common with the Mediterranean diet). In the following chapters, our book will demonstrate how to identify a poor diet, as well as the dietary changes needed to minimize the risk of AD/dementia and memory loss due to a poor diet, diabetes, hypertension, or obesity.

DEPRESSION appears to be a significant risk factor for AD/dementia both midlife and in later life, but the risk heightens with age.[8] Although dementia risk increases by 20% for sufferers of midlife depression, it increases by 80% for those who experience it in later life; for vascular dementia, the risk of AD/dementia increases threefold when depression is experienced both in midlife and later life.

There is compelling data that depression should be treated in order to avoid AD/dementia, especially in later life. Treatment for depression helps improve cognitive function in older adults, but some treatments (such as with anticholinergic drugs) can actually reduce cognitive function,[9] so the treatment method should be carefully chosen in conjunction with your doctor.

Did You Know? Aside from anticholinergic drugs, there are several other commonly prescribed drugs that could increase cognitive decline. These include protein pump inhibitors (PPIs), calcium channel blockers, and androgen-depriving drugs.

PHYSICAL INACTIVITY increases the risk of developing both dementia and AD, but the risk seems to be greater for developing AD. It is unclear why this is so, but since vascular dementia is an important determinant of dementia in general, it may be that the vascular disease that controls vascular dementia is relatively independent of physical activity.

There have been many papers published on the benefits of exercise in reducing the risk of dementia, but one published in March of 2016 can serve as a typical example.[10] This article demonstrated that cognitive decline could be reduced in individuals in their mid 60s by the equivalent of 10 years of aging with moderate-to-intense exercise (e.g., running or swimming) as compared to low-level exercise (e.g., walking). Although moderate-to-intense physical exercise was shown to be superior for preventing cognitive decline, even light exercise performed on a regular basis (at least three times per week for 30–60 minutes each time) will have some benefit.

MIDLIFE OBESITY is also a significant risk factor for both AD and dementia, where obesity is defined by a number called body mass index (BMI) that is equal to or greater than 30. What is interesting is that this risk is primarily for midlife obesity, and that, in later life, being underweight actually is a greater risk factor than being overweight. (This may be because being underweight in later life could be the result of poor health of the individual, which in turn can increase the risk of AD/dementia.)

To minimize obesity as a risk factor, a person should control their food intake to maintain a normal BMI for their height. This is especially important during midlife, when the biggest risk seems to occur.

DIABETES is now a well-established risk factor for AD/dementia, with diabetics being up to three times more susceptible to AD/dementia. And it's not just AD/dementia that's affected. According to the National Institute of Health (NIH) in the US, diabetics also have two-to-four times the risk of having a stroke than non-diabetics, and a much-reduced probability of recovering from the stroke. There are a few compelling theories. First, it is well known that people with diabetes have a greater risk of cardiovascular disease than people without diabetes. Because of this, diabetics would therefore seem more prone to vascular dementia than non-diabetics. Another theory is that the brain itself is sensitive to the debilitating effects of high sugar and impaired insulin function. This effect has been dubbed type 3 diabetes, which is exclusive to the brain and can reduce neuronal function leading to AD/dementia.

Did You Know? Although the brain is only 2% of the body mass, it consumes about 25–33% of the calories absorbed.

WHAT WE CAN DO TO HELP REDUCE THE RISK OF AD/DEMENTIA

In the previous section, we touched on the major risk factors for developing AD/dementia; in this section, we will expand on some of the actions we can take to proactively reduce these risks.

The first thing we need to understand is that there are some risk factors we can do little about, and some lifestyle risk factors where we can make a significant difference. These are summarized in Table 3 below.

Table 3. Risk factors that can and can't be changed.

Risk Factors that Can't Be Changed	Risk Factors that Can Be Changed
Age	Diet
Having one or two copies of the APOE4 gene	Depression
Low education level	Physical exercise
Diabetes	Vascular risks (hypertension, high triglycerides, high cholesterol)
	Mental exercise
	Midlife obesity
	Smoking

Note that some of the risk factors that can't be changed can be controlled to some extent. Although having a higher education level relates to a lower risk of AD/dementia (because of increased cognitive reserve), one can compensate for this to some extent through mental exercise. Similarly, although we cannot reverse diabetes, we can control it with drugs and diet so that it does not get worse. Also, the risk factors that can be changed will have an impact not only on healthy individuals, but also on those who have mild cognitive impairment (MCI)—defined by the Mayo Clinic as the stage between the expected cognitive decline that occurs with normal aging and the more-serious decline of dementia.

The World Alzheimer Report 2014 recommends—and subsequent studies have confirmed—a multipronged approach to reducing the risk of AD/dementia by addressing as many of the controllable risk factors as possible. In total, these risk factors represent approximately 50% of all dementia cases. Below, we'll look at the individual risk factors and what we can do to minimize them. This summary is based on a thorough review of intervention strategies published in 2017 by Gopalkumar Rakesh et al.[11]

DEPRESSION: This is a major risk factor for AD/dementia. The more frequent and severe the depressive episodes, the greater the risk, not only for healthy adults, but also for those with mild cognitive impairment (MCI). Effective treatment of depression has been shown to reduce negative cognitive outcomes, especially when depressed subjects were also subject to stress.

Did You Know? Depression can also double the risk of death in people with coronary artery disease.

There are several treatment options for depression. Historically, anticholinergic drugs and select serotonin reuptake inhibitors (SSRIs) have been used. However, several recent papers have shown that these drugs can actually worsen cognitive function. A review article published in 2017 demonstrated that antidepressant drugs in general can increase the risk of developing dementia twofold.[12] Therefore, it would be wise to consider non-drug treatments for depression.

Did You Know? Drug antidepressants have also been linked to a significantly increased risk of stroke.

Below, we have highlighted some of the non-drug treatments that can fight depression, whilst also having an impact on other AD/dementia risk factors. This way you can kill two birds with one approach.

- Exercise in itself will reduce the risk of AD/dementia. It will also generate endorphins, which temporarily makes a person feel better, thus alleviating depression. There are also indications that exercise has long-term benefits for reducing depression.
- Foods that have been shown to reduce the risk of AD/dementia have also been shown to alleviate depression. These include B vitamin–rich leafy vegetables (e.g., spinach) and Omega-3 rich fats, such as those found in fish (e.g., salmon and sardines).
- Too little sleep is a risk factor for AD/dementia, but can also aggravate the symptoms of depression.

There are many other interventions that can help with depression, such as cognitive behavioral therapy or other lifestyle changes, though many of these are usually conducted in an environment with professional help.

PHYSICAL EXERCISE: Although there is some inconsistency, the majority of studies have shown a reduced risk of AD/dementia with exercise. Part of the reason for these inconsistencies may be the wide range of different protocols for the exercise programs used in the studies, but some things do stand out:

- Information presented by independent Canadian and Danish studies at the Alzheimer's International Conference in Washington DC in 2015 showed that exercise could improve cognition in people who already had dementia. For individuals with mild vascular dementia, a supervised 60-minute exercise program, three times a week, improved memory and attention. (This group also demonstrated lower levels of depression and anxiety.) In another study from the US, individuals with AD who undertook an exercise program had significantly lower levels of tau proteins, which are implicated in the development of AD.
- It appears that moderate to intense exercise (e.g., running, swimming, aerobics, calisthenics) has more impact than none/light exercise (e.g., walking, yoga). The Northern Manhattan Study found a 10-year difference in age-related cognitive decline between moderate/intense exercise versus none/light exercise.[10] To get into the moderate-to-intense category, an individual had to perform an activity that raised their heart rate for more than a few minutes several times a week.

- The type of exercise may also have an effect, but the results are inconsistent, so the best approach is to participate in as many forms of exercise as possible, including endurance aerobics (e.g., running), high-interval intensity training (e.g., treadmills), and resistance training (e.g., weightlifting). The duration of the exercise regimen also varies widely in the studies, but a minimum of 20–30 minutes twice per week would seem to be in order, with three 60-minute sessions per week also recommended, depending on the capability of the person. The bottom line is to do as much as you can, as often as you can.

Did You Know? Exercise is also inversely related to incidence of stroke, vascular disease, and congestive heart failure.

VASCULAR RISKS: These include contributors to metabolic syndrome, which can lead to diabetes, and include hypertension, high triglycerides, and high cholesterol. Other contributors are high blood sugar, inadequate physical activity, smoking, and an unhealthy diet. It is well established that these factors contribute to cardiovascular health problems such as stroke and heart attacks, but it was also shown in the Northern Manhattan Study that they contribute to cognitive decline.[9] Dr. CB Wright, one of the authors of the study, commented that looking after cardiovascular health also benefits cognitive health. In fact, he and others have shown that reducing these risks can improve symptoms even of mild vascular dementia and MCI. This is partially due to the impact of vascular risk factors on vascular dementia, but it also affects other forms of dementia such as AD. It is of interest that the two biggest vascular risk factors with the biggest effect on cognitive decline are high blood sugar and smoking.

Did You Know? High blood sugar and smoking seem to be implicated in many chronic diseases, including heart disease, cancer, and diabetes.

Steps you can take to minimize vascular risks include drug control for hypertension (ace inhibitors, diuretics, beta blockers, etc.) and statins for cholesterol control. Physical activity has already been discussed, and blood sugar control and diet will be discussed in depth in the sections relating to sugars and diet control. Control of smoking risk is self-evident—stop smoking!

MENTAL EXERCISE: There are many short-term studies showing the benefits of mental exercise, especially structured mental exercises on attenuating cognitive decline in older-age subjects, but one of the most important reviews was published in 2016 in the *American Journal of Psychiatry*.[13] This review assessed 17 randomized control trials (RCT—the best kind of investigation) over a period of 20 years involving 700 participants with mild cognitive impairment (MCI, which increases the risk of developing AD/dementia). It found that computerized cognitive training (CCT), such as Mindfit, Lumosity, Nintendo, Braintrain, and others, led to improvements in cognition, memory, learning, and attention in people with MCI (it even helped reduce symptoms of depression). Unfortunately, the results were not as good for those who already had AD/dementia, though even here there was some improvement for subjects engaged in immersive programs such as Wii or virtual reality games.

If you do not want to use CCT, consider any other type of mental stimulation, such as crossword puzzles, chess, or Sudoku. These may not provide stimulation in all brain functions the same way CCT does, but will likely provide some benefit.

MIDLIFE OBESITY: For most people, this is a function primarily of diet, and therefore will be discussed throughout our book. However, be aware that obesity is not just a risk factor for AD/dementia, but also for heart disease and diabetes, as well as for cancer.

DIET: This will be discussed in the next section in depth. Of all the risk factors for AD/dementia, diet probably has the greatest impact. This is because not only does poor diet alone increase your risk of getting AD/dementia by 30–90% (depending on which study you consider), it also can aggravate some of the other major risk factors. Figure 1 below shows schematically how a poor diet can affect certain major risk factors.

Figure 1. Impact of diet on lifestyle risk factors for AD/dementia.

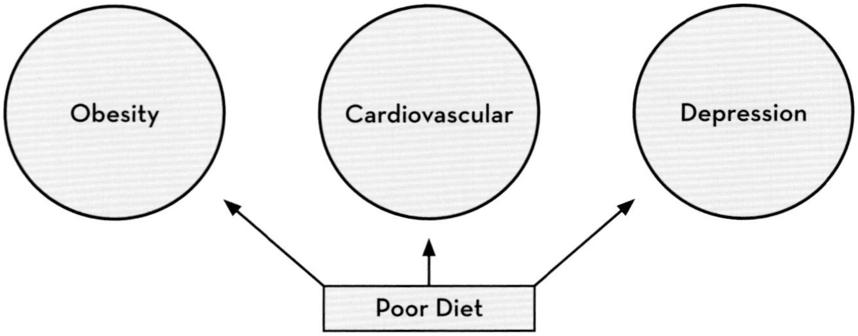

How poor diet affects obesity is relatively straightforward. Our North American diet emphasizes quantity over quality, and with food easily available and thrust on us through clever marketing schemes, it is easy to overeat and become obese. What's more, the food we are urged to buy is often dense in calories and sparse in nutrition.

The impact of diet on cardiovascular risks for AD/dementia is also well known. We tend to eat too much food containing bad elements, such as sugar, salt, and saturated fat, and too little of the good elements, such as fiber, antioxidants, unsaturated fats, and Omega-3 fats. All of this contributes to cardiovascular disease and diabetes, which in turn also contributes to an increased risk of AD/dementia.

3. THE PROBLEMS WITH OUR NORTH AMERICAN DIET: THE THREE DEADLY DIETARY SINS

We have seen in the previous chapter that obesity is a major risk factor for AD/dementia as well as a host of other chronic diseases. Although there are a number of factors that contribute to obesity, including genetics, psychology, depression, and so on, the fundamental reason we gain weight is that we consume more calories than we expend. And it is getting worse. Figure 2 is a dramatization showing portion sizes consumed 50 years ago versus today.

Figure 2. Comparing portion sizes 50 years ago with today.

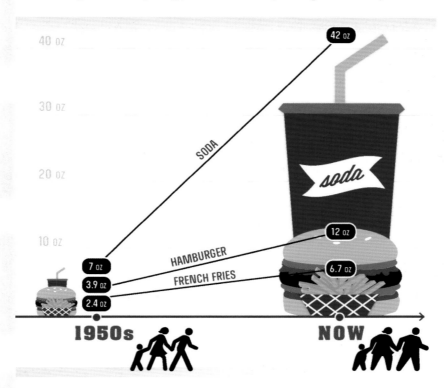

Source: Ellsworth Air Force Base.

The National Heart, Lung, and Blood Institute of the US Department of Health and Human Services has conducted a similar study over a period of 20 years, and some of their data are summarized in Table 4.

Table 4. Comparison of portion sizes 20 years ago versus today.

Food Item	20 Years Ago		Now	
	Calories	Size	Calories	Size
Bagel	140	3" diameter	350	6" diameter
Spaghetti and meatballs	500	1 cup spaghetti + sauce + 3 small meatballs	1025	2 cups spaghetti + sauce + 3 large meatballs
French fries	210	2.4 oz	610	6.9 oz
Turkey sandwich	320		820	

Both of the above studies were carried out several years ago, and there is some variation in portion size depending on the food establishment, but the key takeaway message is that our food portions have increased between two-to-three times in the last 20–50 years. Interestingly enough, although serving sizes have not changed much, the difference between serving size and portion size is getting larger.

The net effect of all this increase in food consumption is that the prevalence of obesity has skyrocketed in North America from 10% of the adult population over 20 in 1990, to 31% in 2017, and it continues to grow despite increased exercise activity. The Center for Disease Control in the US (CDC) estimates that today the total prevalence of overweight individuals and obesity is about 71% of the population. Canada has somewhat lower percentages at 25% for obesity in adults and 62% combined for overweight and obesity, but these are startling numbers that do not bode well for the future.

So why is this happening? There are a number of possible reasons. First and foremost, food is relatively cheap and readily available from all over the world.

Did You Know? There are some professionals who claim that the situation is aggravated by government policy which subsidizes crops such as corn, resulting in an abundance of food of poor nutritional quality.

Secondly, the food industry has developed its marketing skills to such an extent that it knows exactly what is required to get you to buy their products. Unfortunately, what the industry has found is that what people crave are fat, sugar, and salt. So they load up their products with these low-nutrition and obesity-contributing ingredients. On top of that, they have found that big portions sell, and as we have seen in the chart and table above this has resulted in a significant increase in caloric intake.

So how does obesity adversely impact memory and brain health? First, we know obesity is a significant risk factor for cardiovascular disease and diabetes, which themselves are risk factors for AD/dementia. In addition to this, recent studies have shown that obesity can have a directly adverse effect on memory, independent of other risk factors. One study in particular published in 2016 by the Cambridge Center for Ageing and Neuroscience showed that there was less of a type of brain matter called white matter in the brains of obese people as compared with their lean peers, reflecting a brain age difference of 10 years between obese and non-obese people. Researchers at the University of Cambridge showed that non-obese young people performed significantly better on memory tests than their obese counterparts.[1]

A paper published in 2017 attributed the effect of memory loss to inflammation, as measured by C reactive protein (CRP).[2] So, from all aspects, obesity is a major problem for AD/dementia risk.

What We Can Do to Overcome the Deadly Sin of Too Much Food

We eat too much because we eat beyond hunger or physiological need. There are several reasons for this. One reason is that we are constantly exposed to advertising that encourages us to eat more, either because we crave the sugar, fat, and salt contained in much of the processed foods we eat, or because we believe we are getting a bargain by buying super-sized portions. Another reason is that people often eat not because they are hungry, but because they are bored, anxious, or stressed. Finally, we overeat because we don't keep track of what we are eating while we are eating when we are distracted by other activities. This is often called "mindless eating."

With this knowledge in hand, psychologists and researchers have developed some strategies to control our overeating:

- We need to focus on our eating times. Studies have shown that seeing how much food we eat will help reduce our food consumption. So we should try to avoid distracting diversions when we eat. Avoid eating while watching TV, working on a computer, or using your cell phone. Instead, try to set aside a quiet time where you can focus on your food.

- Research has shown that increased portion size correlates to the amount of food eaten. So when eating out, resist going for the super-sized deal and pick the small portion size.
- When you are bored, anxious, or stressed, ask yourself if you are eating because you are hungry, or because you are feeling down. If you suspect that it is not hunger that is driving your eating, then consider other ways to adjust your feelings. Consider going for a walk, contacting a friend or family member, exercising, listening to some music, or reading a book. Before eating always pause a few minutes to ask yourself the real reason for eating.

The above suggestions are just a few of the methods that you can use to control overeating. If they don't work for you then contact a nutritionalist, or you can follow up with other approaches that people have used successfully to lose weight, such as the high-protein-sparing fast diet, the low-carb Atkins diet, or the meal-replacement diet.

An interesting paper from the *Journal of the American Medical Association* (JAMA) in February 2018 showed that as long as a person consumes a healthy diet based on low added sugar, low refined or digestible carbs, and that is low in processed foods, the amount of food is irrelevant for significant weight loss. (More on sugars, refined carbs, and processed foods in the next two sections of this chapter.)

DEADLY SIN #2—TOO MUCH SUGAR AND CARBS

It may sound strange to consider sugar a major risk factor for developing AD/dementia. After all, sugar in the form of glucose is the main energy source for the brain, and the brain uses more glucose than any other organ of the body.

Did You Know? The brain only weighs about 3 lb, but consumes 20% of the body's energy and oxygen.

The problem occurs when the biochemical pathways of the brain are damaged by age or chronic disease in such a way that the brain cannot effectively use all the glucose that is transported across the blood–brain barrier. In such a case, the build-up of unused glucose in the brain can lead to what is now being called type 3 diabetes. In the same way that excessive sugar in the rest of the body leads to insulin resistance and type 2 diabetes, with all its deleterious ramifications, the same thing can happen in the brain. As will be explained below, recent research is increasingly demonstrating that what was once thought to be the harmful effects of too much fat can now be more properly ascribed to too much sugar, and its close cousin, available or easily digestible carbohydrates.

The failure to recognize the damage that sugars cause to general health and the brain is due to two main factors. First of all, scientists are also human, and tend to jump on bandwagons led by the most vociferous among them. Starting in the 50s, and continuing up to the 80s, the conventional wisdom was that fats, especially saturated fats, were bad and carbs were not.

Did You Know? British professor John Yudkin was one of the first to alert the world to the problems of sugar in his 1972 book, *Pure, White & Deadly,* but his voice was drowned out by the powers of the time.

The other major factor is that humans don't eat ingredients, they eat food, and the reality is that many foods are high in both fat and sugar, thus making it difficult to separate the effects of each.

Scientific opinions of the last 10 years have caused a sea change in our attitude toward fat and sugar. The evidence is mounting that sugars (we will explain what we mean by sugars later in this chapter) are the key enemy rather than fats. The change started with how we view fats and carbs as related to cardiovascular disease (CVD). A study by Harvard researchers on a large cohort of over 125,000 people published in 2015 in the *Journal of the American College of Cardiology* showed that replacing saturated fats with refined carbohydrates (which we will show are as bad as, and are precursors to, sugars) did not reduce the risk of CVD.[3] However, replacing the saturated fats with unsaturated fats did significantly reduce CVD risk. And there is ongoing controversy as to whether even saturated fats are harmful or not. A comprehensive review in 2016 in the journal *Progress in Cardiovascular Diseases* concluded that sugars provide a greater risk of CVD than saturated fats, and that a diet high in added sugar causes a threefold increase in risk of death.[4]

How Sugars are Implicated in Cognitive Decline

There are many kinds of sugar, ranging from common table sugar or sucrose, to high-fructose syrups, to milk sugar or lactose. The common element among the most common sugars is that they break down during digestion into the two basic harmful units of glucose and fructose when consumed in large quantity. The main difficulty with these sugar units is that, as the blood levels of these units are increased, they lead to the following problems:

- increased obesity risk;
- increased insulin levels due to high blood glucose, leading to insulin resistance and diabetes;
- increased glycation breakdown products from glucose metabolism, leading to inflammation and impaired immune response.

All of the above problems have been correlated with an increased risk of AD/dementia. The effect of blood glucose concentration on the risk of AD/dementia was shown dramatically in a paper published in 2013 in the *New England Journal of Medicine*.[5] A key table from that paper is reproduced below.

Table 5. Risk of dementia associated with average blood glucose level.

	Glucose Level American Units	Glucose Level Canadian Units	Hazard Ratio for Dementia
Non-diabetics	95 mg/dL	5.3 mmol/L	0.86
	100 mg/dL	5.6 mmol/L	1.0
	105 mg/dL	5.8 mmol/L	1.10
	110 mg/dL	6.1 mmol/L	1.15
	115 mg/dL	6.4 mmol/L	1.18
Diabetics	150 mg/dL	8.3 mmol/L	1.10
	160 mg/dL	8.9 mmol/L	1.0
	170 mg/dL	9.4 mmol/L	1.01
	180 mg/dL	10 mmol/L	1.15
	190 mg/dL	10.6 mmol/L	1.40

Source: Paul Craine et al., *New England Journal of Medicine*, 8 Aug. 2013.

Table 5 shows the impact of blood glucose level on risk of dementia for non-diabetics and diabetics; Canadian units of blood glucose are shown as a reference. The maximum normal blood glucose level of 100 mg per dL is considered as a baseline, and the risk or hazard ratio for this group is 1.00. A number above 1.0 is considered an increased risk, and a number below 1.0 is considered a decreased risk.

There are two important things to understand from the above table. The first is that the risk of dementia increases up to 18% in people without diabetes (and up to 40% in people with diabetes) who experience increases in blood glucose level above the normal maximum. Prediabetes, considered a high-risk factor for diabetes, is when blood sugar is between 100 and 125 mg per dL.

Did You Know? Other studies have shown that high blood sugar is suspect for depression and other mental disorders, in addition to dementia.

The second, which is surprising, is that blood glucose levels slightly below normal result in a 14% reduced risk of dementia for people without diabetes, as compared with normal levels. So, the lower the blood glucose level, the lower the risk of dementia, even when you have normal blood sugar levels.

Linked of course to diabetes and prediabetes is metabolic syndrome, which is an underlying condition characterized by high blood glucose, high blood pressure, abdominal obesity, and decreased HDL cholesterol. Of these metabolic syndrome characteristics, blood glucose and blood pressure are most strongly associated with cognitive decline.

A very important study linking brain glucose with AD was published in November 2017 in the journal *Alzheimer's & Dementia*, and was supported by the Institute on Aging at the National Institute of Health (NIH).[6] By doing autopsies on the brains of people who had participated in cognitive studies, the authors found for the first time that brain blood glucose was directly correlated to the severity and symptomology of AD. Simultaneously, they also found that the protein that is essential in utilizing glucose in the brain was in a much lower concentration in subjects with AD. In addition, they found that high blood glucose in the rest of the body correlated with high brain glucose. This was an elegant study to tie up the connection between blood glucose, diabetes, and AD, and it helped to substantiate that AD and some forms of dementia may be considered as type 3 diabetes of the brain.

And it doesn't stop there. Simple or digestible carbohydrates (i.e., those that do not contain fiber, such as are found in starches, potatoes, rice, white bread, etc.) have been shown to be as harmful as glucose or fructose. The reason for this is that they are quickly converted to glucose in the body. In a paper in the *Journal of Alzheimer's Research* in 2012 and supported by the National Institutes of Health,[7] Rosebud Roberts and his group compared a group of subjects who were either on high-carb or high-fat diets and their risk of dementia and mild cognitive impairment. What the researchers found was that the group in the top 25% of carb intake had an 89% increased risk of dementia or mild cognitive impairment (MCI, a possible precursor to AD/dementia) compared to those at the lowest level of carb intake. What was surprising was that the study also found that those subjects who were in the top 25% of fat intake had a 44% reduced risk of dementia and MCI as compared with those at the lowest level of fat intake.

Did You Know? It actually gets much worse. A large, well-designed study published in late 2017, called the PURE study, found that participants who ate the highest level of carbs had a 28% higher risk of death from all causes as compared to those eating the least carbs.[8]

Interestingly, another group in Denmark in 2017 showed that fat metabolism can detoxify the harmful components of blood glucose metabolism,[9] which could explain the dementia and MCI risk reduction of high fat intake described above.

So it appears from recent research that excess carbs and sugars can be harmful to the brain and health in general. The questions that remain to be answered are what is an excess of sugar and carbs, and what can be done to reduce our intake.

How Much is Too Much Sugar and Carbs?
The American Heart Association (AHA) recommends that added sugars should not be more than 5% of total calories, or 25 g (about 6 tsp) per day, for an average 2000 calories per day. The World Health Organization (WHO) goes a step further and recommends no more than 5% of calories from any sugars. This includes not only sugars added to food, but also sugar naturally occurring in foods such as fruits and some vegetables.

There is no question that North Americans far exceed these guidelines. The average American consumes about 77 g (15% of calories for a 2000 calories-per-day diet) of added sugar per day (about 18 tsp), while the average Canadian consumes less, at about 55 g per day.

Did You Know? The average American male consumes about 84 g of added sugar per day. The average American female consumes somewhat less at about 58 g.

If we include sugars naturally occurring in foods, the Canadian Sugar Institute estimates an increase in consumption of 133 g per day for Americans (27% of caloric intake at 2000 calories per day) and 110 g per day for Canadians (22% of caloric intake at 2000 calories per day). For children and teens, it's just as bad, as American youth consume about 16% of calories as added sugar. A relatively recent review of added-sugar consumption for Americans appeared in 2014 in the American Journal of Clinical Nutrition.[10] It found that the major source of added sugars was from sodas and energy and sports drinks, which represented 34.4% of all added sugars. Grain desserts represented 12.7%, fruit drinks 8%, candy 6.7%, and dairy desserts 5.6%.

Did You Know? Other jurisdictions in Europe and North America have also found that sweetened drinks are a major source of added sugars, and that they contribute significantly to obesity. These bodies have therefore implemented, or have plans to institute, special taxes on these drinks.

Canadian data appearing in a Statistics Canada report in 2004 are even more interesting because they consider major sources of all sugar intake, which includes both added sugars and sugars occurring naturally in foods. The top five sources of total sugar intake for adults according to Statistics Canada are fruits at 17.4% of total sugars, soft drinks at 13.0%, sugars (white and brown) at 11.4%, milk at 10.7%, and fruit juice at 7.6%. This is food for thought, because some foods considered as good nutritional sources such fruit and milk can also be major sources of sugar. It appears that, based on the above data, added sugars only represent 58% of total sugar intake for

Americans and 50% of total sugar intake for Canadians. A summary of major contributors of added and total sugars to the diet are shown in Tables 6 and 7 in the following section.

Further, we need to understand that, in reality, our total consumption of sugars is actually much greater than the numbers above show. This is because many of the carbohydrates we consume, such as rice, bread, pasta, potatoes, and so on, are very easily and quickly converted in the body to sugar in the form of glucose. The 2015 Dietary Guidelines for Americans recommends consumption of 225–325 g per day of carbohydrates, for an average 2000 calories per day, and the actual carb consumption by Americans is estimated to be not far from this target. So, if we assume an average of 275 g of carbs are consumed each day, and conservatively assume that 70% of these carbs are converted to glucose, we end up with an additional 193 g per day of sugar, which represents an increase of more than 100% in total sugar consumption.

An interesting study was published in 2016 by Po-Ju Lin and his group.[11] This study found that decreasing total carb calories consumed, from 60% of total calories to 30% of total calories (which is below the Dietary Guidelines), resulted in a drop of 30% in blood insulin after three meals. Since high insulin levels have been implicated as a risk factor for the development of diabetes and AD/dementia, it would appear that reducing carbohydrate intake could have some benefit for both the brain and general health.

Did You Know? The Atkins diet, which has been used extensively for some time without noticeable harmful effects, recommends an initial reduction of total carbs to 20 g per day for two weeks, with a gradual increase to about 50–100 g per day thereafter.

Now that we have offered reasonable evidence that excess carbs and sugars are harmful to health, and that we as a North American society consume too many carbs and too much sugar, we need to shift our attention to how we can reduce our intake.

What We Can Do to Overcome the Deadly Sin of Too Much Sugar

The simplest way to avoid a lot of sugar intake is to avoid those foods that contribute the most to our added-sugar consumption. We discussed these foods earlier, but they are reproduced below in Table 6 for emphasis.

Table 6. High added-sugar foods to avoid.

High-Sugar Food	% of Added-Sugar Consumption	Alternative Foods to Consume
Sodas and energy/sports drinks	34.4	Water, unsweetened tea, coffee, nut milks, diet drinks
Grain desserts (do-nuts, cake, etc.)	12.7	Sugar substitute grain desserts (with sucralose, maltose, stevia, etc.)
Fruit drinks	8.0	Water, unsweetened tea, coffee, nut milks, diet drinks
Candy	6.7	Candy with maltitol or other sugar substitutes
Dairy desserts	5.6	Unsweetened dairy desserts (e.g., plain yogurt)

The next thing we need to consider is that many foods are high in natural sugar as opposed to added sugar.

Did You Know? Many so-called healthy natural foods are actually mostly sugar—honey, molasses, agave syrup, and so on.

Indeed, added sugars only represent 58% of total sugars consumed for Americans and 50% for Canadians. The top food sources for total sugar consumption, which were described earlier, are summarized in Table 7.

Table 7. High total-sugar foods to control, according to a Statistics Canada study.

Sugary Food	% of Total[a] Sugar Consumption	Alternative Food Possibilities
Fruits	17.9	Lower-sugar fruit options such as berries. Moderate consumption of high-sugar fruits
Soft drinks	13.0	Diet drinks, unsweetened tea, coffee, or nut milks
Brown and white sugar	11.4	Sugar substitutes or unsweetened foods
Milk	10.7	Fortified nut milks or moderate milk quantities
Fruit juice	7.6	Fruit instead of fruit juice

[a] Includes added plus natural sugar.

So, looking at the above tables, we get an idea as to what to cut out. Try to eliminate as many of the added-sugar foods described in Table 6, or try to substitute for the alternative foods described. Eliminating the high natural-sugar foods described in Table 7 is more complex. First, eliminate as much direct sugar as possible (see Table 8), as well as fruit juices, which can be consumed as a more-nutritious alternative in the form of whole fruits. We do not recommend eliminating fruits and milk, because they provide essential nutrients, but choose lower-sugar fruits, and ingest both fruits and milk in moderation. Using this strategy will eliminate a large amount of the harmful excess sugar we consume.

Another way to reduce consumed sugar is to read the nutrition tables on prepackaged foods and note the sugar content of the product (see Appendix 4). You will be amazed at how many prepackaged foods contain added sugar that you never expected (e.g., tomato sauce, peanut butter, salad dressings, etc.)

You will also be amazed at how much sugar is contained in traditional sugary foods like soft drinks and baked goods. For prepackaged foods, we suggest that you read the nutrition tables and ingredient lists and eliminate any foods that contain more than 6–7 g sugar per 100 g or 100 mL. This will go a long way to reducing your total sugar intake.

However, in order to properly read the ingredient declarations on foods, we need to understand what is meant by the term "sugar." It comes in many forms and under different names. So watch out for the following names, among others, that can appear in the ingredient declarations of foods: agave syrup, brown sugar, cane syrup solids, corn syrup, brown rice syrup, dextrose, fruit juice concentrate, fructose, high-fructose corn syrup, honey, lactose, evaporated cane solids, maltose, malt syrup, sucrose, sugar, and molasses.

All of the above are sugars, and all have the deleterious effects of sugar described earlier. Note that the line item for sugar in the Nutrition Facts table should take into account all of the above forms of sugar as well as the sugar naturally contained in the food.

Reduce Foods Containing Carbohydrates and Digestible Carbohydrates

There are two groups of carbohydrates (or carbs). One is the group of digestible carbs, or net carbs, as referred to by Dr. Atkins. These are typically grain or potato products that have been refined to remove complex, undigestible carbs and other constituents for improvement in taste, texture, or shelf life. Typical products in this category are white bread, buns, pastry, pasta, French fries, potatoes, rice—most anything that is white or made from white carbs. The other category is complex carbs, which are carbs that resist digestion and absorption by the body. Typical foods in this category are whole grains and whole grain bread, most vegetables, nuts, and legumes.

Foods that are high in digestible carbs and deficient in complex carbs will quickly convert to basic sugars in the body and result in high blood glucose, which can result in insulin resistance and perhaps diabetes. Foods that contain high levels of complex carbs will slow down the digestion of the digestible carbs and result in lower blood glucose concentration.

The conventional wisdom is that if we eat foods high in complex carbs our blood sugar will be ok. Unfortunately, recent data have shown that this is not quite true. A measure of the volume of complex and total carbs that a food contains is called the glycemic index (GI). Either glucose or white bread, which convert readily to blood glucose, is given an arbitrary reference glycemic index of 100, and all other foods are given a rating compared to this reference value. The lower the number is from a hundred, the more complex carbs in the food (or the lower the carb content is, and supposedly the better it is for you). However, many foods that are thought of as being healthy because they have complex carbs are not that much different in GI from their refined cousins, as can be seen from Table 8 below (which is selected from the 2008 International Glycemic Index tables of the American Diabetes Association).

Did You Know? The glycemic index of foods depends on which reference food is chosen—white bread or glucose—and even within each reference food tabulated values can vary. Therefore, average GIs from several sources are usually used.

Table 8. Glycemic index (GI) of some key
foods with glucose as the reference value 100.

Food	Glycemic Index (GI)	Food	Glycemic Index (GI)
White bread*	75	Whole wheat bread	74
White rice (boiled)	73	Brown rice (boiled)	68
Spaghetti (white)	49	Spaghetti (whole wheat)	48
Instant oat porridge	79	Cornflakes	81
Chickpeas	28	Soya beans	16
Sucrose (table sugar)	65		

*When white bread is used as a reference instead of glucose,
its GI is taken as 100.

Table 8 highlights some interesting observations. Based on table sugar having a GI of 65 with reference to glucose, we can estimate that any food with a GI of 65 or higher is considered high. The other thing we notice is that there is not much difference in GI between refined grain and whole grain foods, and that both have a high GI. Also notable is that some of the lowest GIs occur in beans and legumes.

Further evidence that some complex carb foods may not be that much better than purely digestible carb foods appeared in the *Journal of the American Medical Association* in 2014,[12] showing that there was no difference in insulin sensitivity, lipid levels, or systolic blood pressure between high GI (GI of 65) and low GI (GI of 40) foods. Another randomized crossover trial published in 2017 in the journal *Gut* showed that a whole grain diet did not affect insulin resistance when compared with a refined grain diet that included pasta and white bread.[13] So, even foods with high complex carb content and low GI may not be that good for you when they also come with high digestible carb content. Based on the above information, we recommend the following approach to carb consumption:

1. First, try to eliminate as many refined grains from your diet as possible. This includes white bread, baked goods, white rice, boiled potatoes, and any food products made from refined flour.
2. Second, try to reduce your total intake of carbs. Foods with complex carbs may not be much better for you than foods made from refined carbs, but they do contain important nutrients such as fiber and vitamins and minerals that refined flours may not. Therefore, your required carb intake should emphasize a moderate intake of this type of food. Beans and legumes, as well as other vegetable sources, are probably among the best in this category because they have very low GIs.

Set Targets for Total Sugar and Carbohydrate Consumption

By any measure, North Americans are consuming way in excess of the recommended intake. We recommend that you set a target of 25 g per day for total sugars (several health organizations recommend a maximum of 25 g or 6 tsp/30 mL of added sugar per day) and control your intake using the methods suggested above. Setting targets for digestible and total carb intake is more controversial. A very low-carb diet is usually defined as being less than 50 g per day (1 cup/250 mL of rice or two bread slices), but low carbs in the range of 20–50 g per day can put the body into what is called a state of ketosis, whereby the body utilizes breakdown products from fats for energy instead of carbs and sugar. This is not necessarily bad, and this type of diet has been used successfully for weight loss and chronic diseases. Generally, this type of diet has proven to be safe, but may be harmful for some people. As well, possible side effects such as bad breath may preclude it as an option for many. So, before starting a ketogenic diet, it is wise to consult with your doctor.

Did You Know? The Atkins diet is a ketogenic (based on ketosis) diet.

A review paper published in the *Annals of the New York Academy of Sciences* in 2016 found that there was a moderately beneficial effect on subjects with mild cognitive impairment or mild-to-moderate AD who adhered to a ketogenic diet.[14] This was because the brain was able to use the fat breakdown products called ketone bodies for energy, even though utilization of glucose was impaired.

Did You Know? One study found that having people eat 20–70 g per day of a special fat from coconut or palm kernel oil (called medium-chain triglycerides, or MCT) had the same beneficial effect on AD and MCI subjects as putting them on a ketosis diet.

Nevertheless, not everybody wants to adopt a ketosis diet, for reasons mentioned above, so we recommend a total carb target of 150 g per day made up primarily of complex carb foods. Average carb intake in the US is approximately 296 g per day for men and 224 g per day for women.

DEADLY SIN #3—TOO MUCH PROCESSED FOODS

Processed foods are foods that have undergone a change in a manufacturing facility. According to Dr. Larry McLeary, a neurosurgeon and author, 80% of the food on supermarket shelves today did not exist 100 years ago. Unfortunately, in the process of developing and marketing these foods, companies have chosen a path that has resulted in many food products that can be harmful to your health and mind. Not all processed foods are harmful, but many are. The profit motivation of the manufacturer is to get you to buy their product, and the food components that get you to buy the products are primarily fats, sugars (including refined carbs), and salt—all ingredients that have been shown to cause harm in one way or another but that taste and make you feel good.

Did You Know? Historically, all fats were thought to be the primary food component to limit. However, scientific opinion has now changed to a belief that only saturated fats are harmful, and even this is controversial.

Processed food products contain differing quantities of fats, sugars, and salts, but there is a category of processed foods called ultra-processed foods with exceptionally high levels of these components. An example of this type of product is shown in Figure 3 below.

Figure 3. Conversion of natural
food to ultra-processed food (wheat sugar puffs).

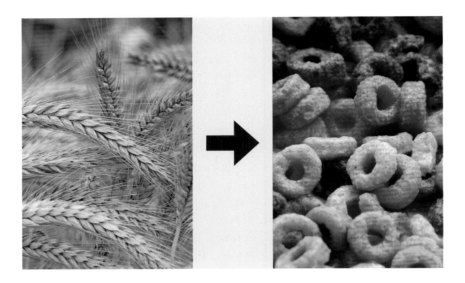

In the example shown, the problem with this type of conversion is that, in the manufacturing process, the natural food (wheat) is stripped of most of its nutrients (such as fiber, vitamins, and minerals) and left with refined or digestible carbs supplemented with added sugar, salt, and/or fat, such as the sugary breakfast cereal shown in the example. Some manufacturers try to add back some of the lost nutrients, but it is impossible to go back to the product's original state, and many of the original product's components, such as antioxidants, are left out.

Did You Know? It can get worse than this—during the manufacturing process, potentially harmful chemicals such as BPA and acrylamide may be incorporated into food.

These ultra-processed foods, such as soda pop, candies, cakes, pretzels, chips, and so on, contribute 90% of added sugars and 50% of calories to our diet, according to the Nutrition Insight website, because they are the products we primarily consume. The empty calories and high content of sugars, salt, and fat in these foods increases the risk of AD/dementia as explained earlier, as well as the risk of heart disease and other chronic diseases such as diabetes and cancer.

Processed Meats

There is a sub-category of processed foods called processed meats that includes ham, bacon, sausages, deli meats, and hot dogs. Most are based on red meats such as pork and beef. Although there is not much data on their influence on AD/dementia, these products have been shown in studies to increase the risk and mortality of several major diseases including heart disease, diabetes, kidney disease, liver disease, respiratory disease, and cancer. For this reason, and because of their impact on heart disease and diabetes (which indirectly increases AD/dementia risk), we include them as processed foods to avoid.

How to Choose Wisely

The best choice when it comes to processed foods is simple—avoid them by preparing as many of your meals yourself from natural foods or ingredients. Having said that, we also realize that it is difficult to avoid consuming processed foods. They are convenient, usually taste good, and are readily accessible. Besides, some processed foods can be nutritionally good for you. So rather than avoid them completely we should pick and choose which to avoid and which to consume.

The best tool to use in selecting processed foods, which you might want to use, is the Nutrition Facts tables that are required by law to be on all prepackaged foods sold in both Canada and the US. The nutrition facts tables are somewhat different in Canada than they are in the US, but they are generally the same. Both the current Canadian and US table formats are shown in Appendix 4, along with proposed changes that are targeted to be implemented by 2021. By way of example, we have reproduced the Canadian nutrition facts tables in Figure 4 as well.

Figure 4. Canadian Nutrition Facts tables.

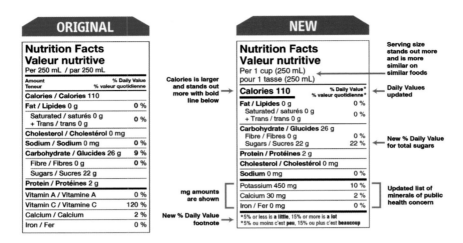

Source: Health Canada.

The original Nutrition Facts table is what appears on food products today. The new table is what will be required by 2021. Use the above tables to identify processed food products. Here are some some suggestions on how to use the tables for the maximum benefit:

- Look at the serving size first and use this as a basis for referencing other nutrients. Knowing the serving size used for calculation of nutrient content will help you measure nutrient intake at different consumption levels. The serving size of drinks is usually 1 cup (250 mL); the serving size of solid foods is expressed in grams and can vary from food to food.
- Mind your calories. An average adult will consume approximately 2000 calories daily, so monitor the calorie count of the processed food you are eating to determine if it will make a significant impact on your total daily calories.
- Saturated fats in a daily diet should not exceed about 5% of your caloric intake, according to the American Heart Association. This translates to 100 g per day with an average daily adult caloric intake of 2000 calories (or 75 g if you restrict your calories to 1500 calories per day). So, consider how much you are getting from each serving of processed food and decide if that will cause you to exceed the recommended 75–100 g per day.

- Trans fats should be zero, but this will not generally be a problem, since most developed countries have prohibited their use.
- Minimize sugar consumption so that you do not exceed 25 g per day.
- Try to minimize total carbs, and especially refined or digestible carbs, so you do not exceed 150 g per day. Calculate digestible carbs by subtracting the fiber from total carbs.
- Minimize sodium consumption so that you do not exceed 1500–2300 mg per day.
- Maximize the fiber you consume to target 25 g or more per day.
- Maximize the protein you consume—in doing so you will lower the amount of carbs, sugar, salt, and saturated fat you eat.

In the next chapter we will highlight those foods that adhere to these guidelines and those that do not.

4. FOODS THAT HELP

AND FOODS THAT HURT

THE BRAIN

In the previous chapter, we identified the major faults of our North American diet in regards to the risk of developing AD/dementia. Now it is time to determine how to set that right by choosing foods, diet plans, and recipes that help reduce the risk of AD/dementia. We'll try to do this in a simple stepwise manner.

First, we'll identify specific foods that help the brain and foods that harm the brain. With this information, we can proceed to Chapter 5, which will look at establishing eating plans that utilize the good foods we have identified. These eating plans will cater to every reader's preferences with increasing levels of detail. For those who just want a short, quick recommendation, we'll summarize the food groups you should choose from. Others may want to know how many servings of certain foods to eat, and when to eat them. For this group, we will review the well-known Mediterranean and MIND diets, which have been established to help prevent AD/dementia. We will then extend these diets through our own Brain Boosting Diet, which is a natural evolution of the previous beneficial diets. Finally, we'll compare all the diet plans and discuss which you should choose. In Part 2 of the book we will translate our recommended diet plan into specific food recipes.

FOODS THAT HELP THE BRAIN

Foods that have been found to help the brain and reduce the risk of AD/dementia are summarized in Table 9.

Table 9. Foods that help the brain.

Food Group	Especially Look for	The Good Stuff Inside
Leafy greens and other vegetables 	**Leafy greens:** Spinach, kale, collard, mustard **Other vegetables:** Cruciferous (broccoli, cauliflower, Brussels sprouts, etc.), legumes, bell peppers, beans, tomatoes, squash, avocado, mushrooms **Spices:** Cloves, turmeric, rosemary, cinnamon, oregano, ginger	Excellent source of complex antioxidants (phytoantioxidants), simple antioxidants (vitamins A, C, and E), B vitamins (except B12), and fiber. Also minerals (magnesium, manganese, and zinc), and plant Omega-3 fats. Low in fat, sugar, and salt.

(CONTINUED NEXT PAGE)

Table 9. Foods that help the brain. (CONTINUED)

Food Group	Especially Look for	The Good Stuff Inside
Fish	**Fatty (darker color) fish:** Salmon, sardines, herring, anchovies, mackerel, tuna	Excellent source of high-quality Omega-3 fats, vitamin D, vitamin B12, and selenium. Low in sugar and salt.
Fruits	**Berries:** Cranberries, blackberries, blueberries, strawberries, acai, elderberry, kiwi **Other fruits:** Pomegranate, grapes	Excellent source of complex (phytoantioxidants) and simple (vitamin C) antioxidants, manganese, fiber, and B vitamins (except B12). Low in fat and salt.
Liquid fats and oils	Extra virgin olive oil, canola oil, high-oleic sunflower oil, flaxseed oil	Contains unsaturated fatty acids and complex antioxidants. Rich in vitamin E antioxidant. Low in salt and cholesterol.
Nuts and seeds	Almonds, sunflower seeds, walnuts, cocoa beans	Rich in natural vitamin E and monosaturated fatty acids (MUFA), fiber, and complex antioxidants. Low in salt, sugar, and cholesterol.
Beverages (unsweetened)	Red wines (dry), coffee, tea (green or white), vegetable smoothies	Rich in complex antioxidants. Vegetable smoothies also provide the full benefits of vegetables. Low in fat, salt, and sugar.

Food Group	Especially Look for	The Good Stuff Inside
Whole grains 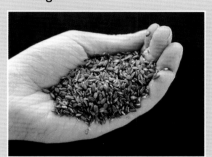	Flaxseed, quinoa, black rice, oats, barley, buckwheat	Contains complex antioxidants, fiber, plant Omega-3 fats, and minerals (selenium, magnesium, manganese, and zinc).

Table 9 provides a summary of the key information on the foods that are beneficial for the brain and indeed for the whole body, and which are constituents of the Mediterranean diet, which has proven to be one of the best diets for the brain and body. The first column identifies the important food groups for a healthy diet, the second column identifies foods in that category that are brain-healthy, and the last column shows the key nutrients in these foods that, by research, have been shown to reduce the risk of AD/dementia and even slow down cognitive decline.

Did You Know? In general, it has been found that foods that are good for the brain are also good for the heart, and vice versa.

All of the above food groupings contribute to a healthy brain and body, but if we were to pick the most important foods from the table based on the amount of research conducted, they would include the following:

LEAFY AND CRUCIFEROUS VEGETABLES: These seem to have one of the best dietary correlations with a reduced risk of AD/dementia.

Did You Know? It is estimated that 96% of Americans do not get their recommended intake of leafy vegetables.

Early data on this phenomenon developed in the late 90s, when spinach was found to have strong cognitive protective properties as compared with strawberries, vitamin E, and red wine.[1,2] More recent studies have investigated leafy vegetables in general,[3] as well as other vegetables, and have confirmed their benefits for brain health. One cohort study by Kang et al. found that leafy vegetables and cruciferous vegetables helped slow cognitive decline in aged women.[4] Another very recent prospective study by Morris et al., which appeared in the journal *Neurology* in early 2018, found that a median of 1.3 servings of leafy vegetables per day reduced cognitive decline to the point that, after 4.7 years, those who consumed this quantity of leafy vegetables had a brain age equivalent to 11 years younger than those who did not consume any leafy vegetables.[5]

Based on research, it is believed that the benefits of leafy vegetables are primarily due to their high content of the B vitamins folate and B6 (especially for people who have high blood levels of a chemical called homocysteine[6]), as well as their very high content of simple and complex antioxidants.

Did You Know? Some studies have shown reduced levels of depression, as well as dementia risk reduction, to be associated with leafy vegetables containing high B vitamin content.

A randomized double-blind study by A. David Smith et al. in 2010 tested the B vitamins found in leafy greens and the vitamin B12 usually found in animal food sources or supplements.

It was discovered that, as compared to taking a placebo, brain atrophy was reduced by 30% over a period of 24 months, which could be correlated with reduced cognitive decline.[7]

Although there is some inconsistency, other studies have also found benefits with dietary B vitamins. One study in 2016 in France found a 50% dementia risk reduction for those consuming a minimum of 375 mcg of folate per day as compared with those consuming the least folate (less than 168 mcg per day).[8]

Did You Know? Recent studies have shown that the best results with B vitamins occur when Omega-3 fats are consumed at the same time.

Leafy vegetables are also very rich in antioxidants. Morris has highlighted some of these antioxidants, such as lutein (which has also been shown to be effective in reducing macular degeneration of the eye) and kaempferol, as being especially good for the brain.[5]

Did You Know? Plants are the world's richest sources of antioxidants. From an evolutionary perspective this can be traced back to the fact that plants generate large amounts of oxygen during photosynthesis, and they developed their antioxidants as protection against this oxygen.

The USDA Human Nutrition Research Center on Aging has shown that lutein is preferentially taken up by the brain. Several papers, including one from the USDA Human Nutrition Research Center on Aging and one from the Irish Longitudinal Study on Ageing, have shown cognitive protection and reduction in cognitive decline in older-age subjects.[9,10] Leafy greens also contain simple antioxidants such as vitamin C, A, and E.[11,12] Furthermore, they contain nitrates, which help maintain blood flow in the vascular system.

FATTY FISH: Many papers have been published on fish consumption and AD/dementia risk reduction—and even one fish meal per week can reduce risk.[13, 14,15,16,17,18]

Did You Know? The health aspects of fish were first discovered when it was observed that the Inuit, who ate a lot of fish, had relatively little heart disease even though they ate copious amounts of fat.

Two important things seem to stand out from these studies. The first is that several papers have found that there is a dose-response effect to the benefits of fish consumption—i.e., the more you eat, the better the effect.[17,18] Nurk et al. in 2007 found that a minimum of 10 g per day of fish was required to see an effect, and that an optimum intake was 75 g per day, which represents about one fish meal per day.[17] The second important point is that it doesn't seem to matter whether the fish is fatty or not—you still get a benefit.[17,18] Although most of the benefits of fish are ascribed to a special fat in fatty fish called Omega-3, the observed benefit of fish with lower Omega-3 means that there are other factors in fish not yet identified that also help maintain cognitive health. What this means is that you should get your Omega-3 fats from fish, preferably fatty fish, rather than from supplements.

The two most important Omega-3 fats for the brain are called EPA and DHA, of which DHA is considered to be the more important. These Omega-3 fats make up a large part of nerve cell membranes, are involved in neuron and synapse formation, and have anti-inflammatory properties. They have also been shown to reduce cholesterol build-up through control of triglyceride fat in the body, and thus help in the control of vascular dementia.

Did You Know? The brain is 60% fat on a dry basis and DHA makes up about 30% of the phospholipids in the brain cell membranes.

Studies carried out on consumption of Omega-3 fats EPA and DHA have had mixed results, primarily because not all studies used adequate levels of fats. One paper summarized many trials with DHA according to their results and the dose of DHA used.[19] It was found that the best positive results were obtained when DHA levels ranged between 750 and 1500 mg per day, and that the studies showed no benefit for doses below 500 mg per day.

Common fatty fish have DHA content ranging from 500 to 1500 mg per 3-oz (90 g) serving. So, in order to get a strong benefit from fish based on DHA alone, one would need to consume at least one fatty fish meal per day. However, since we indicated earlier that there are other components in fish that may be beneficial, we can probably reduce the fish meal and fish DHA intake somewhat.

A number of studies with higher doses of DHA have shown significant brain benefits for mild cognitive impairment and a reduction of AD/dementia risk.[20,21,22] One Japanese study in 2016 even indicated a benefit with 1.7 g per day of DHA for people who already had AD, indicating the importance of this fish fat component for cognition.[23]

Did You Know? North America, Europe, and Latin America have very low blood EPA and DHA when compared to the recommended levels for good health, and these low blood levels also correspond with low fish intake.

Appendix 1 provides a list of fatty fishes along with their Omega-3 content, so you will have the basis for choosing which fish to eat. We recommend sticking to fatty fish that are not bottom feeders, especially smaller fatty fish (e.g., sardines, herring, salmon, mackerel—but not king mackerel), rainbow trout, and anchovies, to avoid the possibility of ingesting PCBs, mercury, and other contaminants. Caviar and fish roe are also very rich sources of Omega-3s.

Note also that although you may read that you can get your Omega-3 fats from plant sources such as flaxseeds, black walnuts, or canola oil, the reality is that these Omega-3 fats are very poorly converted into the active forms of Omega-3 fats that the brain needs, which are EPA, and especially DHA. So, stay primarily with fish as your source of Omega-3 fats whenever possible, and supplement with fish oil or DHA capsules only when this is not feasible.

Did You Know? In addition to Omega-3 fats, fatty fish are also excellent sources of high-quality protein, B12, vitamin D, and the antioxidant selenium.

BERRIES AND GRAPES: These are the most studied fruits to show benefits for preventing cognitive decline. Their positive impact is most probably due to their high antioxidant concentrations, both in simple antioxidants, such as vitamin C, and complex antioxidants, such as polyphenols. Berries in particular have been extensively studied, and animal tests have repeatedly shown a slowing of cognitive decline with increased consumption.[30,31,32,33,35] A large human study in 2012, called the Harvard Nurses Study, found that higher consumption of blueberries and strawberries resulted in an effective delay in cognitive aging of 2.5 years.[34] Blueberries in particular have been heavily studied.[24,25,26,27,28] These studies, performed over short terms no longer than 3–4 months, have demonstrated cognitive and memory improvement in both healthy and MCI (mild cognitive impairment) subjects, with visible benefits for both whole blueberries and blueberry juice.

Did You Know? The general rule that one can use is that the darker the color of the fruit, the greater the concentration of antioxidants.

Although grapes are not berries, they also have a significant impact on slowing or reducing cognitive decline. They contain large quantities of polyphenol antioxidants and improve blood flow to the brain by reducing inflammation and increasing artery flexibility. Grapes and their components have been shown to improve cognitive, memory, and motor skills in both healthy middle- and older-age subjects, and have even shown the possibility of slowing cognitive decline in AD subjects.[36,37,38]

Berries and grapes tend to have high levels of soluble fiber, which help control sugar absorption and benefit the immune system. Within this group, berries such as raspberries, blackberries, blueberries, and strawberries seem to have the greatest effect on lowering the risk of AD/dementia. Except for blueberries, they also all have an added advantage in that they tend to be lower in sugar than other fruits. If you choose strawberries, buy organic, since strawberries are in the top three foods to contain pesticides (as seen on the Dirty Dozen list published by the Environmental Working Group, a non-profit environmental activist group).

Did You Know? A bonus of eating berries is that studies have demonstrated a reduced risk of death from cardiovascular disease.

LIQUID FATS AND OILS: In the liquid fats and oils category, olive oil is important for cognition. The brain is 60% fat and relies on essential fats such as Omega-3s, as well as on unsaturated fats containing linoleic and linolenic fatty acids, which it can only obtain from food sources. Olive oil is a key ingredient of the Mediterranean diet and its derivative diets. Other oils, such as canola, have a similar profile to olive oil in saturated and mono- and polyunsaturated fat content, but olive oil seems to have other qualities that distinguish it in brain benefits from the other oils.

Did You Know? Olive oil is embedded in antiquity and was the oil used to consecrate the ancient temple in Jerusalem as well as its equipment and priests.

In a randomized clinical trial called PREDIMED published in 2015, the authors found that a Mediterranean diet plus a liter of extra virgin olive oil (EVOO) per week resulted in improved global cognition as compared with the control diet.[39] This improvement was attributed to the antioxidant profile of the olive oil, and other studies in mice confirmed the effect. One study at the University of Florence with EVOO found strong improvements in coordination, memory, and anxiety-related behavior in aged mice.[40] In another study at Temple University in 2017, researchers used mice susceptible to AD and found that those that had EVOO added to their diet displayed reduced manifestations of AD, including a reduction of amyloid plaques, tau proteins, adverse neuronal integrity, and adverse behavior.[41] Other studies confirmed that frequent users of olive oil showed improved cognition.[42] We note that the recent trials used extra virgin olive oil in order to maximize antioxidant content, and we therefore recommend that whenever possible you use extra virgin first cold-pressed olive oil.

Many oils are extracted from their fruit or seeds using solvents that tend to leave behind important natural antioxidants. First cold-pressed olive oil physically squeezes the oil out of the fruit at a cold temperature and, if it is unfiltered, you will get the maximum content of antioxidants and the oil in its natural state.

Did You Know? Olive oil contains a natural chemical called oleocanthal that causes cancerous cell death, and studies with extra virgin olive oil have shown a reduction in breast cancer risk.

NUTS AND SEEDS: We recommend walnuts, almonds, and sunflower seeds as the most important choices in the group of nuts and seeds; they have been identified as key components of the Mediterranean diet and its derivatives. Nuts and seeds are powerhouses of nutrition, not only because of their important nutrient contents, but also because these nutrients are concentrated in an environment with little moisture to dilute them. Most studies have focused on heart health, and there have been many studies demonstrating the positive impact of nuts and seeds on cardiovascular health.

Did You Know? The FDA has approved a health claim for nuts that 45 g per day may reduce the risk of heart disease. Peanuts, which are legumes, are usually added to the nuts and seeds category because of the similarity of their nutritional profiles.

One large study involving 210,000 people found that five or more servings per week of nuts (one serving = 1 oz/30 g) was associated with a 20% lower risk of coronary heart disease.[43] This is important because what is good for the heart has been found to also be good for the brain. Good heart health also means less vascular dementia, which is the second most prevalent form of dementia. What is even more important is that one study found that nuts in excess of 20 g per day (five servings per week) reduced all-cause mortality, and especially mortality from neurodegenerative disease and diabetes.[44]

Did You Know? An interesting recent study from Yale showed that survival of stage 3 colon cancer patients could be increased by 57% if they consumed 60 g of nuts per week. Most of this benefit was from tree nuts, not peanuts.

There have also been some cognitive function studies with nuts. One study over 11 years with older-age subjects found that nuts were associated with higher cognitive functioning.[45] Another study found that nut consumption of at least five servings per week in older-age women improved cognition significantly.[46] Finally, the paper mentioned earlier as showing improved global cognition with olive oil added to a Mediterranean diet also demonstrated improved cognition with nuts.[39]

When it comes to specific nuts, most studies have been carried out with walnuts, with a few using almonds. Several papers have shown improved cognition in both the young and the old, especially in working memory.[47,48,49] One paper using mice bred to be susceptible to AD found that 1–1.5 oz (30–45 g) per day of the human equivalent dose of walnuts improved cognitive function and behavior in the AD mice to the point that they behaved similarly to the normal mice controls.[48]

Did You Know? Walnuts contain 1.9 g per 1 Tbsp (15 mL) Omega-3 fatty acids, which have been shown to be beneficial in the prevention of brain deterioration.

Almonds have also demonstrated cognitive benefits.[50] A study of rats in 2010 significantly reversed memory loss at a low dose of 6 g per day of the human equivalent of almonds, and also lowered triglycerides and cholesterol, which are considered risk factors for AD.[51]

Although all nuts are beneficial, our recommendation is to focus on walnuts, almonds, and sunflower seeds. Each of these nuts and seeds have unique characteristics that, in combination, should maximize their benefits. Almonds and sunflower seeds have the highest concentrations of natural vitamin E in any food, and this vitamin in food form (not as a supplement) is considered one of the most important components in staving off AD/dementia.[52]

Did You Know? A single ounce of almonds provides 37% of the daily recommended value of vitamin E.

Both almonds and sunflower seeds also have the typical nut and seed profile of low sugar and digestible carbs, high fiber, antioxidants, magnesium, and B vitamins, all of which are important to the brain. Walnuts are unique in that they contain very large amounts of a polyunsaturated fat called alpha-linolenic acid, which is in the category of Omega-3 fats that are critical for the brain. Walnuts also contain the same nutrients as almonds and sunflower seeds, with a combination of nuts providing a variety of antioxidants unique to each of the foods. We recommend a target consumption of 1–1.5 oz (30–45 g) total nuts per day from all varieties discussed.

Did You Know? Walnuts and almonds have very hard shells, which makes it difficult for toxins and pesticides to penetrate to the nut core. Peanuts, which have a softer shell, are much more susceptible.

WHOLE GRAINS: Flaxseed, Quinoa, and Oats belong to the family of whole grains that have been shown to be an important component of the Mediterranean diet and its derivatives, and studies have demonstrated their benefits against cognitive impairment and risk reduction for AD/dementia as well as heart disease.[45,53,54] Nevertheless, whole grains still contain high levels of digestible carbohydrates, and although they do reduce blood glucose concentration because of their fiber content, it is not by much, as shown by their glycemic index (described in Chapter 3).

Did You Know? Grain carbohydrates are primarily made up of starches, which are just chains of sugar (glucose). The body breaks the starches down into glucose during the digestion process.

That said, when used in moderation (in conjunction with a healthy diet), whole grains do offer nutritional benefits for the brain, including fiber, B vitamins, magnesium, zinc, and antioxidants. Many of these nutrients are significantly diminished during the processing of whole grains to refined flours and grains such as bread, pasta, French fries, refined rice, and so on, so based on our discussion of carbs in Chapter 3 we recommend a target of 150 g per day for whole grains, which represents approximately 30% of calories for a person consuming 2000 calories per day.

We recommend three specific whole grains to focus on, because of their unique health properties. Flaxseeds stand out in the category of whole grains because of their very high content of alpha-linolenic acid (ALA), an essential fatty acid belonging to the Omega-3 family that has been shown to be very important to cognitive function. They also contain high antioxidant levels, and one polyphenol antioxidant they contain, called lignan, occurs in a higher concentration than in any other plant.

Another whole grain to consider is oats, which have the highest concentration of soluble fiber of any grain and provide several benefits. Soluble fiber is filling and low in calories, which makes it helpful in weight control. Oats also decrease LDL (bad) cholesterol and reduce overall risk of death.[55,56] Finally, a recent study found that an extract of oats increased cognitive function in a randomized control trial.[54]

The last whole grain to be recommended is quinoa. Quinoa is unique because, unlike most plant proteins, its protein is similar to animal-based proteins, which are more complete in essential amino acids and therefore better for you. In addition, recent studies on animals have shown that quinoa contains a particular phytonutrient called hydroxyecdysone, which increases lifespan and reduces inflammatory markers, glycation products, and blood sugar that can accelerate cognitive decline.[57,58]

BEVERAGES: Red wine, coffee, and tea have all been studied and shown to reduce the risk of AD/dementia. Red wine in particular, and Cabernet Sauvignon specifically, seems to top the list.[59] Some studies have shown a reduction risk of up to approximately 50% for dementia, mainly because of the antioxidants.[60] Some words of caution when imbibing red wine or any alcohol, however: First, you should limit your consumption to one medium glass per day. Although it is considered light drinking, it can still reduce AD/dementia risk by approximately 30%.[60] Wine in amounts greater than that can adversely lead to certain cancers, such as breast cancer, and in older brains (age 40 and up) can actually worsen memory and cognitive function and cause a threefold increase in brain atrophy, even with moderate drinking levels.[61,62] Furthermore, excessive drinking in older people can increase inflammation and reduce the ability to fight infection.[63] Secondly, if you do decide to drink wine, make sure it is a dry wine so that you do not consume too much sugar. Finally, if you decide not to consume wine, you can still get benefits from both grapes and grape juice, though they will not contain the alcohol content that provides an added benefit.

Coffee recommendations over the years have been a bit of a roller coaster. Early studies and ancient folklore thought that coffee was harmful, but the pendulum has swung to the other side in recent years.

Did You Know? In the 1600s coffee was thought to cause impotence, and in the early 1900s it was thought to stunt growth and cause heart attacks.

Recent data have shown coffee to be helpful in reducing the risk of all kinds of diseases, including Parkinson's, asthma, depression, diabetes, liver disease, and inflammation. Most major health associations now recognize its health benefits.

Did You Know? A study published in September 2017 found that drinking four cups of coffee daily could decrease the risk of all-cause mortality by 64%. Another paper in 2017 in the *Annals of Internal Medicine* showed that two to three cups per day could reduce mortality by 18%.

Studies have shown that more than six cups per day can reduce the risk of diabetes by 30%, and two to five cups per day can reduce death from cardiovascular disease by 20%, all while contributing to cognitive maintenance.[64,65] For cognitive health, a review of several studies by Wu L. et al. in 2016 found that one to two cups per day was optimum for the reduction of cognitive disorder risks, including AD/dementia, cognitive decline, and cognitive impairment.[66] Overall, for all cognitive disorders, the risk reduction was approximately 18%. These benefits are thought to be due to a combination of the caffeine in the coffee and the natural antioxidants that it contains—both regular coffee and caffeine-free coffee can reduce cognitive disorders.

Tea, like coffee, has been found to be beneficial for general health, and has been found to reduce blood pressure, diabetes risk, harmful cholesterol, inflammation, and all-cause mortality.[67,67] Tea consumption has also been shown to benefit the brain. A mouse study using a green tea antioxidant extract found that memory impairment and brain insulin resistance could be improved.[68] A cohort study of older-age Chinese subjects in Singapore, published in late 2016, showed that frequent tea drinkers (three to four cups per day), primarily women, had a 50% reduction in cognitive disorders and dementia risk compared to non-tea drinkers, and those who were genetically predisposed to AD had an 86% risk reduction.[69]

Interestingly enough, the type of tea did not matter. Black, green, or oolong all had the same effect. This effect of tea is probably due its content of antioxidant polyphenols, but another impact on AD was demonstrated in a study published in Japan that showed a 33% reduction in diabetes risk for those who consumed six or more cups of green tea per day as compared to those who consumed less than one per day.[70] In another paper published in the *American Journal of Medicine* in 2016, people who consumed more than one cup per day had a 30% lower incidence of cardiovascular events when compared with non-tea drinkers.[71] Vascular dementia is the second most common cause of dementia after AD, so anything that can improve heart health will have an effect on overall dementia risk.

FOODS THAT HURT THE BRAIN

Foods that can increase the risk of AD/dementia are summarized in Table 10.

Did You Know? Just as foods that are good for the brain are good for the heart, foods that hurt the brain also hurt the heart.

Table 10 highlights the food groups and foods that we should avoid to help reduce the risk of AD/dementia. Many of these foods have been discussed in Chapter 3, but we will quickly review the major problems with these foods.

Table 10. Foods that hurt the brain.

Food Category	Especially Avoid	The Bad Stuff Inside
Sweets and high-carb foods	**Sweets:** Cakes, cookies, candies, ice cream, sodas, juices **Starchy foods:** Pasta, bread, cereal, pizza, French fries, chips	Sugar, digestible carbs, partially hydrogenated fats, saturated fats, gluten, salt
High-fat red meats, processed meats, and dairy	**Red Meats:** Beef and pork* **Processed Meats:** Sausage, deli meats, ham*, bacon*, hot dogs, hamburgers	Saturated fats, inflammatory proteins, excess iron, carcinogens
High-salt foods	Chips, processed soups, salt-added foods (e.g., salty nuts)	Sodium
Saturated fats and trans fats	Partially hydrogenated fats/oils, lard*, butter, other animal fat	Saturated fats, trans fats

*Please note: Pork products are not acceptable in a halal or kosher kitchen.

SWEETS AND HIGH-CARB FOODS: We discussed this topic extensively in Chapter 3 because we believe that high blood glucose levels resulting from these foods are one of the major contributors to memory loss and AD/dementia through the build-up of insulin resistance, inflammation, and obesity. In addition to the problems with high carbs and sugar, many of these foods have negligible nutrients and contain other deleterious components such as salt and saturated fats, so we recommend minimizing intake.

The top priority should be on cutting back on added sugars, which appear in many processed foods, but especially in sweets such as cakes, cookies, candies, ice cream, sodas, and juices. Fruits also should be eaten in moderation—even though they have significant nutritional benefits—because they are the number-one contributor of total sugars to the diet, even more than soft drinks. After sugars, look at cutting back on high-carb foods, especially refined grain foods such as pasta, white bread, rice, French fries, chips, and so on. Guidelines for doing so are also presented in Chapter 3.

RED MEATS AND PROCESSED MEATS: There seem to be consistent studies showing an association of red meat and processed meat consumption with increased all-cause mortality, as well as increased death from several diseases, including heart disease, diabetes, kidney disease, liver disease, respiratory disease, stroke, and cancer—but not AD/dementia. Nevertheless, because of the dangers presented by this group of foods and because they are indirectly related to AD/dementia through their impact on heart disease and diabetes, we recommend avoiding these foods as much as possible.

Did You Know? The World Health Organization (WHO) issued a statement in 2015 declaring that processed meat is carcinogenic to humans, and that all red meats (i.e., all mammalian meats) are probably carcinogenic to humans.

A European cohort study found a 15% increase in all-cause mortality for red meat consumption of 10–20 g per day, and an even higher increase of 44% for processed meat consumption of 10–20 g per day.[72] A review paper in 2016 covering 17 group studies also found an increased risk of death of 15% associated with red and processed meats.[73] A more recent study in 2017, following 537,000 AARP members aged 50–71 over 16 years, found an increase in all-cause mortality and eight disease-related mortalities of 26% for total red meat and processed meat consumption.[74] It is thought that several factors could account for these observations, including increased meat iron, salt, nitrates, and nitrites added to processed meats and saturated fat. This effect was not observed, however, with white meats. Based on the above data, we therefore recommend minimizing consumption of red and processed meats and substituting with chicken or fish instead.

Did You Know? The evidence continues to mount—in 2018, another study found that red and processed meats increase insulin resistance and damage the liver.

HIGH-SALT FOODS: These primary sources of sodium in the body are harmful not only to the body but also to the brain. Risk factors associated with salt are especially high for people over 50, for diabetics, and for those with high blood pressure—all of which also have a higher risk of AD/dementia. We all know that salt increases blood pressure (BP), which leads to heart attacks and strokes, but even without a rise in BP it has been shown that elevated sodium can damage the heart, kidneys, and brain.[75]

Did You Know? People who have had a stroke are three times as likely to develop AD as those who have not had a stroke.

Taking all the potential damage caused by excess sodium into account, one investigation found that risk of death from all causes increased by 20% for the highest sodium consumers versus the lowest, and that this risk of death was 46% higher when potassium was low in combination with high sodium.[76]

Did You Know? Fruits and vegetables tend to be high in potassium and low in sodium.

In another recent study published in 2018, it was discovered that high salt consumption resulted in inflammation, which caused behavioral and cognitive impairment in mice.[77] Interestingly enough, these impairments were reversed when the mice returned to their normal diets.

We consume too much salt and it has been estimated that we eat 50% more than is recommended by health authorities. A large source of this excess salt is in snacks such as chips, pretzels, and so on. Other sources are processed soups, which tend to have very high salt levels. Also, just like added sugars, many foods you would consider healthy and would not suspect do in fact contain added salt—for example, cheese and nuts. So, as with sugars, look at the nutritional labels of foods to be aware of how much salt they contain.

SATURATED AND TRANS FATS: In the past, many of our chronic ailments stemming from diet were attributed to fats. However, in recent years, the pendulum has started to shift. As explained in Chapter 3, it is becoming more and more apparent that sugars and digestible carbs are the real culprit and not fats. Certainly there is consensus today that trans fats are bad for the heart and brain, and that unsaturated fats (mono- and polyunsaturated fats) are good for the heart and brain. However, there is still an ongoing controversy with saturated fats.

Did You Know? Trans fats are on the way out, as most Western countries have adopted legislations to ban them. However, some foods, especially imported foods containing partially hydrogenated fats, may still contain trans fats.

In the fall of 2017, a major study called PURE was published in *The Lancet*, which followed the diet of 135,000 people in 18 countries.[78] It demonstrated that those who consumed the highest levels of fat, independent of the type of fat, were 26% less likely to die from any cause compared to those who consumed only 10% of calories from fat. Furthermore, those who had the highest intake of carbs (77% of calories) were 28% more likely to have died than those who consumed the least (46% of calories).

Another comprehensive review paper published in 2016 concluded that a high-sugar diet was much more harmful for cardiovascular disease than a high–saturated fat diet, and that you were three times as likely to die from a high-sugar diet than a high–saturated fat diet.[79] Finally, a well-known and healthy diet, the DASH Diet (to reduce blood pressure and other symptoms of cardiovascular disease), was amended to replace carbohydrates with saturated fats. The results obtained were comparable or better for the saturated fat diet, indicating that saturated fats are not harmful.[80]

Nevertheless, there are also many papers that point to saturated fats as unhealthy—the American Heart Association has issued an advisory against saturated fats and recommends replacing them with polyunsaturated fats.[81] As well, a reputable review of the matter, referred to as a Cochrane review, concluded that saturated fats did slightly increase the risk of cardiovascular disease.[82]

The saturated fat controversy is not limited to heart disease but also to the risk of AD/dementia. One Finnish study following a group of 2000 people, starting at an average age of 50 and ending when they were 65 or older, found that saturated fat from dairy significantly increased the risk of AD/dementia and mild cognitive impairment, but that this risk did not exist with unsaturated fats from fish or vegetables.[83] Another study on mice found that excess saturated fat caused an immune reaction and inflammation that destroyed nerve synapses.[84]

On the other hand, there have been reports that indicate the opposite for brain health. One paper published in 2016 as a part of the Nurses' Health Study included over 3000 subjects aged 30–75 and found that the highest quartile of dairy saturated fat resulted in reduced obesity and a 44% lower risk of diabetes as compared with the lowest quartile.[85] Both obesity and diabetes are high risk factors for AD/dementia. Another trial testing triglyceride (TG) levels in older-age Chinese subjects found that higher TG levels, which result from higher saturated fat intake, actually improved cognition.[86] Finally, a paper published in July of 2018 in the *American Journal of Clinical Nutrition* found that consumption of saturated dairy fats did not result in increased mortality or cardiovascular disease, and could even protect against certain types of stroke.[87]

On the whole, we believe that the current weight of evidence still indicates that saturated fats may be detrimental to brain health and the risk of AD/dementia, and therefore we include these fats in the list of foods to limit. At this point, it would be wise to limit saturated fats to the US government recommendation of 10% of calories, or about 22 g per day, in an average 2000 calorie-per-day diet.

5. PULLING IT ALL

TOGETHER: MENU PLANS

The previous chapters gave us a firm grounding by identifying those foods that are good for the brain and those that are bad for the brain, and the reasons for their benefits or harm. Now we can use this information to develop good eating habits and plans that will slow cognitive decline and reduce the risk of AD/dementia. In helping to develop a good diet plan for the brain, an interesting review paper published in 2016 (and in general agreement with our tables in Chapter 4) determined the key components of dietary risk factors in 10 counties that most affected cognitive function.[1] It found that diets high in whole grains, fruits, vegetables, and fish were associated with a lower risk of AD, but could not counter the effects of meat, eggs, and high-fat dairy consumption. Therefore, it is just as important, or even more important, to reduce consumption of harmful foods as it is to increase consumption of beneficial foods.

Did You Know? The importance of diet was demonstrated in Japan. As Western dietary habits became more mainstream in Japan, AD rates also rose: from 1% in 1985, to 7% in 2008.[2]

A diet plan that incorporates the information from the previous chapters can be something very simple and general or very detailed, depending on the interest of the reader. Of course, the more detailed we get, the more effective the diet plan will be.

If we just want a basic guideline to follow, then the simplest one is from Michael Pollan's book *In Defense of Food*. His basic rule is to "eat food, not too much, mostly plants."

What he means by food is food that is minimally processed. It's a great mantra, but it doesn't offer us much guidance as to which specific foods to eat and which to avoid, nor does it tell us how much of each food to eat. So, over the last several years, researchers followed the diets of population groups, called cohorts, and determined which food groups reduced the risk of AD/dementia and cognitive decline, and which increased the risk. The 2017 Alzheimer's International Conference reviewed the results available up to that time.[3] Basically, what it found was that diets that were rich in the good foods and low in the bad foods significantly reduced the risk of AD/dementia and cognitive impairment. It also found that diets that were deficient in these good foods and their corresponding nutrients, such as Omega-3 fatty acids, polyunsaturated fatty acids, B vitamins, and vitamins D and E, increased inflammation, which is believed to be a contributing factor to AD/dementia.

At its 2017 conference, the Alzheimer's Association focused its attention on three diet plans for reducing the risk of AD/dementia and cognitive decline. One was a Swedish plan called the Healthy Nordic Diet, which followed 2200 dementia-free adults in Sweden over six years and found that those who adhered to the diet had significantly improved cognitive function over those who did not. They also found that the Mediterranean and MIND diet plans reduced the risk of cognitive decline.

Did You Know? In general, any of these diets will be an improvement for brain health over the current North American diet. The objective is to continue to refine these diets as new science is developed and maximize their benefits.

In keeping with our general recommendations in Chapter 4, these diets emphasize the consumption of non-root vegetables, certain fruits (such as apples, pears, and peaches), fish and poultry, vegetable oils, tea, and light-to-moderate wine consumption. They also suggest a less-frequent intake of refined grains/cereals, butter/margarine, sugar, sweets/pastries, and fruit juices. The Mediterranean and MIND diet plans are probably the most studied diet plans for cognitive function, and exhibit the most evidence for their efficacy. For this reason, we will concentrate on these plans as a lead-in to our own Brain Boosting Diet plan.

MEDITERRANEAN DIET PLAN (MED): The Mediterranean diet was originally found to reduce the risk of cancer, obesity, hypertension, coronary heart disease, and abnormal glucose metabolism. In recent years it has also been found to reduce the risk of AD and MCI. The MED is based on the premise that a combination of beneficial foods with a reduction of detrimental foods associated with AD/dementia is better than boosting individual foods with additive effects and synergistic interactions. The original MED was characterized by a high consumption of beneficial foods such as vegetables, fruits and nuts, legumes, cereals, grains, fish, unsaturated fats, and moderate wine consumption with a low consumption of meats and dairy products. Over the years, as the science developed, the MED was revised and beneficial foods were adjusted so that olive oil was emphasized as an unsaturated fat, only whole grains (as opposed to refined grains) were considered good, herbs and spices were added as good foods, and poultry was considered acceptable. As for harmful foods, red meats were emphasized as well as junk foods and sweets.

The MED is a work in progress, and is reflecting more and more the good and bad foods described in Chapter 4.

Scarmeas was one of the best-known pioneers who demonstrated the cognitive benefits of the original MED.[4] He applied a nine-point score for adherence to the diet and found that the highest third had a 60–68% (depending on the population group) reduced risk of AD as compared with the lowest tertile. In a separate study, Scarmeas also found that the highest tertile of MED adherence had a 28% lower risk of MCI (which can lead to AD/ dementia).[5] Subsequent researchers confirmed the benefits of the MED, and several authors reviewed selected studies considered acceptable, concluding that the MED was indeed beneficial not only for decreasing the risk of AD/ dementia, but also for slowing cognitive decline and mild cognitive impairment. Singh et al. selected five studies out of 664 that met their eligibility criteria and, in the summary results, concluded that those who were in the highest third of the MED had a 33% reduced risk of mild cognitive impairment (MCI) or AD/dementia, and that the risk of progressing from MCI to AD also decreased.[6] Hardman et al. reviewed 18 eligible cohort trials in 2016 and came up with the same conclusions, that a higher adherence to a MED diet is associated with slower rates of cognitive decline, reduced conversion to Alzheimer's disease, and improvements in cognitive function.[7] Petersson and Philippou, also in 2016, reviewed five randomized control trials and 27 observational studies that met their criteria and found that the majority of studies showed that the MED was associated with improved cognitive function, a decreased risk of cognitive impairment, and a decreased risk of dementia or AD.[8] So, there is a weight of evidence surrounding the benefits of the MED.

One difficulty with the MED is that it is not clearly defined, and this has resulted in some inconsistency in trial results. As mentioned above, it is a work in progress, and continues to be modified as new science is developed to improve it. This is not surprising, since the MED is defined by general groups of foods, although one paper that tried to define the MED based on the averages of other authors' definitions came up with the following general recommended servings per day:[9]

- 3–9 servings of vegetables;
- ½–2 servings of fruit;
- 1–13 servings of cereals;
- up to 8 servings of olive oil;
- 37% of calories as total fat, 18% as monounsaturated fat, 9% saturated, 33 g fiber.

The above information goes a long way to explaining why different authors had different efficacies with the MED, because their definitions of what a MED actually is varied so much. By the same token, it also shows that the MED is quite robust, and significant benefits can be obtained even in large variations of its components. It also demonstrates that there is room for improvement, and optimization of the MED and its improvements are demonstrated in the MIND and Brain Boosting Diet plans.

MIND DIET PLAN: The MIND Diet is a diet developed by Martha Clare Morris and colleagues at the RUSH institute in Chicago. It is a combination of the MED and DASH (Dietary Approach to Stop Hypertension) diets, with particular emphasis on dietary components shown to be neuroprotective. The original MED and DASH diets were developed for reducing the risk of cardiovascular disease and based on consuming primarily plant foods with a limited intake of animal foods and saturated fat. This has also proven effective for reducing the risk of AD/dementia, with risk reductions of approximately 37% and 54% for the DASH and MED diets, respectively.

The basic elements of the MIND Diet, which essentially follow the good and bad foods listed in Tables 9 and 10, include an optimum of:

- at least 3 servings per day of whole grains;
- at least 6 servings per week of green leafy vegetables;
- more than 1 serving per day of other vegetables;
- 1 glass of wine per day;
- more than 5 servings of nuts per week;
- at least 3 servings of beans per week;
- at least 1 serving of fish per week;
- a minimum of 2 servings of berries per week (with an emphasis on blueberries);
- olive oil as the primary oil consumed.

The MIND Diet also limits butter or margarine to 1 Tbsp (15 mL) per day, fried food and cheese to one serving per week, pastries and sweets to less than five servings per week, and red and processed meats to less than five servings per week.[10] Using a scoring system based on these optimum values, Morris followed 960 older-age individuals over an average of 4.7 years and found that the third who adhered most closely to the MIND Diet slowed their cognitive decline to a point that it seemed they were 7.5 years younger than the third who least adhered to the diet. It should be noted, however, that the risk reduction for AD/dementia within this group that most closely adhered to the MIND Diet was the same as for those that most closely adhered to the MED diet. The difference was that the MIND Diet also had a 35% risk reduction for those who only moderately adhered to it, compared to no risk reduction for moderate adherents to the MED diet.

BRAIN BOOSTING DIET (BBD): This diet uses the MIND Diet as a basic platform and optimizes it based on the latest scientific findings as summarized in Tables 9 and 10. The BBD maintains the positive elements of the MIND Diet, such as the importance of fish, olive oil, nuts, green leafy vegetables and other vegetables, beans, wine, and berries. It also minimizes the consumption of red and processed meats, saturated fats such as butter, fried foods, pastries, and sweets.

Where the BBD differs from the other brain-healthy diets is in two key areas of developing science. The first has been discussed in Chapter 3, and has to do with the impact of sugars and digestible carbohydrates on brain and heart health. We concluded, based on updated research, that sugars and carbohydrates are a greater threat for cognitive decline than fats, and that AD/dementia could be considered the type 3 diabetes of the brain. Because of this, we have modified the MIND Diet to reduce those foods with added sugar, such as sweets and pastries, and to restrict other processed foods even further. In addition, we have also recommended a reduction in the consumption of foods that are high in naturally occurring sugars, such as fruits and even berries (especially blueberries). Instead, we emphasize consuming berries containing relatively low sugar, like strawberries, blackberries, and raspberries. We also reduce the amount of refined and starchy grains, and vegetables like rice, potatoes, and white flour, because they are easily converted into sugars by the body. Beyond this, we also de-emphasize the consumption of whole grains, since they contribute significantly to blood sugar levels, and because the benefits they offer can also be provided by legumes, other vegetables, seeds, and nuts.

The other major area of developing science affecting our diet recommendations is the observation that many foods that benefit the brain are dose dependent. What this means is that the more of that food you eat, the greater the effect. So, for example, at least 10 g of fish per day (about 1/10th serving) is required to see any effect, but 75 g per day (about one serving) is required for optimum effect.[11] Additionally, a key paper explaining inconsistencies in fish and Omega-3 effects showed that that best results were obtained between 750 and 1500 mg per day of DHA, a key Omega-3 fat found in fish, and that no effect was obtained below 500 mg per day.[12] Considering that most fatty fish contain 500–1500 mg of DHA per serving, it would appear that a serving of one meal per week of fish, as recommended in the MIND Diet, may not be enough. What's more, a Japanese paper found that even higher doses of DHA (at 1.7 g per day) could actually benefit people who already had AD.[13] Other key foods also showed dose-response effects. For example, a randomized control trial—the PREDIMED trial—found that when an extra liter of olive oil was added to a MED diet each week, and 30 g per day of nuts was added to a separate MED diet, both significantly improved cognitive ability.[14] As a result, we recommend the increased consumption of those beneficial foods, which have shown a dose-response effect.

Finally, within each food group, and wherever possible, we have emphasized the specific foods that have been shown to contain the highest concentrations of beneficial nutrients. Thus, in the nuts and seeds group we have focused on almonds, sunflower seeds, and walnuts, because almonds and sunflower seeds have the highest concentrations of natural vitamin E of any food, and this vitamin, in its natural form, is important for brain health. Walnuts have the highest concentration of plant-based Omega-3 fat of all nuts. In the case of fish, we have tried to emphasize fatty fish because they contain the highest concentration of Omega-3 fish oils, including DHA, which is so important for cognition.

Which Diet Should I Choose?

We have summarized the important characteristics of four major diet plans for the brain (and heart), each one increasingly following the latest nutritional recommendations for reducing the risk of AD/dementia and slowing cognitive decline. A comparison of the different plans, along with recommended serving sizes per week or day, is shown in Table 11. The question now is which diet should the reader follow?

The reality is that all the diets mentioned above will reduce your risk of AD/dementia as well as heart disease, but the likelihood, based on recent research, is that the effectiveness of the diet will improve as you go from the MED to the MIND, and ultimately to the BBD, and that as you go from the MED to the BBD you should increasingly be able to reduce your risk of cognitive decline even if you only partially adhere to the diet.

Table 11. Comparison of MED, MIND, and BBD diets.

	MED Diet and Servings	MIND Diet and Servings (major changes with MED in italics)[1]	BBD and Servings (major changes with MIND in bold)
High-intake consumption	Whole grains: >4/day Vegetables: >4/day Potatoes: >2/day Fruits: >3/day Fish: >6/wk Legumes and nuts: >6/wk Olive oil: >1/day	Whole grains: >3/day *Green leafy: >6/wk* *Other vegetables: >1/day* *Berries: >2/wk* *Nuts: >5/wk* Olive oil: primary	**Fish: >6/wk** Green leafy: >6/wk **Other vegetables (emphasize cruciferous vegetables): >1/day** **Berries (raspberries, blackberries, strawberries): >1/day** **Blueberries: >2/wk** **Nuts (emphasize walnuts, almonds, sunflower seeds): >1/day** Olive oil: primary
Moderate-intake consumption	Poultry: <3/wk Alcohol: <300 mL/day; >0 mL/day Full-fat dairy: <10/wk	Poultry: >2/wk Beans: >3/wk *Fish: >1/wk* Wine/alcohol: 1/day	**Cheese: <2/wk** **Full-fat dairy: <2/wk** **Poultry: <3/wk** Beans: >3/wk Wine/alcohol: 1/day **Whole grains: >1 per day**
Low-intake consumption		*Red meats: <4/wk* *Sweets: <5/wk* *Butter/hard margarine: <1 Tbsp/day* Cheese: <1/wk *Fast/fried food: <1/wk*	**Red/processed meat: <1/wk** **Starchy foods (pasta, rice, bread, potatoes, etc.): <3/wk** **Sweets: <2/wk** Fast/fried food: <1/wk Butter/hard margarine: <1 Tbsp/day

6. OPTIMIZING THE BRAIN BOOSTING DIET (BBD) THROUGH SMART FOOD COMBINATIONS AND PREPARATION

In Chapter 4 we identified those foods and nutrients that slow cognitive decline and reduce the risk of AD/dementia. However, there is substantial research to show that how we combine these foods and nutrients can significantly impact their efficacy. For example, in a paper by F. Jernereu et al. in 2015, it was shown in a placebo-controlled trial that brain atrophy (reduction in brain volume and neurons) could be reduced by 40% in older-age subjects with mild cognitive impairment (MCI) who were supplemented with the B vitamins B12, B6, and folic acid, but only if they had high-plasma Omega-3 levels.[1]

Did You Know? Approximately 5–10% of people with MCI eventually develop AD/dementia, but those who show brain atrophy have a higher rate of cognitive decline.

There was no reduction in brain atrophy with B vitamin supplementation in subjects with low-plasma Omega-3 levels. This could explain some of the inconsistent results obtained with both Omega-3 and B vitamin food interventions, and demonstrates the benefit of combining foods with both nutrients. Practically, this means we should combine foods that are high in each nutrient—for example, we should eat leafy vegetables that are rich in B vitamins with a fish meal. It also means we should obtain our Omega-3 fats through a fish meal rather than as a supplement, because fish contain vitamin B12 as well as Omega-3, whereas Omega-3 supplements may not contain this B vitamin.

Similarly, we earlier identified antioxidants in foods as being important for controlling cognitive decline. What we need to realize, however, is that some antioxidants are water soluble and some are fat soluble. Since humans are a water-based system, this means that those antioxidants that are fat soluble (e.g., carotenoids and vitamin E) may not be well absorbed without fat. For example, studies have found that incorporating some fat with carotenoid-containing foods can increase their absorption severalfold.[2,3]

Did You Know? Carotenoids are a class of fat-soluble antioxidants that give color to vegetables and fruits such as tomatoes, carrots, yams, and spinach. They include lycopene, lutein, and beta carotene.

To get the maximum benefit from fat-soluble antioxidants, we recommend that you add an oil-containing dressing (preferably olive oil) to your salads and vegetables. In this way you get the maximum benefit both from the olive oil and the fat-soluble antioxidants. You should also look for plant foods like avocados, which have significant amounts of fat that can increase the absorption of their fat-soluble antioxidants.[4]

Another example of how different foods can interact to produce different benefits was published recently in 2018 in the journal *Lipids*.[5] In that study it was found that absorption of Omega-3 fats in the diet was reduced by up to 37% when a monounsaturated fat such as soy oleic acid was also added at the same time. Although the study was carried out in chickens, the implication for humans is significant because fat digestion and absorption is similar in both species.

Did You Know? Nutritionists have for a long time advocated for increasing the ratio of Omega-3 to Omega-6 fats in the diet, but high amounts of non-Omega-3 fats can reduce the absorption of Omega-3 fats when both are consumed at the same time.[6]

What this means for our diet is that we should avoid consuming significant amounts of non-Omega-3 oils and fats with our fish (our primary source of beneficial Omega-3 fats).

HOW TO REDUCE DIGESTIBLE CARBS IN HIGH-CARB FOODS

We discussed in Chapter 3 the importance of limiting your consumption of sugars and digestible carbs. The problem is that high-carb foods are ubiquitous, and they often taste good. So, if occasionally you want to consume a high-carb food, there are forms of that food that will help reduce the content of digestible carbs:

RESISTANT STARCH: There is a phenomenon in starchy foods like potatoes and bread called resistant starch. This is starch that is structured in such a way that it becomes resistant to digestion and acts like a fiber.[7]

Did You Know? Once starch is converted to resistant starch it acts like a soluble fiber, which is beneficial for heart health, diabetic management, and metabolic syndrome.

There are several ways this can happen. Starch can be bound to the cell wall of a plant so that if you consume whole or large particle grains, seeds, or legumes, a portion of the starch will be trapped in the plant matrix and be unavailable for digestion.

Foods that have not yet ripened, such as green bananas, tend to have significant quantities of resistant starch, so if you want a banana that is normally very high in sugars go for a green banana instead of a ripe one.

Did You Know? Although a very green banana may not be very palatable, a partially ripe banana can be quite tasty.

Another thing you should be aware of is that starches that are not cooked tend to be very high in resistant starch. For example, raw potato starch and high-maize corn starch (which can be used as a thickener or sprinkled on foods) contain 50–70% by weight as resistant starch. Once cooked, however, most of the resistant starch is converted to digestible carbs. There are some high-carb foods, such as beans, lentils, and cassava, that can contain about 5% resistant starch even after cooking (especially if the food is allowed to cool several hours after cooking).

Finally, if you have a craving for bread, choose pumpernickel, rye, or Italian bread, and preferably hard dry or toasted, which will have the highest amount of resistant starch. For those of you who are interested in further information about resistant starch and lists of foods with their content of resistant starch, we have included some references at the end of this chapter.[7,8,9] Keep in mind that picking foods with resistant starch does not give you a license to binge on them. This is because the content of resistant starch in most foods, with the exception of raw potatoes or high-maize starch (which have limited use), is modest.

SLOWING DOWN CARB DIGESTION: Although we do not recommend eating high-carb foods on a regular basis for the reasons outlined in Chapter 3, an occasional high–digestible carb food should not be harmful, and you can reduce the impact by eating it together with fat, soluble fiber, or vinegar.[10] Fat and soluble fiber tend to slow down the absorption of the carbs, and an easy way to incorporate these with high-carb foods is to also eat a salad with chia, flax, or nuts, all of which are rich in both fiber and fat. Similarly, vinegar inhibits the enzymes that convert carbs into sugar,[11] and 1–2 Tbsp (15–30 mL) can easily be added in the form of a vinaigrette salad dressing. There is also some initial evidence that in consuming these combinations the high-carb foods should be eaten last, for the maximum effect.[12]

ANTIOXIDANT CONSUMPTION: MAXIMUM IMPACT

Antioxidants are important in your diet because they help control the harmful effects of oxidative stress. The primary dietary sources of these antioxidants are plants, and include fruits, vegetables, and beverages derived from sources such as tea (preferably green tea, which has higher antioxidant levels than black tea), coffee, wine, cocoa (and high-cocoa chocolate without sugar), and beer.

The major classifications of dietary antioxidants are polyphenols and carotenoids, and the number of antioxidants identified to date is staggering. In the polyphenol category alone scientists have so far identified over 9000 different molecules, and many plant sources contain large numbers of different antioxidants. Because of this, we have not been able to study these antioxidants, save for the very simple ones such as vitamin C, vitamin E, vitamin A, and beta carotene. It is therefore impossible currently to determine which of the complex plant antioxidants are most beneficial for brain health, and the best approach is to consume a wide variety of antioxidants from different plant sources.

Did You Know? Plants consume large quantities of oxygen for their growth, and to protect them against high oxidative stress evolution has provided them with a complex system of antioxidants.

There are also other things to consider. Some plant antioxidants are fat soluble (e.g., carotenoids in tomatoes and carrots) and some are water soluble (e.g., many polyphenols from leafy vegetables). Since human digestion is essentially a water-based system, this means that in order to better absorb the fat-soluble antioxidants we should eat antioxidant rich foods with a small amount of fat, such as olive oil or butter, or a food that is rich in fat like cheese or nuts.

Another problem is that some antioxidants like lycopene (from tomatoes) are bound very tightly to the tomato matrix, and in order to release them we need to macerate and cook them—you will get much more lycopene from tomato sauce or paste than from fresh tomatoes. Finally, for antioxidants that are easily released from the plant matrix, cooking may destroy many of the antioxidants, and therefore steam cooking or raw consumption is recommended. However, it is not just cooking that can reduce antioxidant efficacy. Extensive processing of any kind can affect antioxidants and produce harmful constituents. For example, although coffee is a rich source of antioxidants, over-roasting can form acrylamides that not only have been shown to accelerate cognitive decline, but can also cause cancer.[13] Therefore, you should choose a mild- or medium-roast coffee.

The following guidelines will help you maximize the benefits of antioxidants:

- eat a variety of different antioxidant-containing foods from fruits, vegetables, tea, coffee, wine, and cocoa;
- add small amounts of fats such as olive oil (e.g., in a salad), butter, cheese, nuts, and so on when eating fruits or vegetable or high-antioxidant beverages that are low in fat;
- vary your preparation procedures to maximize antioxidant impact—cook tomatoes, onions, and cabbage to release more antioxidants, and steam heat carrots, broccoli, and asparagus, or eat them raw, to minimize antioxidant degradation;
- avoid extensively processed foods.

A summary of what has been discussed in this chapter is shown in Table 12.

Table 12. Preparation techniques to optimize the BBD.

Preparation Category	Recommended Preparation	Examples
Combining foods	Combine B vitamin–rich foods with Omega-3–rich foods.	Leafy vegetables (B vitamins) with fatty fish (Omega-3 fat).
	Combine carotenoid antioxidant–containing foods with fat.	Yams, spinach, carrots, tomatoes (carotenoids) with oily salad dressing or butter (fats).
	Avoid monounsaturated fats when consuming Omega-3 fats.	Oily fats or salad dressings (monounsaturated fats) with fatty fish (Omega-3 fats).
Reducing digestible carbs in high-carb foods	Choose resistant starch foods.	Whole or large particle grains, seeds and legumes, unripe bananas and fruits, uncooked starches, cooked and cooled beans, lentils, cassava.
	Slow carb digestion.	Eat high-carb foods with vinegar, fiber, and/or fat.
Maximize antioxidant impact	Spread antioxidant intake over many plant sources.	Eat a variety of vegetables and fruits.
	Vary preparation procedures of plant food.	Cook tomatoes, onions, and cabbage to release antioxidants. Steam cook other vegetables to minimize antioxidant degradation.
	Consume low-fat antioxidant foods with fat.	Consume low-fat vegetables and fruit with oily salad dressings (olive oil), nuts, or cheese.
	Don't overcook or over-process foods.	Use light- or medium-roast coffees.

7. SUPPLEMENTS

Up to this point our book has focused on how different foods and diet plans can help reduce the risk of memory loss and the development of AD/dementia based on the key nutrients that these foods contain. The question that arises, however, is whether we can improve our chances of maintaining memory and avoiding or treating AD/dementia by taking supplements of key nutrients shown to have a beneficial effect. This is the question we will try to answer in this section.

THE ROLE OF SUPPLEMENTS

There are three major areas where supplements may play a beneficial role in brain health:

1. Situations where a diet is insufficient in providing key brain nutrients, or where total ingestion is sufficient but means consuming too much of another food component that is less desired.
2. Situations where the body can better absorb the supplement version of a nutrient over the nutrient naturally present in a food.
3. Situations where the nutrient comes from a non-traditional food source or plant.

Let's explore some examples for the situations described above. In the first situation, the provision of Omega-3 fatty acid DHA is a good example. We know from the previous chapters in this book that DHA is an important Omega-3 fat for the brain, and we know that it is dose-responsive—the more you take, the more effective it is. The potential problem here is that the best source for DHA is fatty fish, and the recommended intake of six servings per week in our Brain Boosting Diet. Some people may not want to consume that much fish, or have an aversion or allergy to fish, or adhere to a vegan diet. For this group, a supplemental source of DHA may be advisable. One available source of supplemental DHA that is also suitable for a vegan diet is an algae-based DHA.

In the second situation, a good example is in B vitamins—folic acid and vitamin B12. Supplemental folic acid is absorbed with 70% more effectiveness than food folic acid, possibly because it is difficult to break apart and digest the natural matrix of the folic acid from the food complex. Since there is evidence of the effectiveness of folic acid in reducing AD/dementia risk, it may therefore be logical to use this supplement. Vitamin B12, which is also important for cognitive maintenance, is another nutrient that may be a candidate for supplementation, especially in older-age individuals. To be absorbed, the B12 must first be separated from the protein with which it is bound in the food. This usually requires acids found in the stomach and saliva, which tend to decrease with age. The use of protein pump inhibitors (PPIs) or other antacids commonly used by older-age people can aggravate the problem. Add to this the fact that most sources of B12 are animal-based and we have an extra problem for vegetarians. Supplemental sources of B12 can overcome both these issues, as they are not bound to proteins and can be obtained from vegetarian sources.

Finally let's look at the third situation. There are many supplements under investigation that either do not exist in traditional foodstuffs or are there in too low a quantity for effectiveness. Although most of these supplements have very little proof of efficacy and will not be discussed in this book, there are a few, such as synthetic alpha lipoic acid and carnitine, that show some promise.

SUPPLEMENTS TO CONSIDER

We have reviewed many supplements that are touted for cognitive health and have rejected most because the evidence just wasn't there, or was of poor quality, or the data were highly inconsistent. However, there are several supplements with considerable research behind them that have shown some efficacy. We have divided these supplements into two categories: "worth taking" and "worth considering." The "worth taking" supplements have solid science behind them, adhere to at least one of the three major areas discussed above where supplements are warranted, and have minimal side effects. The "worth considering" supplements are on a lower rung because of inconclusive evidence, inconsistency in the data, or side effects. Nevertheless, they are included because the positive studies conducted demonstrate significant potential for reducing AD/dementia risk. In the following paragraphs below we will review those supplements which are either in the "worth taking" or "worth considering" category.

SUPPLEMENTS WORTH TAKING

VITAMIN B12: We have established earlier in this book that the B vitamin group has been shown time and again to be beneficial in preventing cognitive decline. The main B vitamins that have been noted for their efficacy are folic acid, vitamin B6, vitamin B12, and niacin. All of these, except for vitamin B12, can be consumed in good quantities using one of the diet plans recommended in our book, and one of them, folic acid, is often used for the fortification of food products.

Vitamin B12, on the other hand, presents several barriers to adequate consumption. As we age, our ability to absorb vitamin B12 diminishes significantly, and it has been found that healthy people in the age range of 61–80 years have three times less vitamin B12 in their brains compared to healthy younger subjects.[1] One paper estimated that up to 43% of community-living older adults suffer from B12 deficiency.[2] There are several reasons for these observations.

Older adults have less capability of separating B12 from the protein to which it is bound in foods, either because of naturally or medically diminished acid production. Additionally, most natural B12 comes from animal-based foods, which means that B12 consumption could be reduced with our emphasis on plant-based food. For these reasons, and for the added bonus that supplemental B12 is not bound to protein (and is therefore easier to absorb), we believe that B12 supplementation is warranted. Recommended dosage of 100 mcg per day.

VITAMIN D: Although vitamin D has not been studied as extensively as B vitamins, there are sufficient positive data both for general health and brain health to merit a closer look. In 2016, two major Asian studies were published that showed an association between low vitamin D levels in an older Korean adults and an extent of cognitive decline.[3] In another study, low vitamin D levels predicted future cognitive decline and impairment in older Chinese adults.[4] The latter results were later replicated in a US study.[5]

It appears that vitamin D has many of the same availability problems vitamin B12 suffers from, and one estimate is that 42% of the US population could be deficient.[6] The major source of vitamin D is from exposure to the sun on the skin, but for older adults the synthesis of sunlight to vitamin D is impaired, a problem that is aggravated for those living outside the sunbelt, or those who wear protective sun screening. Diet is a relatively small contributor of vitamin D, which is sourced mostly from fortified dairy foods, eggs, fatty fish, and meat. People who emphasize plant-based foods in their diet are likely to have reduced levels of vitamin D. For these reasons, we recommend vitamin D supplements. The recommended dosage is 1000 IU per day.

Did You Know? Vitamin D is necessary for the proper functioning of your muscles, nerves, and immune system, and is thought to reduce the risk of severe diseases such as MS and cancer. It is a fat-soluble compound and is therefore better absorbed when taken with a fatty food.

CURCUMIN: Curcumin and its related curcuminoids are the major components of a spice called turmeric, which is used as a main ingredient in curry and some mustards. Curcumin has a characteristic yellow color and is often used as a coloring agent in cheese, butter, and other fatty foods. For many centuries it has been used as both a food and medicine, and medicinally it has been used in the treatment of liver and respiratory ailments, skin diseases, wound healing, abdominal pain, and tumor suppression. Many papers have been published on its medical use, and most of these ascribe its effectiveness to its strong antioxidant and anti-inflammatory properties. More recently, papers have been published on its benefits for cognitive health. These papers indicate its potential for preventing cognitive decline in a number of ways.

There are limited clinical trial data demonstrating the direct effectiveness of curcumin on AD/dementia, but one study found that in combination with vitamin D, beta amyloid (protein associated with AD) clearance was enhanced in Alzheimer's patients.[7] In another double-blind placebo-controlled trial in healthy subjects aged 60–85 years, a bioavailable form of curcumin was found to significantly improve alertness and working memory compared to subjects receiving the placebo both short term (one to three hours) and long term (four weeks).[8] It was also observed to reduce stress in the subjects.

There are other ways that curcumin can prevent cognitive decline. We discussed in Chapter 3 how AD can be considered the type 3 diabetes of the brain because of reduced insulin sensitivity and increased inflammatory glycation products resulting from high sugar intake. In a randomized double-blind placebo-controlled trial of 270 subjects with pre-diabetes over nine months, it was found that 16% of the placebo group developed diabetes and 0% of the curcumin group developed diabetes.[9] In addition, other papers showed that curcumin reduced complications in human subjects with type 2 diabetes such as neuropathy, retinopathy, and hepatic fibrosis,[10] and increased insulin sensitivity in a rat study.[11]

Cardiovascular disease (CVD) is another risk factor for AD/dementia, and is the primary risk factor for vascular dementia. Many publications have shown the beneficial effects of curcumin in reducing the risk of CVD. In one study with healthy volunteers, curcumin decreased serum cholesterol and lipid peroxide levels, and increased high-density lipoprotein, at a relatively low dose of 500 mg per day for seven days.[12] Similar results were obtained in patients with acute coronary syndrome.[14] These effects are comparable with the statin drug atorvastatin (or Lipitor).[15]

The data presented above are probably sufficient to put curcumin in the category of supplements "worth considering," but there are other factors that push it into the "worth taking" realm. Most of the health studies we have described for curcumin are based on the compound itself, but it is very poorly absorbed by the body. Despite this, positive results have been generated in attenuating many chronic diseases. In the last few years, several technologies have emerged to dramatically improve the absorption of curcumin, and we believe, therefore, that its true potential is just beginning to develop. Add to this that it is very safe, even in large doses, and that as a spice and coloring agent it is not available in significant quantities in our diet, and we conclude that it is a supplement worth recommending at a dose of 2 g per day.

Did You Know? There is a compound in black pepper called piperine that can significantly increase the absorption of curcumin. An extract of black pepper is now added to many commercial formulations of curcumin.

PHOSPHATIDYLSERINE (PS): This is a fat-based compound found extensively in brain cell membranes. It is thought to maintain cell membrane fluidity for efficient nutrient uptake and for cell survival and communication. Although it is found naturally in foods, especially in fatty fish and meats, the average dietary intake is below levels that have been found to be efficacious for brain health.

Many double-blind placebo-controlled trials have been conducted on the effects of supplemental PS on brain health. Although these studies have been mostly short term and small, they have generally been positive both in reducing the risk of dementia and in reducing cognitive dysfunction in those that already have dementia.

Did You Know? PS is the only cognitive supplement approved by the FDA with the following qualified health claim: "Consumption of phosphatidyl serine may reduce the risk of dementia and cognitive dysfunction in the elderly."

There have been many controlled studies carried out showing the beneficial effects of PS on subjects who are cognitively impaired but do not suffer from dementia.[16,17,18,19] The weakness of these studies is that they were all of short durations, performed over a duration of months, and that the number of participants were generally below 100. Nevertheless, they were positive and reproducible, and one study found that the effects of PS were enhanced when combined with Omega-3 DHA.[20]

Perhaps more importantly, PS was found in a number of controlled studies to improve cognitive dysfunction in people who were already suffering from AD/dementia.[21,22,23] This is important because few dietary components or supplements have been efficacious in this regard. Granted that these studies suffered from the same short times and low subject numbers as the studies linked to risk reduction of AD/dementia, and that one of them hinted at the interventions not being long lasting.[21] Nonetheless, these studies have shown positive results in a field where only a handful of drugs have been demonstrated to even slightly improve AD symptoms. For all of these reasons, we recommend taking PS at a dose of 300 mg per day.

A summary of the supplements we recommend as "worth taking" is collected in Table 13.

Table 13. Supplements worth taking.

Supplement	Dosage	Comments
Vitamin B12	100 mcg/day	Dietary deficiency in older adults.
		Poorly absorbed at an older age.
		Dietary source mainly from animal foods.
Vitamin D	1000 IU/day	Low levels associated with cognitive decline.
		Deficiency in the general US population.
		Poor conversion of sunlight to vitamin D at an older age.
		Animal-based foods are the main dietary source.

(CONTINUED NEXT PAGE)

Table 13. Supplements worth taking. (CONTINUED)

Supplement	Dosage	Comments
Curcumin	2 g/day	In combination with vitamin D it helps clear beta amyloid (plaque protein). Improves memory. Reduces risk and complications of type 2 diabetes and heart disease. Strong antioxidant and anti-inflammatory. Look for enhanced absorption formulations.
Phosphatidyl serine	300 mg/day	Dietary sources of fish and meat insufficient for an effective dose. Only cognitive supplement approved by the FDA for a health claim. Many well-controlled studies of short durations with small enrollments have shown positive effects on cognition.

SUPPLEMENTS WORTH CONSIDERING

There are a number of other supplements worth mentioning with substantial research behind them that have not been included as "worth taking" in our list of supplements because results have been very inconsistent, or because they have potentially significant side effects. However, they may over time become "worth taking," either by themselves or with modifications, and we offer them below for your consideration.

GINKGO BILOBA (GB): Ginkgo biloba (GB) is not commonly found in the diet and is usually consumed as an extract. According to the Alzheimer's

Drug Discovery Foundation, GB extract is probably the most studied of all the supplements with respect to AD/dementia. Unfortunately, the results are extremely inconsistent. The definitive study of whether GB can prevent cognitive decline in older adults, called GEM, concluded that there was no effect to GB when compared with the placebo.[24] This was a very large (3069 people, 72–96 years old) randomized double-blind placebo-controlled trial conducted in six medical centers in the US over a period of six years.

As opposed to not preventing cognitive decline, however, there is some evidence that GB may slightly improve memory and cognitive function and slow down cognitive decline, at least in the short term, for people who have shown signs of cognitive impairment or dementia. That said, even this information is controversial. One review paper carried out by the respected Cochrane Group concluded that the effects of GB were inconsistent and unreliable,[25] while another more recent meta-analysis (review paper) showed that there was improvement in cognitive scores after 24 weeks for people with mild cognitive impairment or AD when they took GB with conventional medication as opposed to conventional medications alone.[26]

So, as seen from the above discussion, the evidence is very inconclusive, and for this reason we have left it off the "worth taking" list until more-sufficiently consistent data are obtained.

SOY ISOFLAVONES: Soy isoflavones belong to the polyphenol group of plant antioxidants and are found primarily in soy products.

Did You Know? Because soy isoflavones interact with estrogen receptors, they have been called phytoestrogens and have been used to reduce the symptoms of menopause in women.

As polyphenols, they exhibit strong antioxidant and anti-inflammatory properties, and the clinical trials that have been conducted do seem to show cognitive improvement in older adults without dementia. One relatively recent review paper concluded that out of 10 randomized controlled trials, isoflavones improved overall cognitive function and memory in post-menopausal women.[27] There are fewer studies on the effect of soy isoflavones on people with AD/dementia, and one randomized controlled study on a small sample of AD patients found no effect as compared with the placebo.[28]

There appears to be a fair amount of consistent evidence that soy isoflavones can improve cognitive function in healthy older adults. However, we have not included these supplements in our "worth taking" list primarily because they are phytoestrogens, and there is controversy as to whether phytoestrogens may pose a risk for breast cancer.

OMEGA-3 OIL CAPSULES: Omega-3s can be obtained in sufficient quantity from fish; however, there are those that are averse to consuming fish, or who are vegan, and vegetable sources of Omega-3s are thought to be inefficiently converted to EPA and DHA. For these people, fish or algae oil capsules, at 2 g per day, can be helpful.

Did You Know? Algae produce large quantities of the Omega-3 fatty acids EPA and DHA, and are suitable for vegans.

POTENTIAL PROBLEMS TO CONSIDER WHEN TAKING SUPPLEMENTS

We have seen that some of the supplements have a significant weight of evidence associated with them being effective in preventing cognitive decline or even treating AD/dementia. So, in addition to choosing the proper diet, it may make sense to take the supplements rated as "worth taking." However, we should keep in mind potential downsides to taking these supplements:

- Although some supplements show a significant effect on brain protection when studied on their own, their impact may not be as great if a person is already subscribing to a brain-healthy diet. The first action you take to improve your cognition will have the biggest effect. Each intervention you take after that will likely have smaller and smaller impacts when measured as a percentage improvement over the last measure.
- Supplements are not drugs and are not as rigorously supervised by the government, so you may not actually be getting what the label says. This is especially true for herbal or food extracts, which are not well defined, but it could also be the case with pure compounds such as vitamin B12. Always look for the USP logo on these products to ensure that they adhere to very strict testing standards.
- In the case of extracts, you may not be getting the same extract that was tested in clinical trials. For example, when ginkgo biloba has been tested and procured positive results, this is because it was prepared in a special extraction procedure from a selected part of the ginkgo plant.

You would have to make sure that any supplement you purchased was prepared in the same way as the extract used in the positive clinical trials to be sure that it could provide similar benefits. Check the label for information to verify if the product has been processed in the same way as the positive clinical material.

- Herbal or plant extracts depend on the location that the plant or herb was sourced from. Soil conditions, weather, time of harvest, and other factors could affect the active components in the extract. Unless there is a specific analytical test for the active component(s), you don't really know if you are getting what you are supposed to be getting. Look for the amount of active component contained in the product on the package label.

The approach we recommend is to try one or two of the "worth taking" supplements in addition to your diet. If you see no improvement after several months, then replace them with one of the others.

REFERENCES

Chapter 2

1. Scheltens P, Blennow K, Breteler MBM, et al. (2016) "Alzheimer's Disease." *The Lancet.* 388 (10043): 505–517.

2. Burnham SC, Bourgeat P, Doré D, et al. (2016) "Clinical and Cognitive Trajectories in Cognitively Healthy Elderly Individuals with Suspected Non-Alzheimer's Disease Pathophysiology (SNAP) or Alzheimer's Disease Pathology: a Longitudinal Study." *The Lancet Neurology.* 15 (10): 1044–1053.

3. Troncone L, Luciani M, Coggins M, et al. (2016) "Abeta Amyloid Pathology Affects the Hearts of Patients with Alzheimer's Disease." *Journal of the American College of Cardiology.* 68 (22): 2395–2407.

4. Goodman RA, Lochner KA, Thambisetty. (2011–2013) "Fee-for-Service Beneficiaries." *Alzheimer's & Dementia.* 13 (1): 28–37

5. Brenowitz WD, Hubbard RA, Keene CD, et al. (2017) "Mixed Neuropathologies and Estimated Rates of Clinical Progression in a Large Autopsy Sample." *Alzheimer's & Dementia.* 13 (6): 654–662.

6. Barnes DE, Yaffe K. (2011) "The Projected Impact of Risk Factor Reduction on Alzheimer's Disease Prevalence." *The Lancet Neurology.* 10 (9): 819–828.

7. Norton S, Mathews FE, Barnes D, et al. (2014) "Potential for Primary Prevention of Alzheimer's Disease: An Analysis of Population-Based Data." *The Lancet Neurology.* 13 (8): 788–794.

8. Barnes DE, Yaffe K, Byers AL, Whitner RA. (2012) "Midlife vs. Late-Life Depressive Symptoms and Risk of Dementia Differential Effects for Alzheimer's Disease and Vascular Dementia." *Archives of General Psychiatry.* 69 (5): 493–498.

9. Campbell NL, Perkins AJ, Pamela Bradt P, et al. (2016) "Association of Anticholinergic Burden with Cognitive Impairment and Health Care Utilization Among a Diverse Ambulatory Older Adult Population." *Pharmacotherapy.* 36 (11): 1123–1131.

10. Wiley JZ, Gardener H, Caunca MR, et al. (2016) "Leisure-Time Physical Activity Associates with Cognitive Decline." *Neurology.* 86 (20): 1897–1903.

11. Rakesh G, Szabo ST, Alexopoulos GS, Zannas AS. (2017) "Strategies for Dementia Prevention: Latest Evidence and Implications." *Therapeutic Advances in Chronic Disease.* 8 (8-9): 121–136.

12. Moraros J, Nwankwo C, Patten SB, Mousseau DD. (2017) "The Association of Antidepressant Drug Usage with Cognitive Impairment or Dementia, Including Alzheimer Disease: A Systematic Review and Meta-Analysis." *Depression and Anxiety*. 34 (3): 217–226

13. Nicole TM, Mowszowski L, Naismith SL, et al. (2017) "Computerized Cognitive Training in Older Adults with Mild Cognitive Impairment or Dementia: A Systematic Review and Meta Analysis." *The American Journal of Psychiatry*. 174 (4): 329–340.

Chapter 3

1. Cheke LG, Jon S, Simons JS, Nicola S, Clayton NS. (2016) "Higher Body Mass Index is Associated with Episodic Memory Deficits in Young Adults." *The Quarterly Journal of Experimental Psychology*. 69 (11): 2305–2316.

2. Bourssa K, Sbarra DA. (2017) "Body Mass and Cognitive Decline are Indirectly Associated via Inflammation Among Aging Adults." *Brain, Behaviour and Immunity*. 60 (February): 63–70.

3. Li Y, Hruby A, Bernstein AM, et al. (2015) "Saturated Fat as Compared to Unsaturated Fats and Sources of Carbohydrates in Relation to Risk of Coronary Heart Disease: A Prospective Cohort Study." *Journal of the American College of Cardiology*. 66 (14): 1538–1548.

4. DiNicolantonio JJ, Lucan SC, O'Keefe JH. (2016) "The Evidence for Saturated Fat and for Sugar Related to Coronary Heart Disease." *Progress in Cardiovascular Diseases*. 58 (5): 464–472.

5. Crane PK, Walker R, Hubbard RA. (2013) "Glucose Levels and Risk of Dementia." *New England Journal of Medicine*. 369 (6): 540–548.

6. National Institutes of Health, National Institute on Aging. "Higher Brain Glucose Levels May Mean More Severe Alzheimer's." NIH, NIA news release, 6 Nov. 2017.

7. Roberts RO, Lewis A, Roberts LA, Geda YE. (2012) "Relative Intake of Macronutrients Impacts Risk of Mild Cognitive Impairment or Dementia." *Journal of Alzheimer's Disease*. 32 (2): 329–339.

8. Deghan M, Mente A, Xhang X, et al. (2017) "Associations of Fats and Carbohydrate Intake with Cardiovascular Disease and Mortality in 18 Countries from Five Continents (PURE): A Prospective Cohort Study." *The Lancet*. 390 (10107): 2050–2062.

9. Salomón T, Sibbersen C, Hansen J, et al. (2017) "Ketone Body Acetoacetate Buffers Methylglyoxal via a Non-Enzymatic Conversion During Diabetic and Dietary Ketosis." *Cell Chemical Biology*. 24 (8): 935–943.

10. Drewnowski A, Rehm CD. (2014) "Consumption of Added Sugars Among US Children and Adults by Food Purchase Location and Food Source." *American Journal of Clinical Nutrition*. 100 (3): 901–907.

11. Lin PJ, Borer KT. (2016) "Third Exposure to a Reduced Carbohydrate Meal Lowers Evening Postprandial Insulin and GIP Responses and HOMA-IR Estimate of Insulin Resistance." *PLOS ONE*. 11 (10): Published online. Article e0165378 DOI: 10.1371/journal.pone.0165378.

12. Sacks FM, Carey VJ, Anderson CAM, et al. (2014) "Effects of High vs. Low Glycemic Index of Dietary Carbohydrate on Cardiovascular Disease Risk Factors and Insulin Sensititvity." *The Journal of the American Medical Association*. 312 (23): 2531–2541.

13. Roager HM, et al. (2019) "Whole Grain-Rich Diet Reduces Body Weight and Systemic Low-Grade Inflammation Without Inducing Major Changes of the Gut Microbiome: A Randomised Cross-Over Trial." *Gut*. 68 (1): Published online. DOI: 10.1136/gutjnl-2017-314786.

14. Cunnane SC, Courchesne-Loyer A, St-Pierre V, et al. (2016) "Can Ketones Compensate for Deteriorating Brain Glucose Uptake During Aging? Implications for the Risk and Treatment of Alzheimer's Disease." *Annals of the New York Academy of Sciences*. 1367 (1): 12–20.

Chapter 4

1. Joseph JA, Shuktt-Hale B, Denisova, NA, et al. (1998) "Long-Term Dietary Strawberry, Spinach, or Vitamin E Supplementation Retards the Onset of Age-Related Neuronal Signal-Transduction and Cognitive Behavioral Deficits." *The Journal of Neuroscience*. 18 (19): 8047–8055.

2. Cao G, Russell RM, Lischner N, Prior RL. (1998) "Serum Antioxidant Capacity is Increased by Consumption of Strawberries, Spinach, Red Wine or Vitamin C in Elderly Women." *The Journal of Nutrition*. 128 (12): 2383–2390.

3. American Academy of Neurology. "Will a salad a day keep memory problems away?" AAN press release (2017). Reterieved from: https://www.aan.com/AAN-Resources/Details/press-room/current-press-release/

4. Kang JH, Ascherio A, Grodstein F. (2005) "Fruit and Vegetable Consumption and Cognitive Decline in Aging Women." *Annals of Neurology*. 57 (5): 713–720.

5. Morris MC, Wang Y, Barnes LL, et al. (2018) "Nutrients and Bioactives in Green Leafy Vegetables and Cognitive Decline Prospective Study." *Neurology*. 90 (3): e214–e222

6. Setien-Suero E, Suarez-Pinilla M, Suarez-Pinilla P, et al. (2016) "Homocysteine and Cognition: A Systematic Review of 111 Studies." *Neuroscience & Biobehavioral Reviews*. 69 (October): 280–298.

7. David Smith AD, Stephen M. Smith SM, de Jager CA, et al. (2010) "Homocysteine-Lowering by B Vitamins Slows the Rate of Accelerated Brain Atrophy in Mild Cognitive Impairment: A Randomized Controlled Trial." *PLOS ONE*. 5 (9): Published online. Article e12244 DOI: 10.1371/journal.pone.0012244.

8. Lefevre-Arbogast S, Feart C, Dartigues JF, et al. (2016) "Dietary B Vitamins and a 10-Year Risk of Dementia in Older Persons." *Nutrients*. 8 (12): Published online. Article 761 DOI: 10.3390/nu8120761.

9. Johnson EJ. (2012) "A Possible Role for Lutein and Zeaxanthin in Cognitive Function in the Elderly." *American Journal of Clinical Nutrition*. 96 (5): 1161S–1165S.

10. Feeney J, O'Leary N, Moran R, et al. (2017) "Plasma Lutein and Zeaxanthin are Associated with Better Cognitive Function Across Multiple Domains in a Large Population-Based Sample of Older Adults: Findings from the Irish Longitudinal Study on Aging." *Journals of Gerontology Series A—Biological Sciences and Medical Sciences Impact Factor*. 72 (10): 1431–1436.

11. Basambombo LL, Carmichael PH, Côté S, Laurin D. (2016) "Use of Vitamin E and C Supplements for Prevention of Cognitive Decline." *Annals of Pharmacotherapy*. 51 (2): 118–124.

12. Mangialasche F, Xu W, Kivipelto M, et al. (2012) "Tocopherols and Tocotrienols Plasma Levels are Associated with Cognitive Impairment." *Neurobiology of Aging*. 33 (10): 2282–2290.

13. Van de Rest O, Wang Y, Barnes LL, et al. (2016) "APOE E4 and the Associations of Seafood and Long-Chain Omega-3 Fatty Acids with Cognitive Decline." *Neurology*. 86 (22): 2063–2070

14. Morris MC, Evans DA, Bienias JL, et al. (2003) "Consumption of Fish and N-3 Fatty Acids and Risk of Incident Alzheimer Disease." *Archives of Neurology*. 60 (7): 940–946.

15. Morris MC, Evans DA, Bienias JL, et al. (2003) "Consumption of Fish and N-3 Fatty Acids and Risk of Incident Alzheimer Disease." *Archives of Neurology*. 60: 940–946.

16. Huang TL, Zandi PP, Tucker KL, et al. (2005) "Benefits of Fatty Fish on Dementia Risk are Stronger for Those Without APOE e4." *Neurology*. 65 (9): 1409–1414.

17. Nurk E, Drevon CA, Refsum H, et al. (2007) "Cognitive Performance Among the Elderly and Dietary Fish Intake: The Hordaland Health Study."*American Journal of Clinical Nutrition*. 86 (5): 1470–1478.

18. Zhang Y, Jingnan Chen YJ, Qiu J, et al. (2016) "Intakes of Fish and Poly-unsaturated Fatty Acids and Mild-to-Severe Cognitive Impairment Risks: A Dose-Response Meta-Analysis of 21 Cohort Studies." *American Journal of Clinical Nutrition*. 103 (2): 330–340.

19. Raji CA, Erickson KI, Lopez O, et al. (2014) "Regular Fish Consumption and Age-Related Brain Gray Matter Loss." *American Journal of Preventive Medicine*. 47 (4): 444–451.

20. Ismail A. (2015) "Omega-3s and Cognition: Dosage Matters" *GOED Omega-3*. Published online: www.goedomega3.com/index.php/blog/2015/08/Omega-3s-and-cognition-dosage-matters

21. Yurko-Maro K, McCarthy D, Rom D, Nelson EB, et al. (2010) "Beneficial Effects of Docosahexanoic Acid on Cognition in Age Related Cognitive Decline." *Alzheimer's & Dementia*. 6 (6): 456–464.

22. Bo Y, Zhang X, Wang Y, et al. (2017) "The N-3 Polyunsaturated Fatty Acids Supplementation Improved the Cognitive Function in the Chinese Elderly with Mild Cognitive Impairment: A Double-Blind Randomized Controlled Trial." *Nutrients*. 9 (1): Published online. Article 54 DOI: 10.3390/nu9010054.

23. Yurko-Mauro K, Alexander DD, Van Elswyk ME. (2015) "Docosahexaenoic Acid and Adult Memory: A Systematic Review and Meta-Analysis." *PLOS ONE*. 10 (3): Published online. Article e0120391 DOI: 10.1371/journal.pone.0120391

24. Hashimoto M, Kato S, Tanabe Y, et al. (2017) "Beneficial Effects of Dietary Docosahexaenoic Acid Intervention on Cognitive Function and Mental Health of the Oldest Elderly in Japanese Care Facilities and Nursing Homes." *Geriatrics & Gerontology International*. 17 (2): 330–337.

25. Krikorian R. (2016) "Blueberrries May Boost Memory in Mild Cognitive Impairment." American Chemical Society 251st National Meeting and Exposition as reported in *Medscape*. 15 Mar. 2016.

26. Boespflug EL, Eliassen JC, Dudley JA, et al. (2018) "Enhanced Neural Activation with Blueberry Supplementation in Mild Cognitive Impairment." *Nutritional Neuroscience*. 21 (4): 297–305.

27. Bowtell JL, Aboo-Bakkar Z, Conway ME, et al. (2017) "Enhanced Task-Related Brain Activation and Resting Perfusion in Healthy Older Adults After Chronic Blueberry Supplementation." *Applied Physiology, Nutrition & Metabolism*. 42 (7): 773–779.

28. Johnson SA, Figueroa A, Navael N, et al. (2015) "Daily Blueberry Consumption Improves Blood Pressure and Arterial Stiffness in Postmenopausal Women Pre- and Stage1-Hypertension: A Randomized Double-Blind, Placebo-controlled Clinical Trial." *Journal of the Academy of Nutrition & Dietetics*. 115 (3): 369–377.

29. Krikorian R, Shidler MD, Nash TA, et al. (2010) "Blueberry Supplementation Improves Memory in Older Adults." *Journal of Agricultural & Food Chemistry*. 58 (7): 3996–4000.

30. Miller MG, Thangthaeng N, Scott TM, Shukitt-Hale B. (2016) "Dietary Strawberry Improves Cognition in Older Adults: A Randomized, Double-Blind, Placebo-Controlled Trial." *Experimental Biology*. 2016 meeting. Abstract only.

31. Shukitt-Hale B, Lau FC, Joseph JA. (2008) "Berry Fruit Supplementation and the Aging Brain." *Journal of Agricultural & Food Chemistry*. 56 (3): 636–641.

32. Joseph JA, Shukitt-Hale B, Lau FC. (2007) "Fruit Polyphenols and Their Effects on Neuronal Signaling and Behaviour in Senescence." *Annals of the New York Academy of Science*. 1100 (1): 470–485.

33. Shukitt-Hale B, Carey AN, Jenkins D, et al. (2007) "Beneficial Functions of Fruit Extract on Neuronal Behaviour in a Rodent Model of Accelerated Aging." *Neurobiology of Aging*. 28 (8): 1187–1194.

34. Lauren M. Willis ML, Barbara Shukitt-Hale B, Joseph JA. (2009) "Recent Advances in Berry Supplementation and Age-Related Cognitive Decline." *Current Opinion in Clinical Nutrition & Metabolic Care*. 12 (1): 91–94.

35. Devore EE, Kang JH, Breteler MMB, Grodstein F. (2012) "Dietary Intakes of Berries and Flavonoids in Relation to Cognitive Decline." *Annals of Neurology*. 72 (1): 135–143

36. Basu A, Rhone M, Lyons TJ. (2010) "Berries: Emerging Impact on Cardiovascular Health." *Nutrition Reviews*. 68 (3): 168–177.

37. Ho L, Yemul S, Wang J, Pasinetti GM. (2009) "Grape Seed Polyphenolic Extract as a Potential Novel Therapeutic Agent in Tauopathies." *Journal of Alzheimer's Disease*. 16 (2): 433–439.

38. Wang J, Ho L, Zhao W, et al. (2008) "Grape-Derived Polyphenolics Prevent Abeta Oligomerization and Attenuate Cognitive Deterioration in a Mouse Model of Alzheimer's Disease." *Journal of Neuroscience*. 28 (25): 6388–6392.

39. Lamport DJ, Lawton CL, Merat N. (2016) "Concord Grape Juice, Cognitive Function, and Driving Performance: A 12-Wk, Placebo-Controlled, Randomized Crossover Trial in Mothers of Pre-Teen Children." *American Journal of Clinical Nutrition*. 103 (3): 775–783.

40. Valls-Pedret C, Sala-Vila A, Serra-Mir M, et al. (2015) "Mediterranean Diet and Age-Related Cognitive Decline: A Randomized Clinical Trial." *Journal of the American Medical Association Internal Medicine*. 175 (7): 1094–1103.

41. Luceri C, Bigagli E, Pitozzi V, Giovannelli L. (2017) "A Nutrigenomics Approach for the Study of Anti-Aging Interventions: Olive Oil Phenols and the Modulation of Gene and Microrna Expression Profiles in Mouse Brain." *European Journal of Nutrition*. 56 (2): 865–877.

42. Elisabetta Lauretti E, Iuliano L, Pratico D. (2017) "Extra-Virgin Olive Oil Ameliorates Cognition and Neuropathology of the 3xtg Mice: Role of Autophagy." *Annals of Clinical and Translational Neurology*. 4 (8): 564–574.

43. Berr C, Portet F, Carriere I. (2009) "Olive Oil and Cognition: Results from the Three-City Study." *Dementia & Geriatric Cognitive Disorders*. 28 (4): 357–364.

44. Guasch-Ferré M, Liu X, Malik VS, et al. (2017) "Nut Consumption and Risk of Cardiovascular Disease." *Journal of the American College of Cardiology*. 70 (20): 2519–2532.

45. Aune D, Keum N3, Giovannucci E, et al. (2016) "Nut Consumption and Risk of Cardiovascular Disease, Total Cancer, All-Cause and Cause Specific Mortality: A Systematic Review and Dose-Response Meta-Analysis of Prospective Studies." *BMC Medicine*. 14 (207): Published online. DOI: 10.1186/s12916-016-0730-3.

46. Wengreen H, Munger RG, Cutler A, et al. (2013) "Prospective Study of Dietary Approaches to Stop Hypertension And Mediterranean-Style Dietary Patterns and Age-Related Cognitive Change: The Cache County Study on Memory, Health and Aging." *The American Journal of Clinical Nutrition*. 98 (5): 1263–1271.

47. O'brien J, Okereke O, Devore E, et al. (2014) "Long-Term Intake of Nuts in Relation to Cognitive Function in Older Women." *The Journal of Nutrition, Health & Aging*. 18 (5): 496–502.

48. Pribis P, Bailey RN, Russell AA, et al. (2012) "Effects of Walnut Consumption on Cognitive Performance in Young Adults." *British Journal of Nutrition*. 107 (9): 1393–1401.

49. Muthaiyah B, Essa MM, Lee M, et al. (2014) "Dietary Supplementation of Walnuts Improves Memory Deficits and Learning Skills in Transgenic Mouse Model of Alzheimer's Disease." *Journal of Alzheimer's Disease*. 42 (4): 1397–1405

50. Poulose SM, Miller MG, Shukitt-Hale B. (2014) "Role of Walnuts in Maintaining Brain Health with Age." *Journal of Nutrition*. 144 (4 Suppl): 561S–566S.

51. Dhillon J, Tan SY, Mattes RD. (2017) "Effects of Almond Consumption on the Post-Lunch Dip and Long-Term Cognitive Function in Energy-Restricted Overweight and Obese Adults." *British Journal of Nutrition*. 117 (3): 395–402.

52. Kulkami KS, Kasture SB, Mengi SA. (2010) "Efficacy Study of Prunus Amygdalus (Almond) Nuts in Scopolamine-Induced Amnsesia in Rats." *Indian Journal of Pharmacology*. 42 (3): 168–173.

53. Morris MC. (2004) "Diet and Alzheimer's Disease: What the Evidence Shows." *Medscape General Medicine*. 6 (1): Published online. Article 48.

54. Ozawa M, Shipley M, Kivimaki M, et al. (2016) "Dietary Pattern, Inflammation and Cognitive Decline: The Whitehall II Prospective Cohort Study." *Clinical Nutrition*. 36 (2): 506–512.

55. Topiwala A, Allan CL, Valkanova V, et al. (2017) "Acute Effects of a Wild Green-Oat (Avena Sativa) Extract on Cognitive Function in Middle-Aged Adults: A Double-Blind, Placebo-Controlled, Within-in-Subjects Trial." *Nutritional Neuroscience*. 20 (2): 135–151.

56. Thies F, Masson LF, Boffetta P, Kris-Etherton P. (2014) "Oats and CVD Risk Markers: A Systematic Literature Review." *British Journal of Nutrition*. 112 (S2): S19–S30.

57. Boffetta P, Thies F, Kris-Etherton P. (2014) "Epidemiological Studies of Oats Consumption and Risk of Cancer and Overall Mortality." *British Journal of Nutrition.* 112 (S2): S14–S18.

58. Graf B, Kamat S, Cheong KY, et al. (2017) "Phytoecdysteroid-Enriched Quinoa Seed Leachate Enhances Healthspan and Mitochondrial Metabolism in Caenorhabditis Elegans." *Journal of Functional Foods.* 37 (October): 1–7.

59. Graf B, Pouley A, Kuhn P, et al. (2014) "Quinoa Seeds Leach Phtoecdysteroids and Other Compounds with Anti-Diabetic Properties." *Food Chemistry.* 163 (November): 178–185.

60. Wang J, Ho L, Zhao Z, et al. (2006) "Moderate Consumption of Cabernet Sauvignon Attenuates Abeta Neuropathology in a Mouse Model of Alzheimer's Disease." *Federation of American Societies for Experimental Biology Journal.* 20 (13): 2313–2320.

61. Anstey KJ1, Mack HA, Cherbuin N. (2009) "Alcohol Consumption as a Risk Factor for Dementia and Cognitive Decline: Meta-Analysis of Prospective Studies." *American Journal of Geriatric Psychiatry.* 17 (7): 542–555.

62. Kennedy DO, Jackson PA, Forster J, et al. (2017) "Current Heavy Alcohol Consumption is Associated with Greater Cognitive Impairment in Older Adults." *Alcoholism: Clinical and Experimental Research.* 40 (11): 2435–2444.

63. Woods AJ, Porges EC, Bryant VE, et al. (2016) "Alcohol Consumption as Risk Factor for Adverse Brain Outcomes and Cognitive Decline: Longitudinal Cohort Study." *British Medical Journal.* 357: Published online. Article j2353 DOI: 10.1136/bmj.j2353.

64. Curtis BJ, Kovacs EJ. (2016) "Alcohol Worsens 'Inflamm-Aging' in the Elderly." 39th Annual Research Society on Alcoholism Scientific Meeting, June 28, 2016, as reported in *Medscape*, 29 June 2016.

65. Pereira MA, Parker ED, Folsom AR. (2006) "Coffee Consumption and Risk of Type 2 Diabetes Mellitus: An 11-Year Prospective Study of 28 812 Postmenopausal Women." *Archives of Internal Medicine.* 166 (12): 1311–1316.

66. Institute for Scientific Information on Coffee. (2016) "The Good Things in Life: Can Coffee Protect Against the Risk of CVD Mortality?" ISIC report.

67. Wu L, Sun D, He Y. (2017) "Coffee Intake and the Incident Risk of Cognitive Disorders: A Dose-Response Meta-Analysis of Nine Prospective Cohort Studies." *Clinical Nutrition.* 36 (3): 730–736.

68. Kuriyama S, Shimazu T, Ohmori K, et al. (2006) "Green Tea Consumption and Mortality due to Cardiovascular Disease, Cancer, and All Causes in Japan: The Ohsaki Study." *Journal of the American Medical Association.* 296 (10): 1255–1265.

69. Kim HM, Kim J. (2013) "The Effects of Green Tea on Obesity and Type 2 Diabetes." *Diabetes & Metabolism Journal.* 37 (3): 173–175.

70. Feng L, Chong MS, Lim WS, et al. (2016) "Tea Consumption Reduces the Incidence of Neurocognitive Disorders: Findings from the Singapore Longitudinal Aging Study." *The Journal of Nutrition, Health & Aging.* 20 (10): 1002–1009.

71. Iso H, Date C, Wakai K, Fukui M, Tamakoshi A, JACC Study Group. (2006) "The Relationship Between Green Tea and Total Caffeine Intake and Risk for Self-Reported Type 2 Diabetes Among Japanese Adults." *Annals of Internal Medicine.* 144 (8): 554–62.

72. Miller PE, Zhao D, Frazier-Wood AC, et al. (2017) "Associations of Coffee, Tea, and Caffeine Intake with Coronary Artery Calcification and Cardiovascular Events." *American Journal of Medicine.* 130 (2): 188–197.e5.

73. Rohrmann S, Overvad K, Bueno-de-Mesquita HB, et al. (2013) "Meat consumption and mortality-results from the European Prospective Investigation into Cancer and Nutrition." *BMC Medicine.* 11: Published online. Article 63 DOI: 10.1186/1741-7015-11-63.

74. Wang X, Lin X, Ouyang YY, et al. (2016): "Red and Processed Meat Consumption and Mortality: Dose Response Meta-Analysis of Prospective Cohort Studies." *Public Health Nutrition.* 19 (5): 893–905.

75. Etemadi A, Sinha R, Ward MH, et al. (2017) "Mortality from Different Causes Associated with Meat, Heme Iron, Nitrates, and Nitrites in the NIH-AARP Diet and Health Study: Population Based Cohort Study." *British Medical Journal.* 357: Published online. Article j1957 DOI: 10.1136/bmj.j1957.

76. Yang Q, Liu T, Kuklina EV, et al. (2011) "Sodium and Potassium Intake and Mortality Among US Adults." *Archives Internal Medicine.* 171 (13): 1183–1191.

77. Farquhar WB, Edwards DG, Jurkovitz CT, Weintraub WS. (2015) "Dietary Sodium and Health More than Just Blood Pressure." *Journal of the American College of Cardiology.* 65 (10): 1042–1050.

78. Giuseppe F, Brea D, Garcia-Bonilla L, et al. (2018) "Dietary Salt Promotes Neurovascular and Cognitive Dysfunction Through a Gut-Initiated TH17 Response." *Nature Neuroscience.* 21 (2): 240–249.

79. DiNicolantonio JJ, Lucan SC, O'Keefe JH. (2016) "The Evidence for Saturated Fat and for Sugar Related to Coronary Heart Disease." *Progress in Cardiovascular Diseases.* 58 (5): 464–472.

80. Dehghan M, Mente A, Zhang X, et al. on behalf of the Prospective Urban Rural Epidemiology (PURE) study investigators. (2017) "Associations of Fats and Carbohydrate Intake with Cardiovascular Disease and Mortality in 18 Countries from Five Continents (PURE): A Prospective Cohort Study." *The Lancet.* 390 (10107): 2050–2062.

81. Chiu S, Bergeron N, Williams PT, et al. (2016) "Comparison of the DASH (Dietary Approaches to Stop Hypertension) Diet and a Higher-Fat DASH Diet on Blood Pressure and Lipids and Lipoproteins: A Randomized Controlled Trial." *American Journal of Clinical Nutrition.* 103 (2): 341–347.

82. Sacks FM, Lichtenstein AH, Wu JHY, et al. (2017) "Dietary Fats and Cardiovascular Disease: A Presidential Advisory from the American Heart Association." *Circulation.* 136 (3): e1–e23.

83. Hooper L, Martin N, Abdelhamid A, Davey Smith G. (2015) "Reduction in Saturated Fat Intake for Cardiovascular Disease." *Cochrane Database of Systematic Reviews.* 6 (6): Published online. Article CD011737 DOI: 10.1002/14651858.CD01173.

84. Eskelinen M. (2014) "The Effects of Midlife Diet on Late-Life Cognition: An Epidemiological Approach." *Publications of the University of Eastern Finland Dissertations in Health Sciences.* Number 220.

85. Hao S, Dey A, Yu X, Stranahan AM. (2016) "Dietary Obesity Reversibly Induces Synaptic Stripping by Microglia and Impairs Hippocampal Plasticity." *Brain Behaviour and Immunity.* 51 (230-9): Published online. DOI: 10.1016/j.bbi.2015.08.023.

86. Yakoob MY, Shi P, WillettmWC, et al. (2016) "Circulating Biomarkers of Dairy Fat and Risk of Incident Diabetes Mellitus Among US Women in Two Large Prospective Cohorts." *Circulation.* 133 (17): 1645–1654.

87. Lv YB, Yin ZX, Chei CL, et al. (2016) "Serum Cholesterol Levels Within the High Normal Range are Associated with Better Cognitive Performance Among Chinese Elderly." *Journal of Nutrition, Health & Aging.* 20 (3): 280–287.

88. De Oliveira MC, Rozenn O, Lemaitre N, et al. (2018) "Serial Measures of Circulating Biomarkers of Dairy Fat and Total and Cause-Specific Mortality in Older Adults: The Cardiovascular Health Study." *The American Journal of Clinical Nutrition.* 108 (3): 476–484.

Chapter 5

1. Grant WB. (2016) "Using Multicountry Ecological and Observational Studies to Determine Dietary Risk Factors for Alzheimer's Disease." *Journal of the American College of Nutrition.* 35 (5): 476–489.

2. Ibid.

3. Alzheimer's Association. (2017) "Healthy Eating Habits May Preserve Cognitive Function and Reduce the Risk of Dementia." Alzheimer's Association International Conference 16–20 July 2017, London, England. Press Release. Retrieved from: www.alz.org/aaic/press.asp.

4. Scarmeas N, Stern Y, Mayeux R, Luchsinger JA. (2006) "Mediterranean Diet, Alzheimer Disease, and Vascular Mediation." *Archives of Neurology.* 63 (12): 1709–1717.

5. Scarmeas N, Stern Y, Mayeux R, et al. (2009) "Mediterranean Diet and Mild Cognitive Impairment." *Archives of Neurology.* 66 (2): 216–225.

6. Singh B, Parsaik AK, Mielke MM, et al. (2014) "Association of Mediterranean Diet with Mild Cognitive Impairment and Alzheimer's Disease: A Systematic Review and Meta-Analysis." *Journal of Alzheimer's Disease.* 39 (2): 271–282.

7. Hardman RJ, Kennedy G, Macpherson H, et al. (2016) "Adherence to a Mediterranean-style diet and effects on cognition in adults: A qualitative evaluation and systematic review of longitudinal and prospective trials." *Frontiers in Nutrition.* 3: Published online. Article 22 DOI: 10.3389/fnut.2016.00022.

8. Petersson SD, Philippou E. (2016) "Mediterranean Diet, Cognitive Function, and Dementia: A Systematic Review of the Evidence. American Society for Nutrition. Advances in Nutrition." 7 (5): 889–904.

9. Davis C, Bryan J, Hodgson J, Murphy K. (2015) "Definition of the Mediterranean Diet: A Literature Review." *Nutrients*. 7 (11): 9139–9153.

10. Morris MC, Tangney CC, Wang Y, et al. (2015) "MIND Diet Slows Cognitive Decline with Aging." *Alzheimer's & Dementia*. 11 (9): 1015–1022.

11. Davis, Bryan, Hodgson, Murphy (2015).

12. Raji CA, Erickson KI, Lopez O, et al. (2014) "Regular Fish Consumption and Age-Related Brain Gray Matter Loss." *American Journal of Preventive Medicine*. 47 (4): 444–451.

13. Yurko-Mauro K, Alexander DD, Van Elswyk ME. (2015) "Docosahexaenoic Acid and Adult Memory: A Systematic Review and Meta-Analysis." *PLOS ONE*. 10 (3): Published online. Article e0120391 DOI: 10.1371/journal.pone.0120391.

14. Lamport DJ, Lawton CL, Merat N. (2016) "Concord Grape Juice, Cognitive Function, and Driving Performance: A 12-Wk, Placebo-Controlled, Randomized Crossover Trial in Mothers of Pre-Teen Children." *American Journal of Clinical Nutrition*. 103 (3): 775–783.

Chapter 6

1. Fredrik Jernerén, Elshorbagy AK, Abderrahim O, et al. (2015) "Brain Atrophy in Cognitively Impaired Elderly: The Importance of Long-Chain V-3 Fatty Acids and B Vitamin Status in a Randomized Controlled Trial." *American Journal of Clinical Nutrition*. 102 (1): 215–221.

2. Uniu NZ, Bohn T, Clinton SK, Schwartz SJ. (2005) "Carotenoid Absorption from Salad and Salsa by Humans is Enhanced by the Addition of Avocado or Avocado Oil." *Journal of Nutrition*. 135 (3): 431–436.

3. Ribaya-Mercado JD, Maramag CC, Tengco LW, et al. (2007) "Carotene-Rich Plant Foods Ingested with Minimal Dietary Fat Enhance the Total-Body Vitamin a Pool Size in Filipino Schoolchildren as Assessed by Stable-Isotope-Dilution Methodology." *American Journal of Clinical Nutrition*. 85 (4): 1041–1049.

4. Scott TM, et al. (2017) "Avocado Consumption Increases Macular Pigment Density in Older Adults: A Randomized Controlled Trial." *Nutrients*. 9 (9): Published online. Article 919 DOI: 10.3390/nu9090919.

5. Elkin RG, et al. (2018) "Dietary High-Oleic Acid Soybean Oil Dose Dependently Attenuates Egg Yolk Content of N-3 Polyunsaturated

Fatty Acids in Laying Hens Fed Supplemental Flaxseed Oil." *Lipids.* 53 (2): 235–249.

6. Ibid.

7. Lockyer S, Nugent AP. (2017) "Health Effects of Resistant Starch." *British Nutrition Foundation Nutrition Bulletin.* 42 (1): 10–41.

8. Murphy MM, Douglass JS, Birkett A. (2008) "Resistant Starch Intakes in the United States." *Journal of the American Dietetic Association.* 108 (1): 67–78.

9. Moongngarm A. (2013) "Chemical Compositions and Resistant Starch Content in Starchy Foods." *American Journal of Agricultural and Biological Sciences.* 8 (2): 107–113.

10. IDM III. (2014) "Understanding Digestion: Why You Should Eat Carbohydrates with Fat, Fiber, and Vinegar" *IDM III.* Retrieved from: idmprogram.com/understanding-digestion-eat-carbohydrates-fat-fiber-vinegar-idm-3-2/

11. Johnston CS, Gaas CA. (2006) "Vinegar: Medicinal Uses and Antiglycemic Effect." *Medscape General Medicine.* 8 (2): Published online. Article 61.

12. Spero D. (2017) "Eat carbs last to reduce after-meal blood sugar spikes." Retrieved from: www.diabetesselfmanagement.com/blog/eat-carbs-last-reduce-meal-blood-sugar-spikes/

13. Liu ZM, Tse LA, Chen B, et al. (2017) "Dietary Acrylamide Exposure was Associated with Mild Cognition Decline Among Non-Smoking Chinese Elderly Men." Nature. 7 (1): Published online. DOI: 10.1038/s41598-017-06813-9. Retrieved from: www.nature.com/scientificreports/

Chapter 7

1. Zhang Y, Hodgon NW, Trivedi MS, et al. (2016) "Decreased Brain Levels of Vitamin B12 in Aging. Autism, and Schizophrenia." *PLOS ONE.* 11 (1): Published online. Article e0146797 DOI: 10.1371/journal.pone.0146797.

2. Pfisterer KJ, Sharratt MT, Heckman GG, Keller HH. (2016) "Vitamin B12 Status in Older Adults Living in Ontario Long-Term Care Homes: Prevalence and Incidence of Deficiency with Supplementation as a Protective Factor." *Applied Physiology, Nutrition and Metabolism.* 41 (2): 1–4.

3. Lee EY, Lee SJ, Kim KM, et al. (2017) "Association of Metabolic Syndrome and 25-Hydroxyvitamin D with Cognitive Impairment Among Elderly Koreans." *Geriatrics & Gerontology International.* 17 (7): 1069–1075.

4. Matchar DB, Chei CL, Yin ZX. et al. (2016) "Vitamin D Levels and the Risk of Cognitive Decline in Chinese Elderly People: The Chinese Longitudinal Healthy Longevity Survey." *Journals of Gerontology* series *A Biological Sciences and Medical Sciences Impact Factor.* 71 (10): 1363–1368.

5. Miller JW, Harvey DJ, Beckett LA, et al. (2015) "Vitamin D Status and Rates of Cognitive Decline in a Multiethnic Cohort of Older Adults." *Journal of the American Medical Association Neurology.* 72 (11): 1295–1303.

6. Forrest KY, Stuhldrehrer WL. (2011) "Prevalence and Correlates of Vitamin D Deficiency in US Adults Nutrition Research." 31 (1): 48–54.

7. Masoumi A, Goldenson B, Ghirmai S, et al. (2009) "1alpha,25-dihydroxyvitamin D3 Interacts with Curcuminoids to Stimulate Amyloid-Beta Clearance by Macrophages of Alzheimer's Disease Patients." *Journal of Alzheimer's Disease.* 17 (3): 703–717.

8. Cox KHM, Pipingas A, Scholey AB. (2015) "Investigation of the Effects of Solid Lipid Curcumin on Cognition and Mood in a Healthy Older Population." *Journal of Psychopharmacology.* 29 (5): 642–651.

9. Chuengsamarn S, Rattanamongkolgul S, Luechapudiporn R, et al. (2012) "Curcumin Extract for Prevention of Type 2 Diabetes." *Diabetes Care.* 35 (11): 2121–2127.

10. Stefanska B. (2012) "Curcumin Ameliorates Hepatic Fibrosis in Type 2 Diabetes Mellitus-Insights into Its Mechanisms of Action." *British Journal of Pharmacology.* 166 (8): 2209–2211.

11. Na LX, Zhang YL, Li Y, et al. (2011) "Curcumin Improves Insulin Resistance in Skeletal Muscle of Rats." *Nutrition, Metabolism & Cardiovascular Diseases.* 21 (7): 526–533.

12. Pari L, Tewas D, Eckel J. (2008) "Role of Curcumin in Health and Disease." *Archives of Physiology & Biochemistry.* 114 (2): 127–149.

13. Pungcharoenkul K, Thongnopnua P. (2011) "Effect of Different Curcuminoid Supplement Dosages on Total in Vivo Antioxidant Capacity and Cholesterol Levels of Healthy Human Subjects." *Phytotherapy Research.* 25 (11): 1721–1726.

14. Usharani P, Mateen AA, Naidu MU, et al. (2008) "Effect of NCB-02, Atorvastatin and Placebo on Endothelial Function, Oxidative Stress and Inflammatory Markers in Patients with Type 2 Diabetes Mellitus: A Randomized, Parallel-Group, Placebo-Controlled, 8-Week Study." *Drugs in R&D*. 9 (4): 243–250.

15. Kato-Kataoka A, Sakai M, Ebina R, et al. (2010) "Soybean-Derived Phosphatidylserine Improves Memory Function of the Elderly Japanese Subjects with Memory Complaints." *Journal of Clinical Biochemistry and Nutrition*. 47 (3): 246–55.

16. Gindin J, Novikov M, Dedar D, et al. (2009) "The Effect of Plant Phosphatidylserine on Age-Associated Memory Impairment and Mood in the Functioning Elderly." The Geriatric Institute for Education and Research and Department of Geriatrics, Kaplan Hospital, Rehovot, Israel. Unpublished report.

17. Crook TH. (1998) "Treatment of Age-Related Cognitive Decline: Effects of Phosphatidylserine." *Anti-Aging Medical Therapeutics, Vol II*, ed. Klatz RM. Health Quest Publications, Chicago: 20–29.

18. Cenacchi T, Bertoldin T, Farina C, et al. (1993) "Cognitive Decline in the Elderly: A Double-Blind, Placebo-Controlled Multicenter Study on Efficacy of Phosphatidyiserine Administration." *Aging, Clinical and Experimental Research*. 5 (2): 123–133.

19. Vakhapova V, et al. (2010) "Phosphatidylserine Containing Omega-3 Fatty Acids May Improve Memory Abilities in Non-Demented Elderly with Memory Complaints: A Double-Blind Placebo-Controlled Trial." *Dementia and Geriatric Cognitive Disorders*. 29 (5): 467–474.

20. Heiss W.D, et al. (1994) "Long-Term Effects of Phosphatidylserine, Pyritinol, and Cognitive Training in Alzheimer's Disease. A Neuropsychological, EEG, and PET Investigation." *Dementia*. 5 (2): 88–98.

21. Engel R.R, Satzger W, Gunther W, et al. (1992) "Doubleblind Cross-Over Study of Phosphatidylserine vs. Placebo Inpatients with Early Dementia of the Alzheimer Type." *European Neuropsychopharmacology*. 2 (2): 149–155.

22. Delwaide PJ, Gyselynck-Mambourg AM, Hurlet A, Ylieff M. (1986) "Double-Blind Randomized Controlled Study of Phosphatidylserine in Senile Demented Patients." *Acta Neurologica Scandinavica*. 73 (2): 136–40.

23. Snitz BE, O'Meara ES, Carlson MC, et al. (2009) "Ginkgo Biloba for Preventing Cognitive Decline in Older Adults: A Randomized Trial." *Journal of the American Medical Association.* 302 (24): 2663–2670.

24. Birks J, Grimley Evans J. (2009) "Ginkgo Biloba for Cognitive Impairment and Dementia." *Cochrane Database of Systematic Reviews.* Issue 1. Article CD00312.

25. Yang G, Wang Y, Sun J, et al. (2016) "Ginkgo Biloba for Mild Cognitive Impairment and Alzheimer's Disease: A Systematic Review and Meta-Analysis of Randomized Controlled Trials." *Current Topics in Medicinal Chemistry.* 16 (5): 520–528.

26. Cheng PF, Chen JJ, Zhou XY, et al. (2015) "Do Soy Isoflavones Improve Cognitive Function in Postmenopausal Women? A Meta-Analysis." *Menopause.* 22 (2): 198–206.

27. Kalaiselvan V, Kalaivani M, Vijayakumar A, et al. (2010) "Current Knowledge and Future Direction of Research on Soy Isoflavones as Therapeutic Agents." *Pharmacognosy Review.* 4 (8): 111–117.

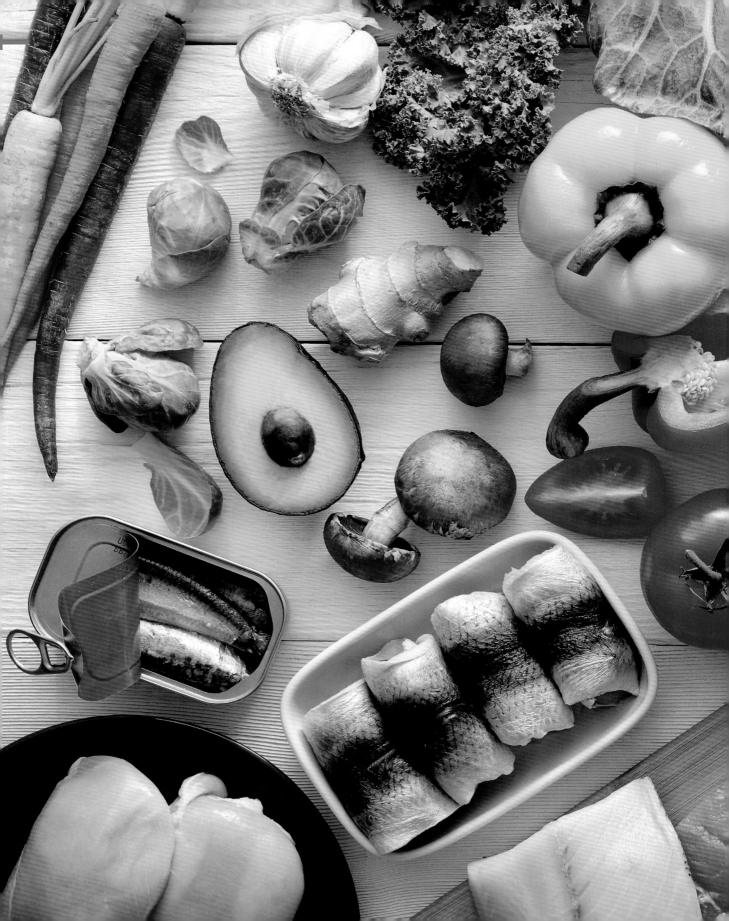

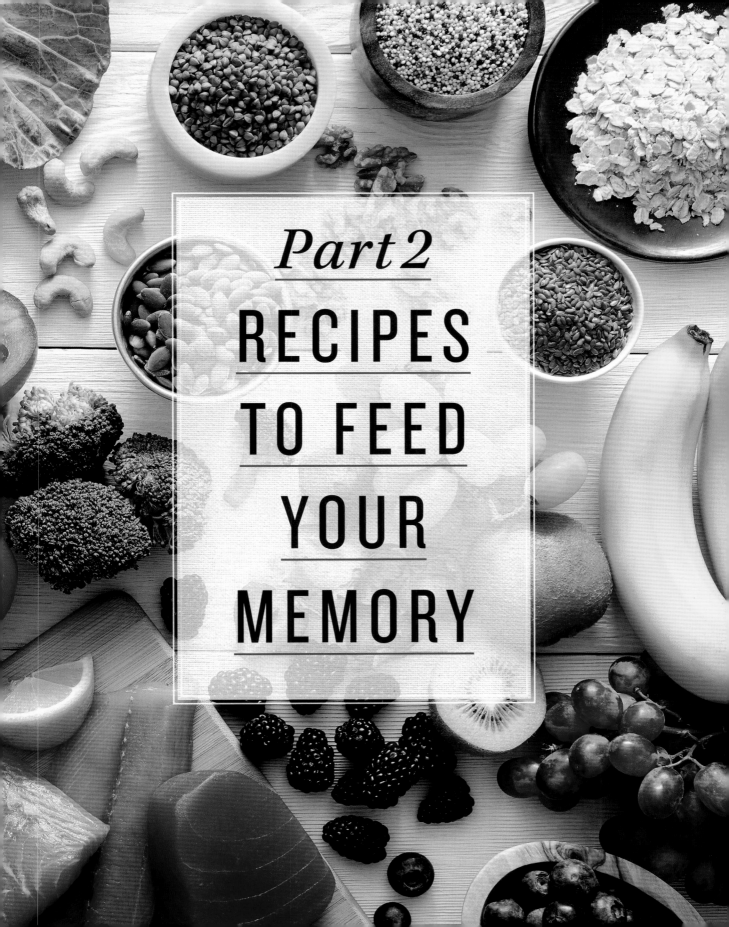

Part 2
RECIPES
TO FEED
YOUR
MEMORY

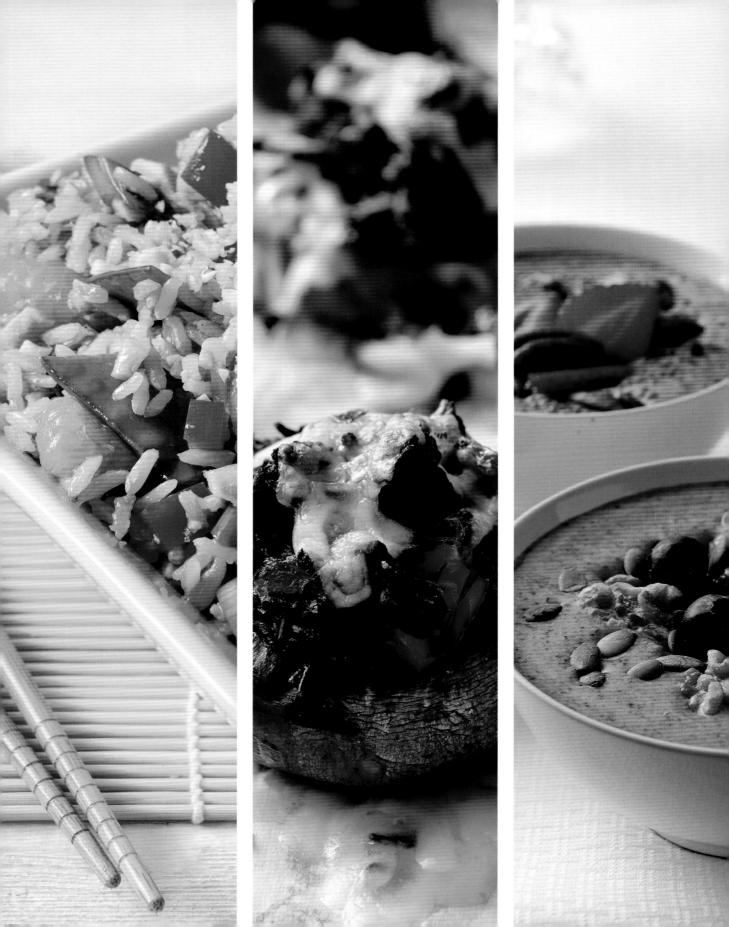

INTRODUCTION

"Food that's good for you should taste good." I firmly believe that no matter how healthy a recipe is, taste always rules. If a dish doesn't appeal to your taste buds, you just won't eat it. The recipes in *The Brain Boosting Diet: Feed Your Memory* have been designed to appeal to a wide range of people with different approaches to getting a meal on the table. People are always hungry for quick, easy-to-prepare meals with a healthy focus. The dishes in this book are fast, fabulous, flavorful, and fun, focusing on smart carbs, smart fats, and smart proteins. Here are some of the few other things to keep in mind as you flip through the book:

- Cook smarter, eat smarter! Learn how to put together memorable meals with minimal fuss and mess, delectable dishes that are lower in sodium, unhealthy fats, chemicals, and additives. They're so much better for you than store-bought or take-out versions.
- Mind your platters! Explore a wide variety of plant-based dishes starring vegetables, fruits (especially berries), beans and legumes, whole grains, nuts, seeds, and dark green leafy vegetables. Fish and lean cuts of poultry are more prominent than red meat, which are best saved for special occasions. I've included a variety of vegetarian dishes, especially mains and sides, that are heart-healthy, diabetes-friendly, and work well with weight loss and low-sugar lifestyles. Many of my desserts focus on chocolate, which comes from the cocoa bean—and we all know that beans are good for you! My recipes use healthier fats, flavorful herbs, and brain-beneficial spices. These simple guidelines are the building blocks of a Brain Boosting Diet.
- Tradition! Discover brain-healthy versions of traditional Jewish dishes—but you don't have to be Jewish to enjoy them. From everyday fare to easy entertaining, you'll find old favorites that have been updated and simplified, along with many new brain-boosting dishes. With simple swaps and switches, it's easy to customize recipes, adapting them to suit your taste and dietary requirements.
- Smart strategies! From singles to families, from children to seniors, from beginners to seasoned cooks, it's time to include meatless mains more often—meals that feature plant-based proteins or incorporate a variety of colorful, fiber-packed vegetables and fruits. Bottom line:

eating healthy has to taste great, or you won't want to make the recipe again.

- It all starts out in your shopping cart! Packaged, processed convenience foods are usually loaded with excess sugar, salt, and unhealthy fats—so focus on natural, unprocessed ingredients. You'll learn how to choose "good-for-you" ingredients that will appeal to your taste buds and those of your family, creating meals that everyone will (hopefully) eat!

- Knowledge is power! My co-author, Edward Wein, PhD, provides the science behind the recipes, highlighting specific ingredients and showing how they benefit the brain. Readers will learn ways to make smarter nutritional choices and how to cook smarter as well. Sharona Abramovitch, RD, provided the nutrient analysis for each recipe, and shared valuable tips.

- Hacks à la carte! I've shared my favorite kitchen hacks to help streamline prep, saving on time and cleanup. I use my food processor, microwave, slow cooker, grill, and other helpful kitchen tools and equipment. There are lots of variations, substitutions, and healthy options to allow for different tastes and availability of ingredients. Bite-sized morsels of information are featured throughout the book, so you'll be able to slowly digest them and apply what you've learned at your own pace. I believe that cooking should be fun, so I've combined puns with pots and pans to help you laugh while cooking your way to better brain health.

Small changes to your daily diet can add up to significant health benefits over time. I strongly believe that the simple choices we make each day have the biggest impact on our health and well-being. Enjoy in good health!

Norene

Nutritional analyses were calculated using data from Food Processor Nutrition and Fitness Software by ESHA Research, Inc., version 11.6, 2018. When reviewing the nutritional information supplied, please note the following:

- If a recipe indicates a range of servings (4–6 servings), it is analyzed with the smaller serving in mind (i.e., 4 servings).
- If there is a choice of ingredients, the first ingredient is analyzed rather than the second (e.g., skim milk is analyzed when a recipe calls for 1 cup skim milk or orange juice). Optional ingredients, and those with no specified amounts, are not factored into the analysis.
- When a range is given, the smaller measurement is analyzed (e.g., ¼ cup is analyzed when a recipe calls for ¼–⅓ cup).
- Nutrient values are rounded off for calories, carbohydrates, sugar, fiber, protein, fat, saturated fat, sodium, and potassium.
- A serving of at least 2 g of fiber is considered a source, 5 g is a high source, and 7 g or more is considered an excellent source of fiber.
- Olive and canola oils are the oils of choice.
- Recipes that give an option of using sugar or granulated Splenda are analyzed using the first listed ingredient option. An equivalent amount of granulated Splenda is used to replace sugar when sugar is listed first.
- Specific measurements of salt are included in the analysis (e.g., 1 tsp salt). When a recipe doesn't give a specific measurement (e.g., "salt to taste"), then salt isn't included in the analysis. If the sodium content of a recipe is very high, lower-sodium products were used for the analysis unless otherwise indicated.
- When cheese is called for, recipes are analyzed using low-fat or reduced-fat cheese (e.g., cheddar, mozzarella, Swiss), light cream cheese or ricotta cheese, or 1% cottage cheese, unless otherwise indicated. Many cheeses are high in salt, so check labels.
- When mayonnaise is called for, the recipe is analyzed using light mayonnaise.
- When sour cream or yogurt are called for, the recipe is analyzed using light sour cream or fat-free yogurt.
- When milk is called for, the recipe is analyzed using skim or 1% milk, unless otherwise indicated.
- When canned products such as tomato sauce, black beans, or corn are called for, low-sodium options are chosen if available.
- Nutrient values are not given for recipe variations.
- Garnishes are not calculated unless a specific quantity is indicated.

SHOP SMART WHEN YOU FILL YOUR CART

The foods you include in your diet are equally as important as the ones that you exclude. Putting these brain-boosting foods into your shopping cart will give you a "head" start on your new journey to better brain health:

- Eat mainly a plant-based diet (i.e., vegetables, fruits) based on foods found in the produce section of the supermarket and at farmers' markets.
- Eat the rainbow! Include a variety of cruciferous vegetables (e.g., cauliflower, cabbage, broccoli), fruits (e.g., berries), and dark green leafy vegetables in your cart.
- Focus on high-quality protein (e.g., skinless white meat chicken/poultry, fish rich in Omega-3 fatty acids, eggs, legumes, and nuts). Eat plant-based proteins more often.
- Eat low- and non-fat dairy products in moderation.
- Choose fresh ingredients over processed ones (i.e., pre-packaged foods that include a list of added ingredients). Fresh produce generally doesn't require an ingredients list!
- Practice portion control.

Following the guidelines above will lead you to a healthier you, but we have gone one step further and selected the best brain-boosting foods that have been shown to be the most beneficial for cognitive function and reducing the risk of AD/dementia:

- **Vegetables** (raw and cooked) especially dark leafy greens (e.g., spinach, kale) and cruciferous veggies (e.g., broccoli, cauliflower).
- **Fruits** (fresh or frozen) especially berries (e.g., blueberries, strawberries, blackberries)
- **Nuts and seeds** (e.g., almonds, walnuts, sunflower seeds, pumpkin seeds)
- **Legumes** (e.g., chickpeas, kidney beans, edamame)
- **Herbs and spices** (e.g., rosemary, oregano, turmeric, cinnamon, cloves)
- **Whole grains and grain alternatives** (e.g., oats, black rice, buckwheat/kasha, quinoa)
- **Fish** mainly fatty fish rich in Omega-3s (e.g., salmon, sardines, trout, mackerel)

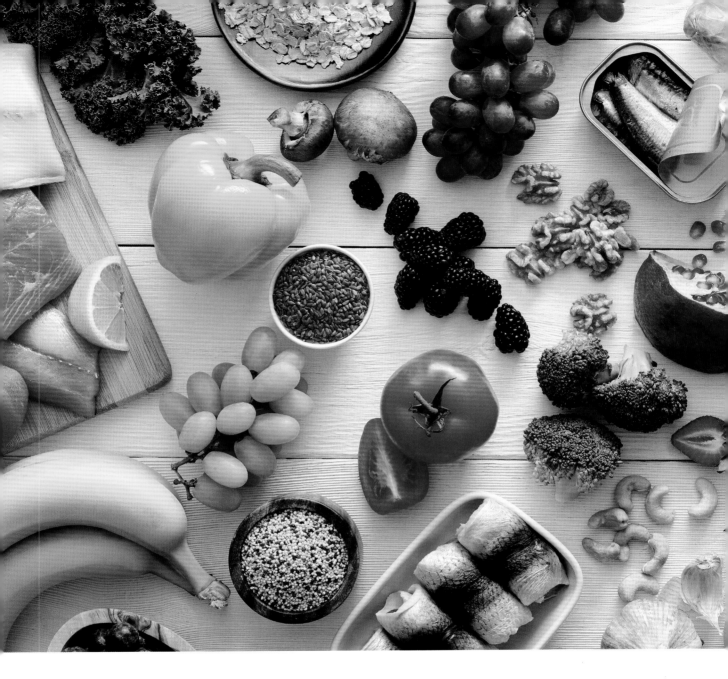

- **Healthy fats** (e.g., extra virgin olive oil, canola oil, flaxseed oil)
- **Beverages** (e.g., red wine such as Cabernet Sauvignon, coffee, green tea, cocoa, water)

The Shopping Cart that follows is a chart of recommended brain-healthy foods, in order of their nutritional benefit.

THE SHOPPING CART TABLE

FRUITS	LEAFY GREENS	LEGUMES	VEGETABLES	NUTS, SEEDS, OILS
Blackberries	Spinach, super spinach mixed greens	Black beans (dried/canned)	Onions	Almonds, almond butter
Raspberries	Kale	Kidney beans (dried/canned)	Yucca/cassava	Sunflower seeds, sunflower seed butter
Strawberries	Arugula	Chickpeas (garbanzo beans) (dried/canned)	Jicama	Wheat germ
Blueberries	Beet/collard greens	Peas (fresh/frozen/canned)	Beets	Walnuts
Kiwi	Parsley/cilantro	Pinto Beans (dried/canned)	Brussels sprouts, cabbage	Olive oil
Unsweetened cranberries	Romaine lettuce	Peanuts	Bok choy	Cashews
Olives	Bibb lettuce	Edamame beans (fresh/frozen)	Broccoli, cauliflower	Pumpkin seeds
Red grapes	Swiss chard	Lentils (dried/canned)	Kohlrabi	Flax seeds
Raisins	Watercress	Tempeh	Butternut squash	Pecans
Cherries	Radicchio	Tofu	Acorn squash	Sesame seeds
Pomegranates			Spaghetti squash	Chia seeds
Lemons			Pumpkin	Pistachios
Tomatoes			Turnips	Brazil nuts
Bell peppers			Radishes	Flaxseed oil, sesame oil, canola oil, and high-oleic sunflower oil

DAIRY, EGGS	FISH, POULTRY, MEAT	HERBS & SPICES	WHOLE GRAINS	BEVERAGE CHOICES
Low-fat and non-fat yogurt (best to use plain)	Salmon (preferably wild) (fresh/frozen/canned), lox (smoked salmon)	Turmeric	Black rice	Dry red wine
Buttermilk, kefir	Sardines	Rosemary	Quinoa	Coffee, tea
Low-fat cheeses	Herring (fresh or marinated)	Oregano	Oats	
Low-fat milk	Mackerel	Other herbs and spices	Whole wheat	
Omega-3 eggs	Anchovies		Kasha (buckwheat groats)	
Eggs	Tuna (bluefin)			
	Whitefish, especially black cod (sablefish)			
	Rainbow trout, arctic char, pollock (boston bluefish)			
	Tuna (canned)			
	Snapper			
	Sole			
	Halibut			
	Lean chicken, turkey			
	Lean beef, veal			

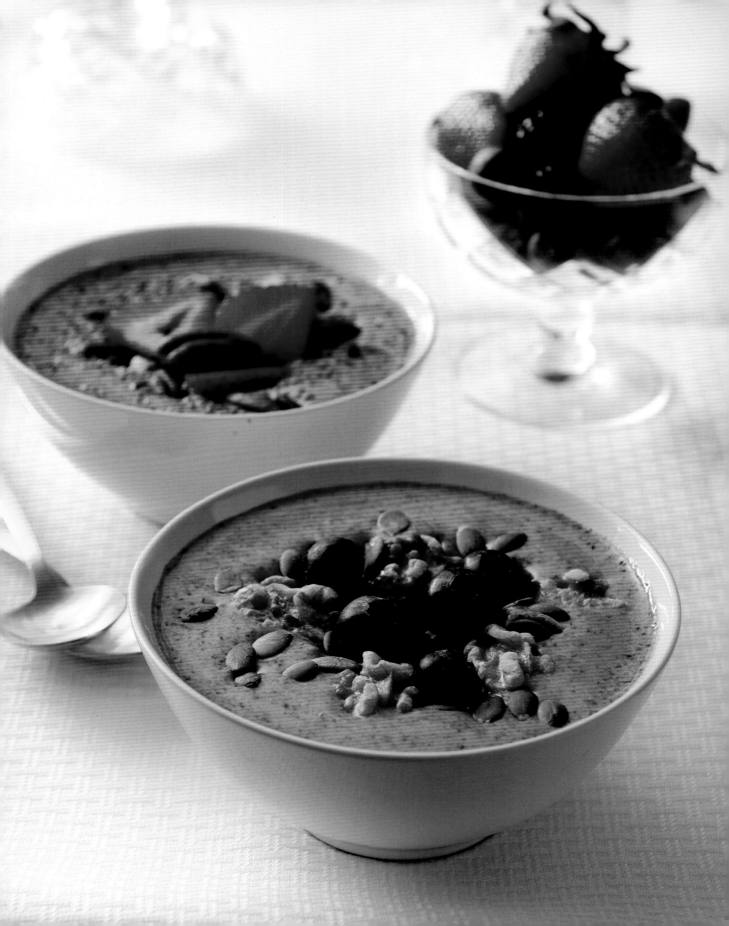

BETTER BREAKFASTS

NO TIME FOR BREAKFAST? Our dietician, Sharona Abramovitch, suggests having a small snack such as yogurt and berries, or a hard-boiled egg and a piece of fruit. If you skip your morning meal, your body and brain will lack fuel and you may be less alert and have more difficulty concentrating. Eating a healthy breakfast is linked to a healthy weight and reduced weight gain over time, as well as improved appetite control and better intake of key brain nutrients, such as calcium, vitamin D, potassium, and fiber.

DRIVE-THRU NO MORE! Prepare breakfast in advance to avoid the drive-thru line in the morning. Make millet, quinoa, or oat porridge in advance and freeze portions (extra toppings can be added before eating). Bake and freeze whole grain muffins or mini frittatas, cook hard-boiled eggs in advance, or keep fruit, yogurt, trail mix, and other ready-to-eat items on hand.

INCLUDE GRAINS AT BREAKFAST: Grains provide carbohydrates, which are essential for your brain! After not eating for about 8–12 hours since the night before, your brain is looking for carbohydrates as a source of energy in the morning. That being said, be careful not to overindulge on grains, especially non–whole grain varieties, as they can cause problems leading to insulin resistance when eaten in excess. Whole grain varieties, such as whole grain oats, quinoa, barley, and bread include the entire grain (the bran, germ, and endosperm) and are better for blood sugar control. Whole grains support cardiovascular health and good blood flow to the brain, which is important for preventing memory decline. For whole grain–rich foods, the first ingredient on a food label should be whole grain, whole wheat flour, whole grain barley flour, or so on, to ensure that all parts of the grain are included in the grain product.

DON'T FORGET FRUIT! Fresh, frozen, or unsweetened fruit can be added to many breakfast items (i.e., cereal, yogurt, pancakes, baked oatmeal, or even a salad), adding a bit of natural sweetness. They contain many brain-healthy nutrients such as potassium, folate, vitamin C, and antioxidants. A banana or apple, in particular, can offer natural flavor to oatmeal. Fun Fact: Fresh fruit is often less nutritious than frozen fruit, as fresh fruit is usually picked before it reaches full maturity, while frozen fruit is picked when fully ripened, allowing for the highest nutritional value. Green or unripe fruits, on the other hand, have less digestible carbohydrates and sugar and more fiber. Antioxidant-rich blueberries help with memory function, but opt for wild blueberries over regular as they often contain double the antioxidants, more fiber, and can contain less sugar. Wild blueberries can also often be purchased frozen for a lower price!

FRUIT VS JUICE: Although fruit juice contains most of the vitamins, minerals, and phytochemicals found in fresh fruit, it contains less fiber, with twice the calories (per unit weight as compared with the original fruit) and sugar. In fact, 2–3 medium oranges are equivalent to 1 cup of orange juice. Fruit juice can also spike blood sugar levels more than whole fruit. It is a good idea to combine fruit with a protein source, such as nuts, milk, yogurt, poultry, legumes, or lean meat, to limit the magnitude of the spike in sugars. Also, only about half the flavonoids (a type of pigment that can aid with inflammation in the body) found in oranges are found in orange juice.

BALANCE YOUR PROTEIN INTAKE THROUGHOUT THE DAY: Use the 30-30-30 g protein rule (30 g protein each at breakfast, lunch, and dinner). Note that 5–10 g protein can be reallocated for a midmorning and/or afternoon snack, such as 10 g from breakfast as your afternoon snack. High-quality protein sources include milk, yogurt, eggs, cheeses, fish, lean meats, poultry, and soy products.

PROTEIN POWDER: Getting tired of consuming protein via eggs or milk at breakfast? Mix protein powder (e.g., whey protein isolate or a plant-based variety) with water/milk and add it to your high-fiber cereal, pancakes, or have it as a beverage. Whey is the byproduct of cheese-making found in milk, and is a mixture of mostly water and lactose, with a small amount of protein and fat. To make whey protein isolate, most of the lactose, carbohydrate, and fat are removed, leaving you with 90% protein.

SUPER SEEDS: Chia, flax, or hemp? Each seed provides varying amounts of protein, fiber, and Omega-3s. It is best to add a variety of them to your food for the maximum benefit. Chia seeds are rated low on the glycemic index (a measure of the rate of sugar absorption—the lower, the better), and most of their carbohydrate content comes from fiber (92% of the total carbohydrates). They also contain calcium (18% of daily needs) and phosphorus (27% of daily needs), which are both brain-healthy nutrients. Mix 1/4 cup (60 mL) chia seeds with 1 cup (250 mL) milk or water and other flavorings (such as vanilla extract) and leave overnight for a quick breakfast! Hemp seeds provide the most protein when compared to the others, helping you stay full longer and making you less likely to overeat. Three Tbsp (45 mL) hemp hearts provide approximately 10 g protein and gives off a nutty flavor. Hemp seeds also contain zinc, which has been linked to improvements in memory. Flax seeds are high in plant-based Omega-3 content, and can aid in brain function as they may help relax blood vessels, leading to better blood flow to the brain. Don't forget to grind them to get the most health benefits. Remember though, the best form of Omega-3s is found in fish and fish oil.

LET'S TALK YOGURTS AND CHEESE: Greek yogurt has about 10 g more protein and is lower in carbohydrates than regular yogurt varieties. If you don't like the tart taste of Greek yogurt, opt for Skyr Icelandic dairy products, which often contain more protein and less sugar than Greek yogurt. Skyr is actually a cheese product that has had the whey and sugars separated from the cheese curd, unlike Greek yogurt, which is only filtered to remove some whey. To reduce sugar intake, choose plain rather than flavored yogurt/dairy products, and add your own flavoring (e.g., cinnamon, peanut butter, or fruit) or stir in 1–2 Tbsp (30 mL) flavored yogurt/dairy product. Yogurt also provides an excellent source of vitamin B12, which is lacking in most plant-derived foods. Vitamin B12 can help slow the process of cognitive decline. Yogurt is also a good source of zinc, a brain-healthy nutrient.

WAKE UP WITH SOME VEGETABLES: Vegetable-based shakes and smoothies provide an on-the-go option, and are an important way to get in some brain-boosting leafy greens at the start of the day! For a quick breakfast, blend baby spinach or kale, a few mint leaves, some lemon juice, half an apple, flax seeds, and some protein powder with ice and water. Some vegetables can also be chopped, steamed, and frozen so that they can easily be added to smoothies (e.g., cauliflower, butternut squash, sweet potato, spinach, kale, and peas). Mint, citrus zests, and/or extracts such as lime, orange, vanilla, and almond can also be added for an extra kick.

TRY A SMOOTHIE BOWL! Want to get in all your brain-healthy foods and super-foods, but not sure how they fit together? Here's how to make a well-balanced, brain-happy breakfast: Blend ½–1 cup (125–250 mL) fruit (brain-healthy choices include berries, kiwi, pomegranate, unsweetened cranberries, or red grapes), a liquid choice (such as dairy or nut milk, water, or even green tea), and thicken with protein sources (e.g., yogurt, tofu, kefir, almond butter, hemp seeds, or protein powder). Additional items such as super seeds, rolled oats, or leafy greens (such as spinach or kale) could also be included. Rolled oats are a good thickener and also contain brain-healthy components such as the antioxidants selenium and zinc. Don't forget to add your favorite toppings to the smoothie to finish the bowl: fresh fruit, shredded coconut, super seeds, nuts, various herbs, zests, and spices (see Smoothie Bowl, p. xx.)

NUTS AND SEEDS: The vitamin E content in almonds, pistachios, pecans, peanuts, hazelnuts, pine nuts, pumpkin seeds, and sunflower seeds can help reduce natural cognitive decline from aging. Eating nuts can also help lower blood pressure and reduce the risk of heart disease and type 2 diabetes, which can all contribute to memory loss and Alzheimer's disease. Walnuts in particular are rich in Omega-3 fatty acids, polyphenols, and other nutrients such as vitamin E, folate, and fiber, which may play a role in improving memory, cognition, and the speed at which our brain functions. Pumpkin seeds provide a good source of antioxidants, phytosterols, zinc, and magnesium, all of which can help preserve memory. All nuts and seeds can be eaten on their own, or sprinkled into cereals, yogurt, salads, desserts, and/or entrees. Eating ¼ cup (60 mL) brain-boosting almonds or walnuts provides approximately 175 calories and 5 g of protein.

CONSIDER A SOURCE OF FAT AT BREAKFAST: Olive oil is an excellent source of monounsaturated fatty acids and antioxidants and helps reduce cognitive decline. Tahini provides high levels of fiber, magnesium, vitamin B6, and folate, which are strongly recommended for cognitive protection. Avocados can be helpful for cognitive health, as they are very low in sugar, and can lower blood pressure. They also provide vitamin B6, potassium, folate, fiber, and vitamin C, and can be eaten as a spread on bread, added to a smoothie, made into a dip, or enjoyed on their own.

SPICE IT UP! Herbs and spices add flavor to foods, allowing you to cut back on butter, oil, and salt. They contain antioxidants and offer many benefits, such as Alzheimer's risk reduction. Cinnamon, which has been shown to be beneficial for cognition, is a good antioxidant and contains high fiber. Cinnamon is rich in manganese (if levels of manganese are low in the blood, it can disrupt cognition). Half a tsp (2 mL) cinnamon each day can also reduce blood sugar, cholesterol, and inflammation, helping to reduce the risk of Alzheimer's disease. Nutmeg can also enhance brain function and boost brain activity. Cinnamon or nutmeg can be added to many breakfast items including yogurt, oatmeal, and so on.

FLOUR POWER: White flour can be replaced in many breakfast items with a combination of other flours to optimize nutrition and brain health. Almond or coconut flour are good alternatives, as they both have more protein and lower carbohydrates than white or whole wheat flours. Almond flour also contains selenium, antioxidants, and vitamin E, which promote brain health. Consider mixing almond or coconut flour with whole wheat/white flour to make homemade pancakes, waffles, or muffins.

NUT-RITIOUS NUT BUTTER

PAREVE | GLUTEN-FREE | PASSOVER | FREEZES WELL | MAKES
1 GENEROUS CUP (250+ ML)

2 cups (500 mL) unsalted
roasted almonds
(see Norene's Notes)

1–2 Tbsp (15–30 mL)
grapeseed oil

Pinch of salt

This scrumptious brain-boosting spread makes a terrific alternative to peanut butter. Make sure that nuts are totally fresh for best results. Spread this nutritious nut butter on whole grain bread (or whole wheat matzo during Passover), or use it as a dip for apple slices or strawberries. Best of all, we've included a chocolate version!

1. In a food processor fitted with the steel blade, process nuts with several quick on/offs to start, then process 30 seconds longer, until coarsely ground.

2. Add 1 Tbsp (15 mL) oil and the salt. Process for 2 minutes longer or until smooth and creamy, stopping the machine several times during processing to scrape down sides of the bowl. If the mixture seems dry, add additional oil and process until smooth.

3. Transfer to an airtight container, cover, and refrigerate.

92 calories per 1 Tbsp (15 mL), 3 g carbohydrates, 1 g sugar, 1 g fiber, 3 g protein, 9 g fat (1 g saturated), 0 mg sodium, 0 mg potassium

NORENE'S NOTES:

- **Go nuts!** Instead of almonds, experiment with different kinds of nuts. Try 1 cup (250 mL) almonds plus ½ cup (125 mL) cashews and ½ cup (125 mL) walnuts or pecans.

- **Chocolate nut butter:** Use 1½ cups (375 mL) nuts and ½ cup (125 mL) chocolate chips (sugar-free or semisweet). Omit oil. Process for 2–3 minutes, until smooth and creamy.

- **Make-your-own almond meal/flour:** Place 2 cups (500 mL) whole blanched almonds in a food processor fitted with the steel blade. Process with quick on/off pulses to start, then let machine run until finely ground, 25–30 seconds. Don't over-process or you'll get almond butter! Refrigerate or freeze. Makes about 2 cups (500 mL).

DR. ED SAYS:

- **You can't go wrong with nuts and seeds** as part of a brain-healthy diet. Low in available carbs and high in fiber, protein, and good fat, they are a great component of any healthy diet as well as being good for the brain.

- **Almond butter,** especially, contains large quantities of the brain-healthy nutrients vitamin E and magnesium.

GOOD FOR YOU GRANOLA

PAREVE | GLUTEN-FREE OPTION | KEEPS ABOUT 3 WEEKS |
FREEZES WELL | MAKES ABOUT 9 CUPS (2.25 L)

3 cups (750 mL) large flake
rolled oats

1 cup (250 mL) unsalted walnut
pieces or slivered almonds

1 cup (250 mL) unsalted
pumpkin seeds

½ cup (125 mL) unsalted
sunflower seeds

½ cup (125 mL) sesame seeds

½ cup (125 mL) unsweetened
shredded or flaked coconut
(optional)

2 tsp (10 mL) ground cinnamon

½ cup (125 mL) canola oil

½ cup (125 mL) pure maple syrup

1 tsp (5 mL) pure vanilla extract

1 cup (250 mL) dried cranberries
or finely chopped dried apricots

Homemade granola tastes so much better than store-bought, and it's better for you too! This combo of oats, nuts, seeds, and dried fruits is great over Greek yogurt or as a topping for your favorite Mix-and-Match Smoothie Bowl (p. 150). Sprinkle some on top of salads for added crunch, or enjoy it as a snack. For a smaller family, make half the recipe.

1. Preheat oven to 325°F (160°C). Line 2 large, rimmed baking sheets with parchment paper.

2. In a large bowl, combine oats with walnuts, pumpkin seeds, sunflower seeds, sesame seeds, coconut (if using), and cinnamon. Add oil, maple syrup, and vanilla. Stir until the oat mixture is well coated.

3. Pour mixture onto the prepared baking sheets and spread out evenly.

4. Bake until golden-brown and dry, about 30 minutes.

5. Remove from oven and let mixture cool on the pan for 20–25 minutes. Stir in dried cranberries.

6. Store in an airtight container in a cool dry place.

130 calories per ¼-cup (60 mL) serving, 13 g carbohydrates, 6 g sugar, 2 g fiber, 3 g protein, 8 g fat (<1 g saturated), 2 mg sodium, 37 mg potassium

NORENE'S NOTES:

- **Gluten-free option:** Use gluten-free oats. Most commercial oats are processed in facilities that also process wheat, barley, and rye.

- **Go nuts!** Use a combo of sliced almonds, chopped pecans, and/or pistachios.

- **Fruity options:** Use your favorite dried fruits (e.g., raisins, dried cherries, finely chopped dried apricots, mangoes, or dates).

- **Savor the flavor:** Instead of maple syrup, use honey. Opt for different spices such as ground cardamom, cloves, or nutmeg . . . the choice is yours!

RECIPE CONTINUED . . .

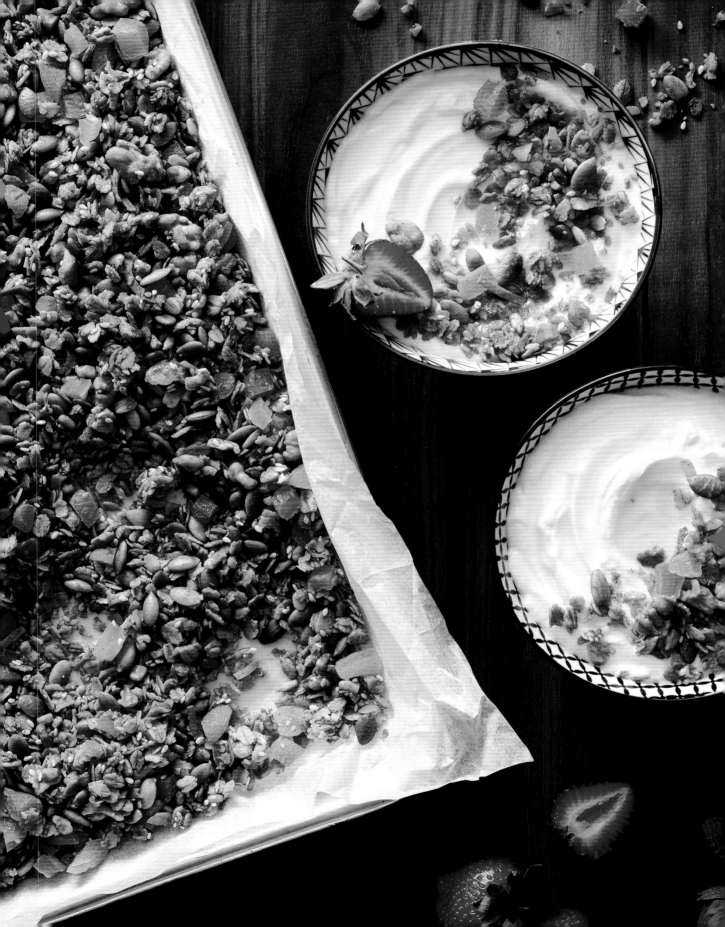

GOOD FOR YOU GRANOLA (continued)

DR. ED SAYS:

- **Nuts** are an essential component of the Mediterranean diet, which has been shown to reduce the risk of AD/dementia. In addition, this recipe contains lots of other goodies for brain health, such as magnesium and B vitamins.

- **Dried fruits, nuts, and seeds** provide antioxidants that reduce oxidative stress; oats provide good amounts of soluble fiber, and walnuts provide some needed Omega-3 fats. Go easy on dried fruits—although they are healthy, they do contain large amounts of sugar. Check online sources for unsweetened dried fruit.

REFRIGERATED OATMEAL

DAIRY | GLUTEN-FREE OPTION | KEEPS ABOUT 3 DAYS | REHEATS
WELL | MAKES 1 SERVING

Sharona Abramovitch, RD, our dietician for this cookbook, shared her recipe for this scrumptious, heart-healthy breakfast that she recommends to her patients. Fiber-packed and protein-rich, it is also great for your brain.

1. Combine oats, milk, yogurt, seeds, sweetener, and cinnamon in a 1-cup (250 mL) Mason jar or container. Cover tightly and shake until well combined.

2. Stir in berries. Store, covered, overnight in the refrigerator.

3. Enjoy chilled or reheated.

194 calories per 1-cup (250 mL) serving, 28 g carbohydrates, 9 g sugar, 7 g fiber, 13 g protein, 4 g fat (<1 g saturated), 78 mg sodium, 125 mg potassium

¼ cup (60 mL) large flake rolled oats

¼ cup (60 mL) milk (skim or 1%)

⅓ cup (80 mL) plain Greek yogurt (skim or 1%)

1½ tsp (7 mL) chia seeds or ground flaxseed

Sweetener to taste (optional)

½ tsp (2 mL) ground cinnamon

¼–½ cup (60–125 mL) blueberries (fresh or frozen)

NORENE'S NOTES:

- **Gluten-free option:** Use gluten-free oats.

- **Peanut butter oatmeal:** Add 1 Tbsp (15 mL) PB2 (dehydrated reduced-fat peanut butter), either chocolate or original, to the basic recipe. Natural peanut butter and Nut-ritious Nut Butter (p. 124) also work well.

- **Very berry oatmeal:** Combine ⅓ cup (80 mL) large flake rolled oats, ½ cup (125 mL) plain Greek yogurt, and 1–2 Tbsp (15–30 mL) low-sugar flavored yogurt. Stir in 1½ tsp (7 mL) chia seeds, ¼ cup (60 mL) blueberries, and ¼ cup (60 mL) diced strawberries. Add ¼ tsp (1 mL) pure vanilla extract, if desired. A satisfying afternoon snack on a long day!

- **Chocolate berry oatmeal:** Mix together ⅓ cup (80 mL) large flake rolled oats, ¾ cup (185 mL) plain Greek yogurt, 1 Tbsp (15 mL) unsweetened cocoa powder, 1 tsp (5 mL) maple syrup or desired sweetener, and ¼ tsp (1 mL) pure vanilla extract. Refrigerate overnight. To serve, top with ½ cup (125 mL) of your favorite berries, preferably lower-sugar berries such as raspberries, blackberries, or strawberries, mixed in with blueberries.

RECIPE CONTINUED . . .

- **Time-saving tip:** Make enough refrigerated oatmeal for 3 days and store it in the refrigerator. Ready when you are!

DR. ED SAYS:

- **Oats** are a great source of soluble fiber, which helps control sugar spikes that can increase AD/dementia risk. They are also high in the brain-healthy minerals magnesium and zinc.

- **Yogurt and milk** provide protein and are good sources of vitamin D and vitamin B12.

- **Chia and flax seeds** provide excellent amounts of needed Omega-3 fats as well as high amounts of fiber.

- **Blueberries** are one of the highest sources of natural antioxidants and have been shown to reduce AD/dementia risk.

- **Overall,** this is a low-sugar, low-fat, and well-balanced mixture of beneficial brain nutrients.

BRAN-ANA CHOCOLATE CHIP LOAF

PAREVE | FREEZES WELL | MAKES 1 LOAF (12 SLICES)

No one will guess that this luscious loaf is made with whole wheat flour and bran. This dairy-free loaf will quickly become a family favorite!

¼ cup (60 mL) canola oil

½ cup (125 mL) sugar

2 large eggs

1 tsp (5 mL) pure vanilla extract

1 cup (250 mL) All-Bran cereal

3 ripe bananas, cut into chunks (or 1½ cups/375 mL mashed)

2 Tbsp (30 mL) water

1 ½ cups (375 mL) whole wheat flour

2 tsp (10 mL) baking powder

1 tsp (5 mL) baking soda

⅔ cup (160 mL) chocolate chips (semisweet or sugar-free)

1. Preheat oven to 350°F (175°C). Spray a 9- × 5-inch (23 × 12 cm) loaf pan with nonstick spray.

2. In a food processor fitted with the steel blade, combine oil, sugar, eggs, and vanilla. Process for 2 minutes, until light.

3. Add bran, bananas, and water. Process until smooth, 18–20 seconds.

4. Add flour, baking powder, and baking soda. Process with quick on/offs, just until combined.

5. Stir in chocolate chips with a rubber spatula.

6. Pour batter into the prepared loaf pan and spread evenly.

7. Bake for 50–60 minutes, or until the top springs back when lightly touched.

8. Let cool in the pan for 15 minutes, then invert onto a serving plate.

226 calories per ¾-inch (2 cm) slice, 36 g carbohydrates, 11 g sugar, 5 g fiber, 5 g protein, 10 g fat (3 g saturated), 134 mg sodium, 297 mg potassium

NORENE'S NOTES:

- **Going bananas!** If you have a lot of ripe bananas, put them in a resealable freezer bag and freeze them. When needed, thaw slightly, about 10 minutes at room temperature. A quick trick to thaw frozen bananas is to put them under hot running water for 20 seconds, then cut away the peel with a sharp paring knife. One large banana yields about ½ cup (125 mL) mashed.

- **Go nuts!** Instead of chocolate chips, substitute chopped walnuts, pecans, pistachios, or your favorite nuts. Toast them first for maximum flavor.

RECIPE CONTINUED . . .

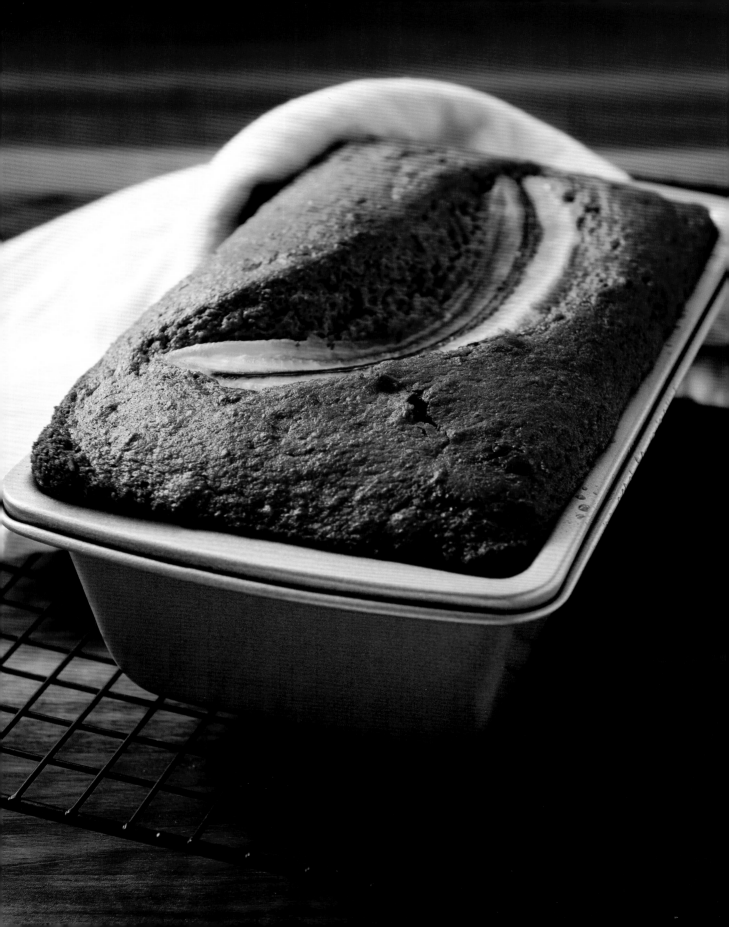

BRAN-ANA CHOCOLATE CHIP LOAF (continued)

- **Mini muffins:** Prepare batter as directed and pour into paper-lined or sprayed mini muffin pans. Bake at 375°F (190°C) for 15–18 minutes. Makes 30–36 minis.

DR. ED SAYS:

- **Whole wheat flour** provides an excellent source of needed B vitamins, which have been shown to reduce AD/dementia risk. It also provides the important minerals magnesium and zinc. In addition, its fiber content will help to reduce sugar spikes.

- **Bananas** provide good levels of vitamin C and zinc, but a higher sugar content as they ripen.

- **Eggs** supply vitamins B12 and D, which are lacking in the other ingredients.

APRICOT ALMOND MUFFINS

DAIRY | FREEZES WELL | MAKES 12 MUFFINS

1 cup (250 mL) large flake rolled oats (quick-cooking is also fine)

½ cup (125 mL) whole wheat flour

½ cup (125 mL) all-purpose flour

1 tsp (5 mL) baking powder

½ tsp (2 mL) baking soda

1 large egg

¼ cup (60 mL) canola oil

½ cup (125 mL) lightly packed brown sugar

1 cup (250 mL) plain yogurt (skim or 1%)

½ tsp (2 mL) pure vanilla extract

⅔ cup (160 mL) dried apricots, cut into small pieces (I use scissors)

12 whole almonds

"Oat cuisine" at its best! This combination of apricots, almonds, and oats makes these muffins A-okay! Cranberries, blueberries, or raisins also make excellent add-ins.

1. Preheat oven to 400°F (200°C). Spray compartments of a muffin pan with nonstick spray.

2. In a food processor fitted with the steel blade, combine oats, flours, baking powder, and baking soda. Process 5 seconds to combine.

3. Add egg, oil, brown sugar, yogurt, and vanilla. Process for 25–30 seconds, or until smooth and blended.

4. Stir in apricots with a rubber spatula.

5. Scoop batter into the prepared muffin pan, filling each compartment about two-thirds full. Top each muffin with an almond.

6. Bake for 20–25 minutes, until tops are golden brown and spring back when lightly touched.

186 calories per muffin, 29 g carbohydrates, 12 g sugar, 3 g fiber, 5 g protein, 6 g fat (<1 g saturated), 82 mg sodium, 100 mg potassium

NORENE'S NOTES:

- **To line or not to line?** Baked muffins may stick to paper liners if your batter is very low in fat. If your batter contains less than ¼ cup (60 mL) fat for 12 muffins, forgo the liners and spray the compartments with nonstick spray. Alternatively, nonstick parchment baking cups are an excellent option.

- **Nuts to you!** Almonds are high in protein, fiber, calcium, vitamin E, and magnesium. A singe cup of almonds contains the same amount of calcium as 1 cup (250 mL) of milk!

- **Almond meal/flour** (finely ground almonds) can replace part of the flour in baked goods. A good starting point is to replace half the flour with almond meal. The carbs will be lower, but the fat and protein content will be higher. See Make-Your-Own Almond Meal/Flour (p. 124).

DR. ED SAYS:

- **Almonds** are one of the best nuts you can choose because of their superior vitamin E content, high magnesium and zinc, high fiber, and low available carbs—all important for warding off AD/dementia. In addition to topping these muffins with whole almonds, consider replacing some of the wheat flour with almond flour.

- **Whole wheat and oat flours** provide fiber, magnesium, and zinc, and contain antioxidants.

- **Dried apricots** provide important antioxidants but are high in sugar and should be used sparingly.

- **Overall,** almonds and whole grains are the focus of this recipe. Since the recipe uses a fair amount of sugar, you may want to experiment with replacing some of it with stevia or sucralose.

BLUEBERRY BRAN CHOCOLATE CHIP MUFFINS

DAIRY | PAREVE OPTION | FREEZES WELL | MAKES 30 MUFFINS

3 cups (750 mL) All-Bran cereal (see Norene's Notes)

⅓ cup (80 mL) canola oil

⅓ cup (80 mL) plain Greek yogurt (skim or 1%)

1 cup (250 mL) hot tea (spice or green tea are great)

2 large eggs

2 Tbsp (30 mL) lemon juice + enough milk (skim or 1%) to equal 2 cups (500 mL)

½ cup (125 mL) firmly packed brown sugar

½ cup (125 mL) molasses or honey

2½ cups (625 mL) whole wheat flour

2 tsp (10 mL) ground cinnamon

2 tsp (10 mL) baking soda

1 tsp (5 mL) baking powder

Zest of 1 orange

1½ cups (375 mL) fresh or frozen blueberries (see Norene's Notes)

½–¾ cup (125–185 mL) chocolate chips (semisweet or sugar-free)

Although this make-ahead batter yields a big batch, leftover batter can be refrigerated up to three weeks, so you can bake as many or as few as you need. As you mix up the batter, brew a big pot of tea—use one cup in the batter, and pour a mug for yourself!

1. In a very large mixing bowl, combine bran with oil and yogurt. Pour hot tea over the mixture and let stand for 5 minutes. Stir well.

2. Add eggs, milk mixture, brown sugar, and molasses. Stir until combined.

3. Add flour, cinnamon, baking soda, and baking powder. Mix until blended.

4. Stir in orange zest, blueberries, and chocolate chips, just until combined.

5. Either let batter stand for 30 minutes, until thickened, or cover and refrigerate up to 3 weeks.

6. Preheat oven to 375°F (190°C). Spray compartments of a muffin pan (or muffin pans) with nonstick spray.

7. Scoop batter into the muffin pan(s), filling each compartment about two-thirds full.

8. Bake 22–25 minutes, or until tops spring back when lightly touched.

135 calories per muffin, 24 g carbohydrates, 12 g sugar, 4 g fiber, 4 g protein, 5 g fat (1 g saturated), 117 mg sodium, 233 mg potassium

NORENE'S NOTES:

- **Bran, baby, bran!** Dare to compare? There are 39 g of fiber in 1 cup (250 mL) All-Bran Buds, whereas 1 cup (250 mL) bran flakes contains just 7 g. A single cup of natural wheat bran or Fiber One cereal contains 28 g of fiber, whereas Original All-Bran cereal contains 17.6 g. Although these are all interchangeable in the above recipe, opt for maximum fiber for maximum health.

- **Frozen berries:** If using frozen berries, toss with 2 Tbsp (30 mL) flour before adding them to the batter—this helps them keep their shape.

- **Mix-ins:** Use mixed berries, fresh or dried cranberries, raisins, or any dried cut-up fruit such mangoes, apricots, or pitted dates.

- **Pareve option:** Replace yogurt with unsweetened applesauce. Use dairy-free milk substitute (e.g., almond, coconut, rice, or soy milk) instead of regular milk.

- **Here's the scoop!** For even-sized muffins, use an ice cream scoop or a ⅓-cup (60 mL) measure, mounding the mixture slightly.

- **Loafing around!** Instead of muffins, bake the batter in two 9- × 5-inch (23 × 12 cm) loaf pans at 350°F (175°C) for 50–60 minutes. When done, a cake tester or toothpick should come out clean when inserted into the centers of the loaves. Each loaf yields 12 slices.

- **Freeze with ease:** Store cooled muffins in resealable freezer bags in the freezer up to 3 months. Frozen muffins take 20–25 seconds to thaw in the microwave, or 20–30 minutes at room temperature.

DR. ED SAYS:

- **Low-sugar chocolate chips** are included in this recipe. The cocoa powder content in these chips has been shown to contain powerful antioxidants to help preserve brain function. These antioxidants are enhanced by the antioxidants found in the berries, cinnamon, and orange zest to result in a more complete and functional antioxidant mix.

- **There is a fair amount** of added sugar, but it will be attenuated somewhat by the fiber in the whole grains, which also supply important minerals and B vitamins. You can experiment with replacing some of the sugar with stevia or sucralose. Also watch out for dried berries or other dried fruits, as they can be high in added sugar (e.g., dried cranberries).

- **Overall,** the main attraction of this recipe is the many and varied antioxidants provided, which reduce oxidative stress and inflammation in the brain.

DOUBLE-GOOD CHOCOLATE MUFFINS

PAREVE | FREEZES WELL | MAKES 12 MUFFINS

¼ cup (60 mL) canola oil

½ cup (125 mL) sugar

⅓ cup + 1 Tbsp (95 mL) water

1 large egg

1 cup (250 mL) mashed ripe
bananas (about 2 large)

1¼ cups (310 mL) whole
wheat flour

1 cup (250 mL) oat bran cereal

¼ cup (60 mL) unsweetened
cocoa powder

2 tsp (10 mL) baking powder

½ tsp (2 mL) baking soda

⅛ tsp (0.5 mL) salt

½ cup (125 mL) chocolate chips
(semisweet or sugar-free)

Enjoy these fiber-packed chocolate muffins instead of cereal and a banana for breakfast. Kid-friendly, guilt-free, dairy-free, and very versatile—they're "oat of this world!"

1. Preheat oven to 375°F (190°C). Spray compartments of a muffin pan with nonstick spray.

2. Combine oil, sugar, water, and egg in a large bowl and beat for 1–2 minutes.

3. Add bananas and mix until blended.

4. Add flour, oat bran, cocoa powder, baking powder, baking soda, and salt. Mix just until blended. Fold in chocolate chips.

5. Scoop batter into the prepared muffin pan, filling each compartment about three-quarters full.

6. Bake for about 20 minutes, or until a cake tester or toothpick inserted into center of a muffin comes out clean.

204 calories per muffin, 34 g carbohydrates, 15 g sugar, 4 g fiber, 5 g protein, 9 g fat (2 g saturated), 80 mg sodium, 227 mg potassium

NORENE'S NOTES:

- **Variations:** Instead of oat bran, use 1 cup (250 mL) natural wheat bran or wheat germ. Instead of chocolate chips, use chopped pecans, walnuts, or almonds.

- **Fiber fact:** Oat bran is high in soluble fiber, whereas wheat bran and wheat germ are high in insoluble fiber.

DR. ED SAYS:

- **Cocoa powder,** which is added to the batter, is a good choice because it provides all the benefits of the cocoa powder antioxidants.

- **Ripe bananas** will increase the sugar in the recipe, so you may want to consider using bananas that are less ripe as they are lower in sugar.

FIESTA CORN MUFFINS

DAIRY OPTION | PAREVE | FREEZES WELL | MAKES 12 MUFFINS

My late mom, Belle Rykiss, often made these colorful savory muffins. With no added sugar, these versatile muffins are lower in carbs and calories. They make an excellent breakfast choice, healthy snack, or are perfect with a salad for lunch. Nibble-it away!

½ red bell pepper, seeded

2 green onions, trimmed

2 Tbsp (30 mL) fresh dill (or 1 tsp/5 mL dried)

1 cup (250 mL) cornmeal (preferably stone-ground whole grain)

1 cup (250 mL) whole wheat flour

2½ tsp (12 mL) baking powder

¾ tsp (4 mL) baking soda

¼ tsp (1 mL) red pepper flakes or cayenne

¼ tsp (1 mL) salt

¼ cup (60 mL) canola oil

2 large eggs

1 Tbsp (15 mL) lemon juice + almond milk to equal 1 cup (250 mL)

½ cup (125 mL) canned corn kernels, well drained

1. Preheat oven to 400°F (200°C). Spray compartments of a muffin pan with nonstick spray.

2. Finely chop red pepper, green onions, and dill (either in a food processor fitted with the steel blade, using quick on/off pulses, or by hand). Place in a small bowl.

3. In a food processor or a large bowl, combine cornmeal, flour, baking powder, baking soda, red pepper flakes, and salt. Mix well.

4. Add oil, eggs, and lemon juice/milk mixture. Blend until smooth.

5. Stir in corn and red pepper/onion mixture with a spatula.

6. Scoop batter into the prepared muffin pan, filling each compartment about three-quarters full.

7. Bake 20–25 minutes, or until golden.

169 calories per muffin, 24 g carbohydrates, <1 g sugar, 3 g fiber, 5 g protein, 6 g fat (<1 g saturated), 151 mg sodium, 156 mg potassium

NORENE'S NOTES:

- **Variations:** Instead of red bell peppers, use ½ cup (125 mL) chopped roasted red peppers or ½ cup (125 mL) chopped sundried tomatoes. Another option is to fold blueberries in instead of adding chopped vegetables and corn.

- **Milk substitutes:** Instead of almond milk, try coconut, rice, or soy milk.

- **Dairy option:** Instead of the lemon juice/milk substitute mixture, use 1 cup (250 mL) buttermilk.

RECIPE CONTINUED . . .

FIESTA CORN MUFFINS (continued)

- **Fiesta corn bread:** Spray a 9- × 5-inch (23 × 12 cm) loaf pan with nonstick spray. Spread batter evenly in the pan. Bake at 350°F (175°C) for 45–55 minutes. When done, a cake tester or toothpick inserted into the center should come out clean.

- **Get stuffed!** Bake muffins or cornbread in advance. Transform them into Cornbread Stuffing Mounds (p. 465).

DR. ED SAYS:

- **Cornmeal, whole wheat flour, and red bell peppers** are the key brain nutrient contributors to this recipe. Whole grains give you the fiber you need, as well as important magnesium and zinc minerals along with needed B vitamins and carotenoid antioxidants. Bell peppers are an excellent source of vitamin C and carotenoid antioxidants.

- **Eggs** provide choline, which some researchers believe is needed for neurotransmitter synthesis in the brain.

- **Overall,** this recipe is low in saturated fat, reasonable in total fat, rich in antioxidants and fiber, and low in sugar and salt.

QUICK COTTAGE CHEESE MUFFINS

DAIRY | FREEZES WELL | MAKES 12 MUFFINS

These are excellent for breakfast or as a snack. They're delicious plain, or topped with plain Greek yogurt and berries or Warm Mixed Berry Sauce (p. 147).

4 large eggs

⅓ cup (80 mL) canola oil

Sweetener equivalent to ¼ cup (60 mL) sugar

2 cups (500 mL) low-fat (1%) cottage cheese (curd-style)

1 tsp (5 mL) pure vanilla extract

½ cup (125 mL) whole wheat flour

½ cup (125 mL) all-purpose flour

2 tsp (10 mL) baking powder

1. Preheat oven to 400°F (200°C). Spray compartments of a muffin pan with nonstick spray.

2. In a food processor fitted with the steel blade (or in a large mixing bowl), combine eggs with oil, sweetener, cottage cheese, and vanilla. Mix well.

3. Add flours and baking powder and mix until fairly smooth.

4. Scoop batter into the prepared muffin pan, filling each compartment about three-quarters full.

5. Bake for about 25 minutes, or until nicely browned. Let cool 10 minutes before removing from the pan.

6. Serve warm or at room temperature. Store leftover muffins in the refrigerator.

153 calories per muffin, 13 g carbohydrates, 2 g sugar, 1 g fiber, 7 g protein, 8 g fat (1 g saturated), 163 mg sodium, 85 mg potassium

NORENE'S NOTES:

- **Variation:** Substitute light ricotta cheese for half the cottage cheese. If desired, use only whole wheat flour rather than a combination.

- **Boost the flavor!** In Step 2, add 1 tsp (5 mL) ground cinnamon or lemon zest. If desired, sprinkle a little cinnamon and grated dark chocolate on top of the muffins just before baking.

- **Add-ins:** At the end of Step 3, fold in ¾ cup (185 mL) of any of the following: blueberries, cranberries, dried cherries, or chocolate chips.

RECIPE CONTINUED . . .

QUICK COTTAGE CHEESE MUFFINS (continued)

DR. ED SAYS:

- **Eggs** provide high-quality protein and a significant amount of choline for neurotransmitter synthesis in the brain, as well as needed vitamin D and vitamin B12. Norene's recommendations to add Greek yogurt and berry topping will enhance the brain nutrient content of the recipe.

- **Overall,** this recipe is low in saturated fat, sugar, and sodium, and contains reasonable total fat and total carbs.

BLUEBERRY CINNAMON PANCAKES

DAIRY OPTION | PAREVE | FREEZES WELL | MAKES ABOUT FOUR-
TEEN 4-INCH (10 CM) PANCAKES

These dairy-free pancakes are "berry" good for the brain! Make extra and freeze them—they'll reheat in moments in the microwave. Check out the scrumptious variations below.

1 cup + 2 Tbsp (280 mL) whole wheat flour

2 Tbsp (30 mL) wheat germ

Sweetener equivalent to 3 Tbsp (45 mL) sugar

1 Tbsp (15 mL) ground cinnamon

1 tsp (5 mL) baking powder

½ tsp (2 mL) baking soda

⅛ tsp (0.5 mL) salt

1⅓ cups (310 mL) dairy-free milk substitute (e.g., almond, coconut, rice, or soy milk)

1½ Tbsp (22 mL) lemon juice

2 Tbsp (30 mL) canola oil

2 egg whites (or 1 large egg)

1½ cups (375 mL) fresh or frozen blueberries (see Norene's Notes)

1. In a large mixing bowl, combine flour, wheat germ, sweetener, cinnamon, baking powder, baking soda, and salt. Whisk together until combined.

2. In a 2-cup (500 mL) glass measure, stir together milk substitute and lemon juice. Add milk mixture, oil, and egg whites to dry ingredients. Whisk together until smooth and blended. Gently stir in berries.

3. Spray a large nonstick skillet with nonstick spray. Heat over medium heat for 2 minutes, or until a drop of water skips on its surface.

4. Drop batter into the hot skillet, using a scant ¼-cup (60 mL) for each pancake (see Norene's Notes). Cook over medium heat until bottoms of the pancakes are lightly browned and small bubbles appear on the top surface. Flip pancakes over and brown the other side.

5. Transfer cooked pancakes to a platter and keep warm. Repeat with the remaining batter, spraying the skillet between batches. Serve warm.

91 calories per 4-inch (10 cm) pancake, 14 g carbohydrates, 2 g sugar, 3 g fiber, 3 g protein, 3 g fat (0 g saturated), 88 mg sodium, 67 mg potassium

NORENE'S NOTES:

- **Flour power:** Adding wheat germ to whole wheat flour boosts the fiber. Flour may vary in moisture content, so if your pancake batter is too thick, dilute it with a little liquid. If the batter is too thin, add a little flour.

- **Dairy option:** Use milk instead of dairy-free milk substitute. Instead of combining it with lemon juice, substitute buttermilk.

RECIPE CONTINUED . . .

- **Measure up:** Fill a ¼-cup (60 mL) measure three-quarters full (about 3 Tbsp/45 mL) with batter. Drop pancake batter into the skillet.

- **Multiply your options:** Fresh or frozen raspberries, blackberries, or strawberries also add flavor and fiber to pancakes. If the berries are frozen, you don't need to thaw them first.

- **Lemon blueberry pancakes:** Omit cinnamon. Choose coconut milk as the dairy-free milk substitute. Stir in zest of a lemon (about 1 Tbsp/ 15 mL) along with the blueberries.

- **Top it up:** Top pancakes with a dairy-free yogurt (e.g., coconut) and fresh berries. For a dairy version, top with plain Greek yogurt (skim or 1%).

DR. ED SAYS:

- **The combination of berries,** wheat germ, and cinnamon provides a varied and significant source of antioxidants to help preserve memory.

- **Dairy option:** I like the idea of substituting buttermilk for the lemon juice mixture and using yogurt as a topping. Both of these substitutes supply probiotics (good bacteria), which are increasingly being shown to benefit the brain and health in general.

- **Overall,** this is a low-fat, low-sugar, low-sodium, and antioxidant-rich recipe. Try using a no-sugar-added version of the dairy-free milk substitute to reduce the sugar level even further, and mix low-sugar berries, such as blackberries and raspberries, with the other berries.

COTTAGE CHEESE PANCAKES

DAIRY | FREEZES WELL | MAKES 10–12 PANCAKES (DEPENDING ON SIZE)

The batter for these moist, protein-packed pancakes can be quickly mixed up in a food processor, so give them a whirl. Leftovers reheat in moments in the microwave, so refrigerate or freeze any leftovers for a future meal.

1 cup (250 mL) low-fat (1%) cottage cheese (curd-style)

1 large egg

⅔ cup (160 mL) whole wheat flour

1 Tbsp (15 mL) wheat germ

¾ tsp (4 mL) baking powder

Sweetener equivalent to 2 Tbsp (30 mL) sugar

⅓ cup (80 mL) milk (skim or 1%)

½ tsp (2 mL) pure vanilla extract

½ tsp (2 mL) ground cinnamon (optional)

1. In a food processor fitted with the steel blade, combine all ingredients and process until smooth, 25–30 seconds.

2. Spray a large nonstick skillet with nonstick spray. Heat over medium heat for 2 minutes, or until a drop of water skips on its surface.

3. Using a scant ¼-cup (60 mL) measure, drop batter into the hot skillet (see Norene's Notes, p. 144). Fry until bottoms of pancakes are lightly browned and small bubbles appear on the top surface. Flip pancakes over and brown the other side.

4. Transfer pancakes to a platter and keep warm. Repeat with the remaining batter.

74 calories per medium-sized pancake, 11 g carbohydrates, 2 g sugar, 2 g fiber, 5 g protein, 1 g fat (<1 g saturated), 92 mg sodium, 51 mg potassium

NORENE'S NOTES:

- **Flour power:** You can also make these with ⅓ cup (80 mL) all-purpose flour and ⅓ cup (80 mL) whole wheat flour (or ⅔ cup/160 mL white whole wheat flour).

- **Top it up:** Serve pancakes with a dollop of plain Greek yogurt or low-sugar flavored yogurt. Top with your favorite berries.

- **Berry good!** For a special treat, serve with Warm Mixed Berry Sauce (p. 147).

RECIPE CONTINUED . . .

DR. ED SAYS:

- **Wheat germ** is an excellent way to provide natural vitamin E intake, which has been linked to decreased AD/dementia risk.

- **Nutrition tip:** In order to include the more-complex antioxidants, I recommend you take up Norene's suggestion to top the pancakes with low-sugar yogurt and berries.

- **Overall,** this is a protein-packed, low-fat, low-sugar alternative, and also provides some vitamin B12 and vitamin D (generally found in animal and dairy products such as milk and eggs.)

WARM MIXED BERRY SAUCE

PAREVE | PASSOVER | FREEZES WELL | MAKES ABOUT 1½ CUPS (375 ML)

This scrumptious sauce is quick and simple to prepare and leftovers keep for 3–4 days in the refrigerator. It's excellent over Cottage Cheese Pancakes (p. 145), hot oatmeal, or your favorite cereal. Add a drizzle to smoothies or spoon it over frozen yogurt (see Berry Mango Sherbet, p. 577).

4 cups (1 L) mixed berries (try equal amounts blueberries, strawberries, raspberries, and/or blackberries)

Sweetener equivalent to 2 Tbsp (30 mL) sugar (or to taste)

1–2 Tbsp (15–30 mL) red wine (optional)

1. In a large nonstick skillet, combine berries with sweetener. Cook over high heat, stirring occasionally, about 2–3 minutes, or until berries start to release their juices but still hold their shape.

2. Stir in wine, if using. Serve warm (although it also tastes delicious when chilled).

24 calories per ¼-cup (60 mL) serving, 6 g carbohydrates, 3 g sugar, 2 g fiber, 1 g protein, 0 g fat (0 g saturated), 1 mg sodium, 63 mg potassium

NORENE'S NOTES:

- **Frozen assets:** When fresh berries are expensive or aren't in season, use frozen mixed berries—they're usually more economical. Cooking time for frozen berries will be 3-5 minutes.

- **So blue-tiful!** Blueberries are a great source of fiber, with almost 3 g per ½-cup (125 mL) serving.

DR. ED SAYS:

- **Berries** have been extensively studied and shown to reduce AD/dementia risk. I can't argue with a recipe that is so rich in simple and complex antioxidants and fiber, and that is so beneficial for the brain. The recipe is also great for heart health. Use the sauce as a topping for breakfast recipes that are deficient in berries where taste will be enhanced.

- **Mix lower-sugar berries** such as raspberries and blackberries with other berries, and avoid berries that have added sugar (e.g., dried cranberries).

BRAIN-BOOSTING SMOOTHIE

DAIRY | PAREVE OPTION | PASSOVER OPTION | MAKES 2½ CUPS (625 ML)

1½ cups (625 mL) frozen blueberries (see Norene's Notes)

½ cup (125 mL) baby spinach

1 cup (250 mL) milk (skim or 1%)

½ cup (125 mL) plain Greek
yogurt (skim or 1%)

1 Tbsp (15 mL) chia seeds or
ground flaxseed (optional)

1 tsp (5 mL) honey, pure maple
syrup, or sugar substitute
(optional)

Ice cubes (optional)

Attention, purple people eaters! This versatile, power-packed smoothie is perfect for breakfast or a snack. Try some of the variations below—different every time! For a single serving, just halve the recipe.

1. Combine all ingredients in a blender or food processor. Blend or process until smooth, 1–2 minutes. For a thicker texture, add a few ice cubes.

2. Serve immediately or cover and refrigerate for a day or two. If you make it ahead, shake or stir well before serving.

176 calories per 1¼-cups (310 mL) serving, 27 g carbohydrates, 20 g sugar, 6 g fiber, 12 g protein, 4 g fat (0 g saturated), 105 mg sodium, 272 mg potassium

NORENE'S NOTES:

- **Frozen assets:** Try frozen strawberries, blackberries, raspberries, or mixed frozen berries. Adding 1 cup (250 mL) frozen mango chunks or banana slices also adds a terrific taste.

- **No frozen berries?** Substitute fresh berries. Add 1 cup (250 mL) ice cubes for a thicker texture.

- **Pareve option:** Use dairy-free milk substitute (almond, coconut, rice, or soy milk). Use coconut or almond yogurt instead of Greek yogurt.

- **Passover option:** Omit chia/flaxseed. Maple syrup requires Passover certification.

- **Protein power:** Add 1–2 Tbsp (30 mL) whey protein isolate powder or peanut butter. Alternatively, enjoy a handful of walnuts or almonds on the side.

- **Grab and go:** Prepare smoothie(s) in advance and store in the refrigerator in a travel mug. Ready when you are!

- **Berries and spinach** have been shown, time and time again, to reduce AD/dementia risk.

- **This recipe combines** the best features of the fruit and vegetable worlds and, as a bonus, incorporates chia or flax seeds, which are very rich in fiber and Omega-3 fats—both of which are brain-healthy nutrients. And for the icing on the so-called cake, we've added Greek yogurt with its beneficial bacteria and vitamins B12 and D. Best of all worlds!

MIX-AND-MATCH SMOOTHIE BOWL

DAIRY | PAREVE OPTION | GLUTEN-FREE | PASSOVER OPTION |
MAKES 2 SERVINGS

BERRY SMOOTHIE BOWL:

1 cup (250 mL) frozen blueberries

1 cup (250 mL) frozen sliced
strawberries

1 cup (250 mL) plain Greek yogurt
(skim or 1%)

Sweetener equivalent to 1 Tbsp
(15 mL) sugar

TOPPINGS:

½ cup (125 mL) blueberries,
raspberries, and/or sliced
strawberries

¼ cup (60 mL) slivered
almonds, walnut pieces, and/
or pecan halves

2 Tbsp (30 mL) pumpkin seeds,
sunflower seeds, or chia seeds
(omit for Passover)

Turn your smoothie into a meal! Smoothie Bowls are thicker than liquid smoothies, so eat them with a spoon. Serve them in a bowl, topped with colorful fruits and crunchy nuts. Have a fun day sundae—any day!

1. In a food processor fitted with the steel blade, combine frozen berries with Greek yogurt and sweetener. Process with several quick on/off pulses, then scrape down sides of the bowl. Process 1–2 minutes, until blended.

2. Transfer mixture to 2 bowls. Arrange toppings in an attractive design overtop each bowl. Serve chilled.

267 calories per serving, 30 g carbohydrates, 18 g sugar, 7 g fiber, 16 g protein, 11 g fat (1 g saturated), 42 mg sodium, 248 mg potassium

NORENE'S NOTES:

• **Berry power smoothie bowl:** Use 2 cups (500 mL) frozen fruit blend (e.g., blueberries, raspberries, blackberries, and/or strawberries).

• **Create your own:** Use 1 cup (250 mL) of your favorite frozen berries or fruit (e.g., mango, peaches) plus 1 banana, cut into chunks. Add ½ cup (125 mL) baby kale or spinach leaves, or 1 avocado. Add a spoonful or two of almond butter, peanut butter, or whey protein powder for a protein boost.

• **Pareve option:** Instead of Greek yogurt, substitute 1 cup (250 mL) dairy-free yogurt (e.g., coconut or almond yogurt). For a thicker mixture, add a handful of ice cubes.

• **Create your own toppings:** Use assorted berries (e.g., strawberries, raspberries, blackberries) and/or sliced fruits (e.g., mangoes, nectarines, pineapple). Crunchy additions can include nuts, seeds, unsweetened coconut, or granola.

DR. ED SAYS:

• **Nutritional benefits:** Although this recipe is not quite as nutritionally complete for the brain as the Brain-Boosting Smoothie (p. 148), it still packs a big punch because of the fiber-loaded berries, the simple antioxidant vitamin C, and other complex antioxidants.

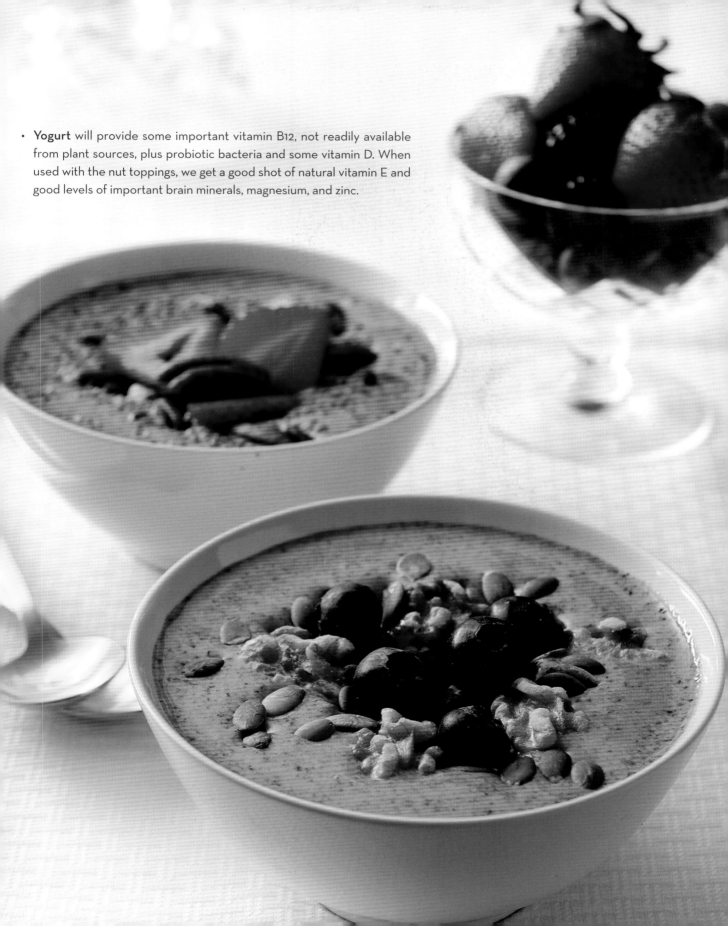

- **Yogurt** will provide some important vitamin B12, not readily available from plant sources, plus probiotic bacteria and some vitamin D. When used with the nut toppings, we get a good shot of natural vitamin E and good levels of important brain minerals, magnesium, and zinc.

SHAKSHUKA

DAIRY OPTION | PAREVE | PASSOVER | SAUCE FREEZES WELL |
MAKES 4–6 SERVINGS

1 Tbsp (15 mL) olive oil

1 large onion, diced

1 red bell pepper, seeded
and diced

4 cloves garlic, minced

1 can (28 oz/796 g) diced
tomatoes (including liquid)

2 Tbsp (30 mL) tomato paste

½ tsp (2 mL) ground cumin

½ tsp (2 mL) sweet paprika

⅛ tsp (0.5 mL) cayenne pepper
or chili powder

Salt and freshly ground black
pepper to taste

1 cup (250 mL) baby spinach,
lightly packed

6 large eggs

¼ cup (60 mL) chopped
fresh parsley

Shakshuka is a popular Israeli dish made with onions, garlic, tomatoes, and eggs. We've added spinach to the traditional recipe to boost brain health. For a delicious dairy version, top with feta or goat cheese. Great for breakfast, brunch, lunch, or even a light supper!

1. Heat oil in a large deep skillet over medium heat. Add onion and red pepper and sauté for 5 minutes, until softened. Stir in garlic and cook until fragrant, about 1 minute longer.

2. Stir in tomatoes, tomato paste, cumin, paprika, and cayenne (or chili powder). Bring to a boil. Reduce heat and simmer, stirring occasionally, until sauce starts to thicken, 6–8 minutes. (If sauce gets too thick, add a little water.) Season with salt and pepper.

3. Stir in spinach and cook 2–3 minutes longer, until wilted slightly.

4. Use the back of a spoon to make 6 indentations in sauce. Crack 1 egg into each hollow.

5. Simmer, covered, until whites are set but yolks are still somewhat runny, 8–10 minutes.

6. Sprinkle chopped parsley overtop. Serve immediately with whole grain bread or pita to soak up the sauce. (Omit bread/pita during Passover, or use Passover rolls.)

205 calories per serving, 16 g carbohydrates, 9 g sugar, 4 g fiber, 11 g protein, 11 g fat (3 g saturated), 135 mg sodium, 630 mg potassium

NORENE'S NOTES:

- **Do-ahead:** Prepare sauce as directed up to the end of Step 2. Once cooled, transfer to a covered container (or containers) and refrigerate or freeze until needed. Makes 4 cups (1 L) sauce.

- **Dairy option:** Sprinkle ½ cup (125 mL) crumbled feta or goat cheese overtop at the end of Step 4.

- **Shakshuka for one:** Pour 1 cup (250 mL) sauce into a small skillet and heat to simmering. If too thick, drizzle in a little water. Stir in a handful of spinach and cook for 2 minutes, until slightly wilted. Crack in 1 or 2 eggs. (Optional: Crumble 2 Tbsp/30 mL feta or goat cheese overtop.) Simmer, covered, for 6–8 minutes, until whites are set but yolks are still slightly runny.

DR. ED SAYS:

- **Vegetables** make their own unique contribution to brain health in this delicious breakfast dish.

- **Spinach** is probably the best among the leafy green vegetables, which, as a category, are one of the leading foods for reducing the risk of AD/dementia. It is a powerhouse in key vitamins and minerals for the brain, contains flavonol antioxidants, and is an excellent source of carotenoid antioxidants as well as vitamin C.

- **Bell peppers** are high in fiber, rich in vitamin C and carotenoid antioxidants, and provide the important B vitamins B6 and folate as well as zinc.

- **Garlic, tomato, spices, and onion** round out the vegetable nutrient contributions, while eggs provide the key nutrients vitamin B12, vitamin D, and choline.

- **Overall,** this recipe is a good representation of important vegetable- and egg-based brain nutrients.

SPINACH & CHEESE FRITTATA

DAIRY | PASSOVER | REFRIGERATE UP TO 2 DAYS | DO NOT FREEZE |
MAKES 4–6 SERVINGS

1 Tbsp (15 mL) olive oil

6 green onions, trimmed and
sliced (or 1 medium onion, diced)

2 cups (500 mL) baby spinach

8 large eggs (see Norene's Notes)

½ cup (125 mL) 1% milk

Salt and freshly ground black
pepper to taste

¼ cup (60 mL) chopped fresh
basil

1 cup (250 mL) grated low-fat
mozzarella cheese

1 tomato, sliced

Some like it hot, some like it cold—so easy, so versatile! Frittata is perfect for breakfast or lunch, or you can even serve it with soup and salad for dinner.

1. Preheat oven to 350°F (175°C). Spray a 10-inch (25 cm) nonstick ovenproof skillet with nonstick spray.

2. Heat oil in the sprayed skillet over medium heat. Sauté onions 3–5 minutes, until softened. Stir in spinach and cook 2–3 minutes longer, until slightly wilted.

3. In a medium bowl, lightly whisk together eggs with milk, salt, and pepper. Stir in basil.

4. Pour egg mixture over cooked vegetables and stir to combine. Let frittata cook till edges start to pull away from the sides of the pan, about 5–7 minutes. Sprinkle with cheese and top with tomato slices.

5. Transfer pan to oven and bake 15–18 minutes, until set. Serve hot or at room temperature.

288 calories per serving, 10 g carbohydrates, 4 g sugar, 2 g fiber, 24 g protein, 20 g fat (7 g saturated), 381 mg sodium, 121 mg potassium

NORENE'S NOTES:

- **Eat the rainbow:** In Step 2, replace baby spinach with your favorite chopped vegetables: asparagus, bell peppers, kale, mushrooms, Swiss chard, and/or zucchini.

- **Perfect pairings:** Match your favorite cheese with the appropriate fresh or dried herbs—feta or goat cheese with dill, Swiss cheese with thyme, Mozzarella cheese with basil or oregano, or Cheddar cheese with parsley and chives.

- **Omega-3 eggs:** Although Omega-3 eggs do provide some Omega-3 fat to your diet, you get more potent amounts from fish and, to a lesser extent, some plant oils such as flax, chia, and hemp. However, Omega-3 eggs are a great alternative for vegetarians and non-fish eaters.

- **Lighter variation:** Use 2 cups (500 mL) liquid egg substitute instead of 8 eggs and reduce cheese to ½ cup (125 mL). One serving of this variation contains 174 calories and 6.9 g fat (2.5 g saturated).

- **Foiled again!** If your skillet doesn't have an ovenproof handle, no problem. Just wrap the handle in aluminum foil before placing the skillet in the oven in Step 5.

DR. ED SAYS:

- **Spinach and eggs** are the main ingredients in this recipe, making it nutritionally similar to Shakshuka (p. 152). You may want to vary your vegetable sources by substituting the recommended kale or asparagus, as mentioned in "eat the rainbow" (p. 154), to obtain a more varied roster of antioxidants.

- **Although Omega-3 eggs** are used, it is much more effective to get your Omega-3 fats from fish rather than Omega-3 eggs.

FLORENTINE CUPCAKES

DAIRY | GLUTEN-FREE OPTION | PASSOVER | REHEATS AND/OR
FREEZES WELL | MAKES 12 CUPCAKES

Half of a 10-oz (300 g) pkg frozen chopped spinach, thawed and squeezed dry

2 green onions, cut into chunks

2 Tbsp (30 mL) fresh dill

2 cups (500 mL, or 1 lb/500 g) cottage cheese (fat-free or 1%; curd-style)

4 large eggs

1 Tbsp (15 mL) vegetable oil

⅓ cup (80 mL) Passover cake meal (regular or gluten-free)

¼ cup (60 mL) grated Parmesan cheese

½ tsp (2 mL) salt

¼ tsp (1 mL) freshly ground black pepper

½ tsp (2 mL) dried basil

Spinach done light! These make a handy grab-and-go breakfast.

1. Preheat oven to 350°F (175°C). Spray compartments of a muffin pan with nonstick cooking spray.

2. In a food processor fitted with the steel blade, process spinach, green onions, dill, cottage cheese, and eggs until smooth and blended, 30–45 seconds, scraping down the sides of the bowl as needed. Add the remaining ingredients and process 15–20 seconds longer, until well mixed.

3. Fill prepared muffin compartments three-quarters full. Bake 40–45 minutes, until golden and set. Cool slightly.

4. Loosen with a flexible spatula and remove carefully.

82 calories per cupcake, 5 g carbohydrates, 1 g sugar, 0.5 g fiber, 8 g protein, 4 g fat (1 g saturated), 308 mg sodium, 107 mg potassium

NORENE'S NOTES:

- **What's your line(r)?** Nonstick parchment baking cups are a less sticky alternative to spraying muffin compartments.

- **Here's the scoop:** For even-sized cupcakes, use an ice cream scoop or ⅓ cup (80 mL), mounding the mixture slightly.

DR. ED SAYS:

- **Spinach:** As I have mentioned throughout this book, spinach is a mainstay of all brain-healthy diet plans, including the Mediterranean diet, the MIND Diet, and our Brain Boosting Diet. It is the most noteworthy of all the dark-green leafy vegetables recommended for these diets because it is an excellent source per 100 g of the brain-healthy nutrients vitamins C, E, and folate. It is also an excellent source of fiber and the important minerals magnesium, potassium, and manganese. Spinach is also very rich in carotenoid antioxidants, especially lutein and zeaxanthin, which have been shown to be important for eye health and cognitive function.

- **Protein:** The cheese and eggs in this recipe end up providing 8 g per serving of high-quality protein. This makes one serving of this cupcake almost a meal in itself thanks to the protein and all the other nutrients of the recipe. Protein is important for all brain and body functions, and we need more of it as we age. Although the RDA (recommended daily allowance) for adults is 0.8 g per kg per day (which works out to about 50 g of protein per day for the average 62.5 kg per 138 lb average adult), this does not take into account the extra needs of older adults, who are less efficient in synthesizing and absorbing protein. Many experts and some countries are now recommending a protein intake of 1–1.3 g per kg per day for adults over 65 years (which translates to 63–81 g per day protein for the average adult).

> **DID YOU KNOW?** Not all proteins are the same. Some are higher quality because they are more efficiently used by the body. In general, the best proteins are egg and whey, and plant proteins are not as high in quality as animal proteins. People who are averse to eating animal protein can overcome this by eating a variety of plant proteins, which have the effect of averaging out the poorer quality of each plant protein to make them more comparable with animal proteins.

PASSOVER ROLLS

PAREVE | PASSOVER | FREEZES WELL | MAKES 10 ROLLS

½ cup (125 mL) olive or vegetable oil

1 cup (250 mL) water

1 tsp (5 mL) salt

1 tsp (5 mL) sugar (optional)

1 cup (250 mL) matzo meal (regular or whole wheat)

4 large eggs

These rolls have a crisp exterior and aren't doughy inside. I've used half the amount of matzo meal and sugar called for in my original Passover recipe, and the sugar is optional. Believe it or not, my Asian homestay students loved these rolls and never complained that they couldn't eat bread during Passover!

1. Preheat oven to 400°F (200°C). Line a large, rimmed baking sheet with parchment paper.

2. In a large saucepan, combine oil, water, salt, and sugar. Bring to a boil over high heat.

3. Remove pan from heat and add matzo meal. Stir vigorously with a wooden spoon until the mixture pulls away from the sides of the pan. Let cool for 5 minutes.

4. Add eggs one at a time, beating well after each addition. (Or, transfer the mixture to a food processor fitted with the steel blade. Drop eggs through the feed tube one at a time while the machine is running. Process for 20–30 seconds, until smooth.)

5. Drop mixture from a large spoon onto the prepared sheet. Wet your hands and shape the mixture into rolls. Leave about 2 inches (5 cm) between rolls, as they will expand during baking.

6. Bake for 15 minutes. Reduce heat to 350°F (175°C) and bake for 30 minutes longer, until nicely browned. (No peeking allowed!)

7. Remove baking sheet from oven and make a small slit on the side of each roll to allow steam to escape. Store in a loosely covered container, or freeze.

168 calories per roll, 9 g carbohydrates, 1 g sugar, 0 g fiber, 4 g protein, 13 g fat (2 g saturated), 262 mg sodium, 28 mg potassium

NORENE'S NOTES:

- **Portion distortion:** These rolls contain half the carbohydrates of my original recipe, but are still high in calories and fat, so control those portions. It's a good thing Passover lasts for only 8 days because these are very addictive!

- **Olive or vegetable oil:** Choose olive oil over vegetable oil, preferably extra virgin, cold-pressed. As part of all the major brain-healthy diets, it has been shown time and time again that olive oil is significant in preventing cognitive decline. Part of this is due to the type of fat (monounsaturated) contained in olive oil, and part is due to its content of antioxidants. And yes, there is a significant amount of fat in this recipe, but don't worry, it is a good fat, and a major study has shown that the more olive oil you consume, the better it is for your brain health.

- **Overall,** due primarily to the olive oil, this recipe is an excellent source of vitamin E and antioxidants, and it also provides good amounts of vitamin B12. Its only drawback is the high carb level, which is mostly digestible carbs. However, the high fat content of the recipe helps to control the resulting blood glucose levels.

> **DID YOU KNOW?** Olive oil contains a natural compound called oleocanthal, which causes cancerous cell death and has been shown to reduce the risk of breast cancer in women.

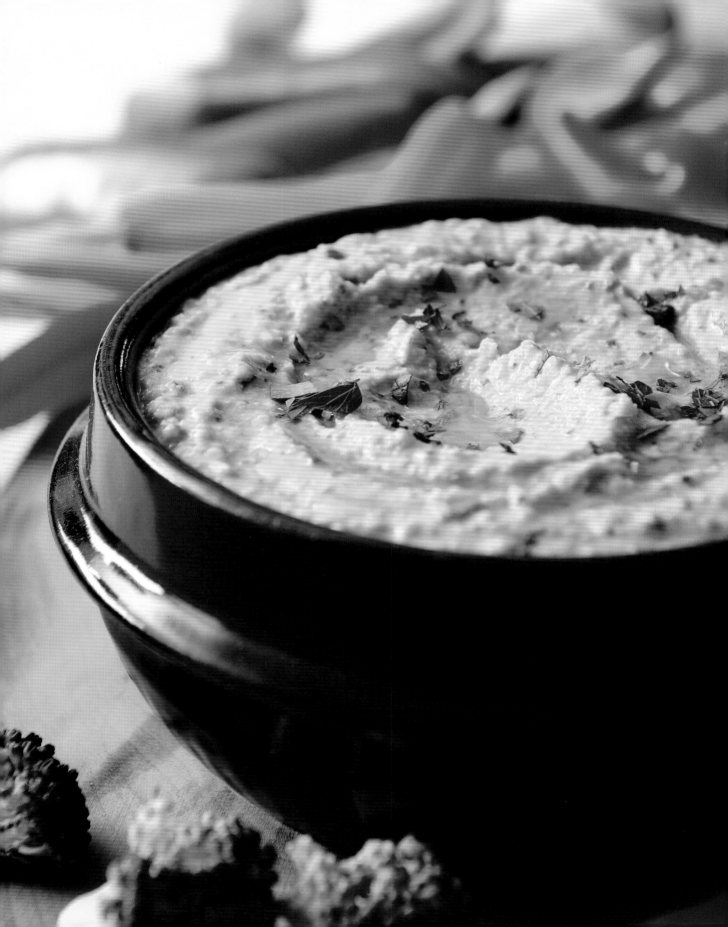

SPLENDID SPREADS & STARTERS

SPREAD IT AROUND: Some dips and spreads, such as Black Bean Dip (p. 164) or Garden Vegetable Hummus (p. 167), can be used instead of butter or mayonnaise as a spread for sandwiches and wraps. Others, such as Roasted Eggplant Spread (p. 172) or Sardine Spread (p. 180), make a terrific topping for salads.

PRESSED FOR TIME? Buy prepared low-fat dips such as hummus, eggplant spread, red bell pepper dip, or tofu spread. Be sure to check labels for fat, calories, and sodium.

FILL 'ER UP! Fill hollowed-out yellow, orange, and red bell peppers, eggplant, or acorn squash with assorted dips or spreads. Perfect party fare!

SUPER BOWL: Cut off the top of a pumpernickel bread. Hollow out the inside, leaving a wall about ½-inch (1 cm) thick on the outside. Cut the bread you've removed into bite-sized chunks and fill the hollowed-out bread with your favorite dip. Surround with bread chunks and assorted veggies.

VEGGIE HEAVEN: Choose a variety of shapes and colors when preparing a vegetable platter. Serve broccoli and cauliflower florets, celery sticks, bell pepper strips, baby carrots, grape tomatoes, lightly steamed asparagus spears, or sugar snap peas . . . the choice is yours. Dip to your heart's content!

LEFTOVER CRUDITÉS? Transform them into soup! Sauté 1 onion over medium heat in 1 Tbsp (15 mL) olive oil until golden. Add leftover vegetables plus enough water, or vegetable or chicken broth, to cover the vegetables by 1 inch (2.5 cm). Season with salt and pepper to taste. Simmer for 30 minutes, then purée using an immersion blender.

STICK 'EM UP! Grilled chicken skewers, such as Chicken Satay (p. 295), make excellent appetizers for a party or barbecue. Marinate chicken in advance and store in the freezer in resealable freezer bags. When needed, thaw overnight in the refrigerator, then thread onto skewers. (Don't forget to soak wooden skewers in water for about 1 hour before using to prevent them from burning.) Allow 2–4 skewers per person as an appetizer.

BOCCONCINI SKEWERS: Marinate miniature bocconcini (soft mozzarella) balls in Power Pesto (p. 492) for 30 minutes. Thread marinated cheese onto wooden skewers, alternating each bocconcini with a grape tomato. For a pretty presentation, place a half melon, flat side down, on a serving platter. Insert bocconcini skewers into the melon.

EASE UP ON CHEESE: Those chunks of cheese can make you chunky too, and crackers aren't all they're cracked up to be—they are often high in carbs and calories.

DOUBLE DUTY: Many appetizers can be served as a main dish and vice versa. A main dish for 4 people will usually serve 6–8 as an appetizer or starter.

PARTY SMART! When faced with temptation, your best choice is a veggie appetizer or starter. If you want to indulge in high-fat fare, eat a small portion—very, very slowly. Adjust for added calories and fat by making lighter choices the rest of the day. Also, increase your activity level. Reaching for a second helping does not count as a stretching exercise!

SHARONA'S CHEESY POPCORN: Toss 3 cups (750 mL) air-popped popcorn with 2 Tbsp (30 mL) nutritional yeast and your favorite spice mix (garlic powder, onion powder, cayenne, no-salt seasoning, etc.).

BLACK BEAN DIP

PAREVE | GLUTEN-FREE | DO NOT FREEZE | MAKES ABOUT 2 CUPS (500 ML)

1 Tbsp (15 mL) extra virgin olive oil

1 small onion, chopped

2–3 cloves garlic, minced

1 can (19 oz/540 g) black beans, drained and rinsed (preferably no-salt-added)

⅓ cup (80 mL) water

1 tsp (5 mL) chili powder

¼ tsp (1 mL) cumin

Salt and freshly ground black pepper

2 tsp (10 mL) lemon or lime juice (preferably fresh)

Finely minced fresh cilantro (for garnish)

Finely minced red bell pepper (for garnish)

This is skinny dipping at its finest! It's delicious as a dip with assorted raw vegetables.

1. Heat oil in a large nonstick skillet over medium heat. Add onion and garlic and sauté for 3–4 minutes, until softened. Stir in black beans, water, chili powder, cumin, salt, and pepper. Simmer uncovered for 5 minutes, stirring occasionally. Stir in lemon juice and remove pan from heat.

2. Using a potato masher or food processor, mash the bean mixture to the desired consistency.

3. Transfer to a serving bowl, cover, and refrigerate until ready to use—it will keep for 3–4 days. Garnish with cilantro and red bell pepper and serve chilled.

20 calories per 1 Tbsp (15 mL), 3 g carbohydrates, 1 g fiber, 0 g sugar, 1 g protein, <1 g fat (0 g saturated), 5 mg sodium, 45 mg potassium

NORENE'S NOTES:

- **Lower-sodium option:** To reduce the sodium content of canned beans, rinse well. Organic brands are lower in sodium than regular brands, but are also usually more expensive. You can also buy no-salt-added canned beans.

- **Using your bean!** Black beans are extremely versatile. Use them in dips, soups, salads, salsas, stews, casseroles, chili, fajitas, and burritos. They have a low GI, which helps to stabilize blood sugar levels. Many people find black beans easier to digest than other types of beans.

- **Black beans** are the major ingredient in this dip and are part of the legume family. They are noteworthy because they are very high in fiber at more than a third of their carbohydrate content. As a result, they have a GI of less than 30, as do many legumes, and their digestible carbs are also low. Black beans are rich in the important polyphenol antioxidants anthocyanins and kaempferols, as well as potassium, folate, and magnesium, and they're also low in sodium. Although black beans are a recommended ingredient, the serving size for a dip is so small that we only get a small amount of the nutrients mentioned.

DID YOU KNOW? In identifying which groups of antioxidants are the best for the heart and mind, researchers have consistently mentioned anthocyanins.

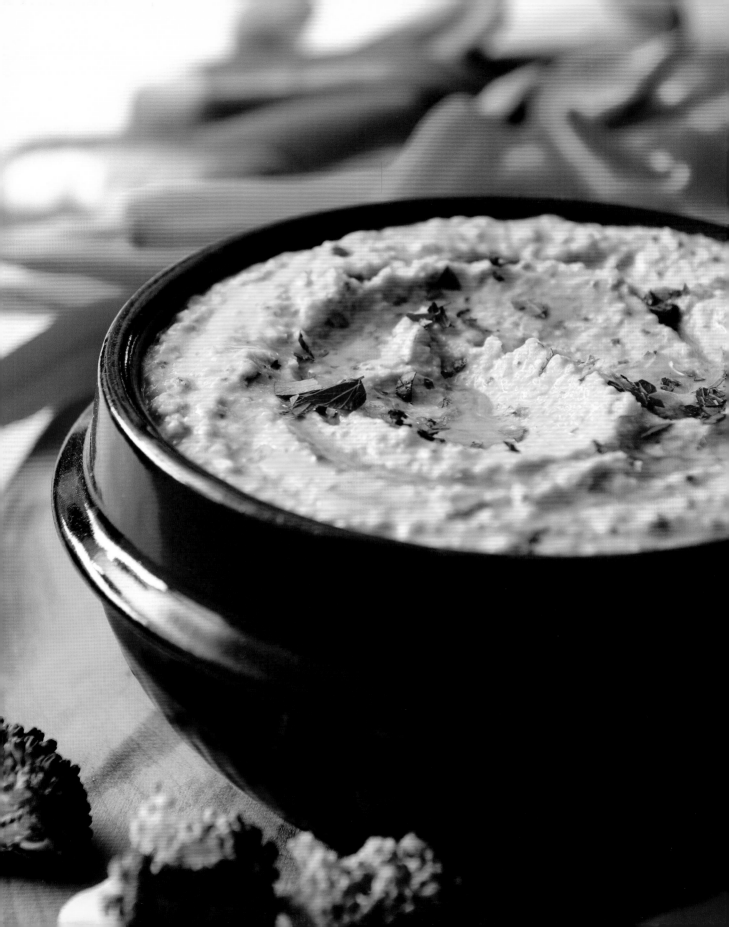

GARDEN VEGETABLE HUMMUS

PAREVE | GLUTEN-FREE | DO NOT FREEZE | MAKES 2½ CUPS (500 ML)

This guilt-free hummus is excellent as a dip with veggies or as a spread on whole wheat pita or wraps. Dip "a-weigh" to your heart's delight!

1 can (19 oz/540 g) chickpeas, drained and rinsed (preferably no-salt-added)

3–4 cloves garlic (about 1 Tbsp/ 15 mL minced)

½ green bell pepper, cut into chunks

½ red bell pepper, cut into chunks

4 green onions (or 1 medium onion, cut into chunks)

¼ cup (60 mL) chopped fresh basil or Italian parsley

2 Tbsp (30 mL) extra virgin olive oil

2 Tbsp (30 mL) lemon juice (preferably fresh)

2–3 Tbsp (45 mL) tahini (sesame seed paste)

Salt and freshly ground black pepper

Chopped fresh parsley (for garnish)

1. Combine all ingredients except parsley in a food processor fitted with the steel blade. Process with quick on/offs to start, then let the motor run until the mixture is very smooth, about 2 minutes, scraping down the sides of the bowl as needed.

2. Transfer hummus to a serving bowl and sprinkle with parsley. Cover and chill for 1–2 hours before serving. (Hummus will thicken when refrigerated.)

26 calories per 1 Tbsp (15 mL), 3 g carbohydrates, 1 g fiber, trace sugar, 1 g protein, 1 g fat (0 g saturated), 4 mg sodium, 40 mg potassium

NORENE'S NOTES:

- **Mediterranean hummus:** Add ½ cup (125 mL) roasted red peppers (p. 188) and a dash of cumin; blend well. For an Italian twist, substitute pesto for the tahini and cumin.

DR. ED SAYS:

- **Chickpeas** are another member of the legume family and have a similar nutritional profile to black beans, although their antioxidant profile is not as well defined.

- **Tahini** (sesame seed paste) is a very nutrient-dense ingredient because it has a very low moisture content. It is an excellent source of mono- and polyunsaturated fats, which are good fats, as well as an excellent source of protein, magnesium, zinc, manganese fiber, and potassium. It is very low in sugar and digestible carbs, and comes with a low GI. It is also very rich in lignin polyphenols.

- **Overall,** if you use this as a meal with whole grain pita instead of as a dip, you will get the most benefit of its nutrient content.

PUMPKIN HUMMUS

PAREVE | GLUTEN-FREE | FREEZES WELL | MAKES ABOUT 3 CUPS (750 ML)

¼ cup (60 mL) fresh flat-leaf parsley

3 cloves garlic (or 1½ tsp/ 7 mL minced)

1 can (19 oz/540 g) chickpeas, drained and rinsed (preferably no-salt-added)

¼ cup (60 mL) extra virgin olive oil

3 Tbsp (45 mL) tahini (sesame seed paste)

Juice of 1 lemon (3–4 Tbsp/45–60 mL)

1 tsp (5 mL) salt (or to taste)

Freshly ground black pepper

½ tsp (2 mL) ground cumin

1 cup (250 mL) canned pumpkin purée (see Norene's Notes)

¼ cup (60 mL) toasted unsalted pumpkin seeds (for garnish)

Here's a different twist on a popular Middle Eastern spread. Pumpkin adds a vibrant hue—it's so "gourd" for you! To make this Hummus even better for your brain, use it in spinach hummus wraps (below).

1. Wash parsley and pat completely dry. In a food processor fitted with the steel blade, process parsley and garlic until finely minced, about 10 seconds.

2. Add chickpeas, olive oil, tahini, lemon juice, salt, pepper, and cumin to the processor bowl. Process until very smooth, about 2 minutes, scraping down the sides of the bowl as needed. Add pumpkin purée and process 30–45 seconds longer.

3. Transfer to a serving bowl. Garnish with pumpkin seeds. Cover and refrigerate 3–4 hours or overnight.

4. Serve chilled with assorted raw vegetables (e.g., broccoli or cauliflower florets, bell pepper strips).

31 calories per 1 Tbsp (15 mL), 3 g carbohydrates, 1 g fiber, 0 g sugar, 1 g protein, 2 g fat (0 g saturated fat), 50 mg sodium, 41 mg potassium

NORENE'S NOTES:

- **Spinach hummus wraps:** Spread ¼ cup (60 mL) Pumpkin Hummus on a whole wheat tortilla. Top with a layer of spinach leaves, red pepper strips, and avocado slices. Roll up tightly into a cylinder and slice in half crosswise. Wrap-sody!

- **Variation:** Instead of canned pumpkin, substitute cooked pumpkin or squash. For additional brain-health benefits, add ½ cup (125 mL) spinach to the original recipe.

- **Fresh or canned:** One can (14 oz/398 g) pumpkin purée is equivalent to 2½ lb (1.1 kg) pumpkin or squash, seeded, peeled, cooked, and puréed. Leftover purée can be added to mashed sweet potatoes or soups.

- **It's a keeper!** Hummus keeps 1 week in the fridge in an airtight container.

- **Freeze with ease:** Freeze Hummus in meal-sized portions. When needed, thaw overnight in the refrigerator. If there is some liquid at the top when you remove the lid, give it a good stir.

DR. ED SAYS:

- **Dark leafy green vegetables** such as spinach and parsley are strongly recommended for reducing the risk of AD/dementia.

- **Chickpeas** are an excellent source of dietary fiber, which helps to slow the release of sugar into the bloodstream.

- **Pumpkin seeds** provide a good source of antioxidants, phytosterols (for cholesterol reduction), vitamin E, and magnesium. Pumpkin seeds offset the pumpkin purée's relatively high carbohydrate content. Both pumpkin seeds and pumpkin purée are low in sodium and sugars, and are very good sources of fiber, which results in a very low glycemic index. Pumpkin seeds are particularly rich in a form of vitamin E (gamma tocopherol) thought to play an important part in preventing cognitive decline.

- **Pumpkin purée** is rich in carotenoid antioxidants, including the important lutein and zeaxanthin.

- **Olive oil,** a part of the Mediterranean diet, is a rich source of mono-unsaturated fat and antioxidants, and helps reduce cognitive decline.

- **Tahini** provides high levels of fiber, magnesium, and vitamins B6 and folate, which are strongly recommended for cognitive protection.

- **Overall,** this tasty snack is rich in fiber and antioxidants, relatively high in magnesium, and low in sodium and sugars. When the ingredients in this recipe are combined with other brain-friendly foods, such as spinach or broccoli, they help optimize cognitive function.

> DID YOU KNOW? Pumpkin seed fat, which makes up about 50% of the seed, is thought to alleviate the symptoms of BPH in men. BPH is a condition of prostate growth that causes frequent urination in men.

SIMPLE SALSA

PAREVE | GLUTEN-FREE | PASSOVER | DO NOT FREEZE | MAKES ABOUT 2 CUPS (500 ML)

2 cloves garlic

2 Tbsp (30 mL) fresh flat-leaf parsley or cilantro

2 Tbsp (30 mL) fresh basil

6 firm, ripe plum (Roma) tomatoes, cut into chunks

1 Tbsp (15 mL) extra virgin olive oil

1 Tbsp (15 mL) lemon juice (preferably fresh)

Salt and freshly ground black pepper

Dash of cayenne pepper

Serve this scrumptious salsa as a dip for assorted veggies or as a topping on toasted whole wheat baguette slices—but not during Passover (see Norene's Notes). It also makes an excellent sauce for fish, chicken, or burgers.

1. Drop garlic through the feed tube of a food processor fitted with the steel blade while the machine is running. Process until minced. Add parsley and basil and process until minced, 8–10 seconds.

2. Add tomatoes, oil, lemon juice, and seasonings. Process with 3 or 4 quick on/off pulses, just until tomatoes are coarsely chopped. Transfer to a serving bowl, cover, and chill.

25 calories per ¼-cup (60 mL) serving, 2 g carbohydrates, 1 g fiber, 1 g sugar, 1 g protein, 2 g fat (0 g saturated), 3 mg sodium, 122 mg potassium

NORENE'S NOTES:

- **Variation:** Stir ½ cup (125 mL) diced avocado and ¼ cup (60 mL) diced red onion into the salsa.

- **Spice it up!** Instead of cayenne pepper, use 1 fresh jalapeno chili pepper, seeded.

- **Easy apps:** Spoon salsa onto slices of toasted whole wheat baguette. Top with grated low-fat mozzarella, Swiss, Monterey Jack, or Parmesan cheese. Broil for 2–3 minutes before serving.

- **To-mato, to-mahto:** Although you can use any kind of tomatoes you have on hand, plum tomatoes (Romas) are best because they have less seeds and juice, making a thicker mixture.

- **Chilling news!** If you refrigerate fresh tomatoes, their texture will become mealy and they will taste watery.

- **Roma tomatoes** are the key ingredient in this recipe. Tomatoes are primarily known for their high content of the carotenoid antioxidant lycopene, which has been linked, without conclusive evidence, to a reduced risk of heart disease and prostate cancer. Some carotenoid antioxidants such as lutein and zeaxanthin have been shown to be beneficial to the brain. Tomatoes are also a good source of vitamin C, vitamin B6, and fiber—not to mention one of the vegetables with the highest contents of sugars. Tomatoes should be cooked to release their lycopene, and be consumed with fat (e.g., olive oil).

DID YOU KNOW? Tomatoes, along with eggplant, bell peppers, avocados, green peas, pumpkins, and olives are technically fruits because they contain seeds. That said, because we commonly consider them as vegetables, they are "fruit vegetables." In general, fruits and "fruit vegetables" contain more sugar than regular vegetables.

ROASTED EGGPLANT SPREAD

PAREVE | GLUTEN-FREE | PASSOVER | FREEZES WELL | MAKES
ABOUT 2¼ CUPS (560 ML)

1 eggplant (about 2 lb/1 kg),
peeled and cut into 2-inch
(5 cm) chunks

1 red onion, cut into 2-inch
(5 cm) chunks

2 red bell peppers, cut into
2-inch (5 cm) chunks

2 Tbsp (30 mL) olive oil

¾ tsp (4 mL) salt (or to taste)

¼ tsp (1 mL) freshly ground
black pepper

1 whole head garlic (trim and
discard the top)

2 Tbsp (30 mL) tomato paste

This scrumptious ruby-red spread comes from Penny Krowitz of
Toronto, who got it from Melissa Adler. I've nicknamed it "Penny's from
Heaven!" If you don't process the roasted vegetables, this recipe does
double-duty as a superb side dish.

1. Preheat oven to 400°F (200°C). Line a large, rimmed baking sheet
with parchment paper.

2. Combine eggplant, onion, and peppers in a large bowl. Drizzle with
oil and sprinkle with salt and pepper; mix well. Spread out vegetables in
a single layer on the prepared baking sheet.

3. Drizzle cut side of the garlic with a few drops of oil, wrap in foil, and
place on the baking sheet next to vegetables.

4. Roast, uncovered, for 40–45 minutes, stirring occasionally, until
vegetables are tender but slightly blackened around the edges. (To
transform this into a delicious side dish, see Norene's Notes).

5. Remove from oven and cool slightly. Transfer vegetables to a food
processor fitted with the steel blade. Squeeze garlic cloves out of their
skins and add to the processor along with tomato paste. Process, using
quick on/off pulses, until coarsely chopped. Transfer to a serving bowl,
cover, and refrigerate to allow flavors to blend.

76 calories per ¼-cup (60 mL) serving, 11 g carbohydrates, 4 g fiber, 6 g
sugar, 2 g protein, 3 g fat (1 g saturated fat), 210 mg sodium, 378 mg
potassium

NORENE'S NOTES:

- **Roasted eggplant and pepper medley:** At the end of Step 4, transfer
the roasted vegetables to a serving bowl. Don't add the tomato paste
or chop the vegetables. Delicious hot or at room temperature.

- **Frozen assets!** Drop tablespoonfuls of leftover tomato paste onto a parchment-lined baking sheet and freeze until solid. Transfer frozen blobs to a resealable plastic bag and used them as needed. Add to soups, stews, and sauces—no need to defrost first.

- **Instant tomato sauce:** Use up leftover tomato paste by mixing it with double the amount of water, turning it into tomato sauce.

DR. ED SAYS:

- **Eggplant** provides a variety of important nutrients for the brain, but in relatively low quantities compared with other vegetables. Because eggplant is actually a fruit, it is relatively high in sugars. It is, however, a good source of fiber. All in all, I would recommend this food primarily for its taste and texture.

- **Bell peppers** are also a "fruit vegetable" and therefore contain significant amounts of sugar. However, they are an excellent source of vitamin C and a good source of fiber, vitamin B6, folate, vitamin E, and carotenoid antioxidants. Therefore, they are more nutritious than eggplant.

- **Overall,** we are getting an excellent amount of vitamin C per serving and good amounts of vitamin E, folate, and vitamin B6, as well as fiber. Sugar is a bit on the high side but acceptable.

TURKISH EGGPLANT SALAD

PAREVE | GLUTEN-FREE | PASSOVER OPTION | FREEZES WELL |
MAKES 6 CUPS (1.5 L)

1 eggplant (about 1½ lb/750 g)

Salt (for sprinkling on eggplant)

2 Tbsp (30 mL) olive oil

2 large onions, chopped

3 cloves garlic (about 1 Tbsp/
15 mL minced)

3 cups (750 mL) tomato sauce

2 Tbsp (30 mL) lemon juice
(preferably fresh)

Sweetener equivalent to
¼ cup (60 mL) sugar

Salt and freshly ground
black pepper

¼ tsp (1 mL) cayenne pepper

½ tsp (2 mL) cumin (omit
for Passover)

½ tsp (2 mL) dried thyme

2 Tbsp (30 mL) minced fresh
cilantro or parsley

This sweet and spicy eggplant dish is served in many Middle Eastern restaurants and everyone I know who tries it loves it. It's absolutely addictive!

1. Cut off both ends from the eggplant but don't peel. Cut eggplant into ½-inch (1 cm) chunks. (You should have about 8 cups/2 L.) Place chunks in a colander and sprinkle with salt to drain out any bitter juices. Let stand for about 30 minutes before rinsing and patting dry.

2. Heat oil in a large pot on medium. Sauté onions and garlic for 5 minutes, until softened. Increase heat to medium-high, add eggplant, and sauté for 5–7 minutes longer, until softened.

3. Stir in tomato sauce, lemon juice, sweetener, salt, pepper, cayenne, cumin, thyme, and cilantro. Bring to a boil; reduce heat to low and cover partially.

4. Simmer for 25–30 minutes, until sauce has thickened, stirring occasionally. Adjust seasonings to taste.

5. Once cooled, cover and refrigerate. Serve chilled.

34 calories per ¼-cup (60 mL) serving, 6 g carbohydrates, 2 g fiber, 3 g sugar, 1 g protein, 1 g fat (0 g saturated), 11 mg sodium, 172 mg potassium

NORENE'S NOTES:

- **Appe-teasers!** This spread makes a delicious addition to any Middle Eastern appetizer platter, including Pumpkin Hummus (p. 168), Garden Vegetable Hummus (p. 167), or Roasted Eggplant Spread (p. 172).

- **Top it up!** This makes a terrific topping for crostini, pita wedges, or toasted whole wheat baguette slices. Sprinkle with low-fat grated mozzarella and broil briefly until the cheese is melted.

- **Eggplant** is not a great source of brain nutrients and has a high sugar content, but leaving the skin on in this recipe helps increase the available antioxidants. Also, the tomatoes (lycopene antioxidant), onions (quercetin antioxidant), and spices provide a good mixture of interactive antioxidants.

DID YOU KNOW? In Turkey there is a famous stuffed eggplant dish called Imam Bayildi, which means the Imam fainted because it was so delicious.

VENEZUELAN GUACAMOLE (GUASACACA)

PAREVE | GLUTEN-FREE | PASSOVER | DO NOT FREEZE | MAKES
ABOUT 3 CUPS (750 ML)

1 can (14 oz/398 g) hearts of palm, well drained

2 Tbsp (30 mL) fresh cilantro

2 Tbsp (30 mL) fresh parsley

1 small onion

1 large clove garlic (about 1 tsp/ 5 mL minced)

½ green or red bell pepper, cut into chunks

1 medium tomato, quartered

1 firm, ripe avocado, peeled and pitted

1 Tbsp (15 mL) extra virgin olive oil

1 Tbsp (15 mL) lemon juice (preferably fresh)

½ tsp (2 mL) salt

Freshly ground black pepper

¼ tsp (1 mL) cayenne pepper or chili powder

The inspiration for this Venezuelan version of guacamole comes from Elena Eder of Miami. Guasacaca (pronounced wasakaka) is usually smoother than guacamole and contains fresh cilantro and parsley. Elena adds hearts of palm to reduce the calories and fat—as a bonus, it keeps the avocado from turning brown. This is traditionally served with grilled fish, chicken or meats, tortillas, pita bread, or flatbread.

---

1. In a food processor fitted with the steel blade, process hearts of palm, cilantro, and parsley with quick on/off pulses, until finely chopped. Transfer to a medium bowl—you should have about 1 cup (250 mL).

2. Process onion, garlic, and bell pepper with quick on/off pulses, until coarsely chopped. Add tomato, avocado, oil, lemon juice, salt, pepper, and cayenne. Process with quick on/offs pulses, until finely chopped.

3. Add mixture to hearts of palm and mix well. Adjust seasonings to taste.

4. Cover tightly with plastic wrap, pressing it directly against the surface. Refrigerate up to 4 days. Serve chilled.

39 calories per ¼-cup (60 mL) serving, 3 g carbohydrates, 2 g fiber, 1 g sugar, 1 g protein, 3 g fat (1 g saturated), 199 mg sodium, 48 mg potassium

NORENE'S NOTES:

- **Hot, hot, hot!** This traditional South American dish is made with red and green chili peppers, but I use green or red bell peppers and kick up the heat with cayenne.

- **Traditional guacamole:** Follow the recipe above, but omit hearts of palm. You can use lime juice instead of lemon juice, and replace cayenne with 2–3 drops of Sriracha. In Step 2, process until desired texture.

- **Avocado purée:** When avocados are plentiful, purée the pulp using the steel blade, adding 1 tsp (5 mL) lemon juice per avocado. Transfer to resealable freezer bags, press out air, seal tightly, and freeze. Great for guacamole!

DR. ED SAYS:

- **Palm hearts,** the edible cores of palm tree stems, are a good source of fiber, vitamin C, magnesium, and folate. They are also very low-calorie, low-fat, and low in digestible carbs. Unlike most vegetables and fruits, however, they tend to be high in sodium (426 mg per 100 g) and low in potassium (177 mg per 100 g). Using avocado instead of palm hearts may be a more nutritious choice, as avocado is a good source of vitamin B6, vitamin E (including the important gamma tocopherol form), and the polyphenol antioxidant group proanthocyanodins, which can lower blood cholesterol. Avocados are an excellent source of fiber, folate, and vitamin C, and are high in potassium, as well as low in sodium, digestible carbs, and sugar.

DID YOU KNOW? Proanthocyanodins, which are also found in cranberry juice, were thought to be an important component in controlling urinary tract infections (UTI) in women, but recent clinical trials have debunked the use of cranberry juice to prevent UTIs. Nevertheless, these compounds are still thought to be important in reducing the risk of cardiovascular disease, and therefore cognitive decline.

MUSHROOM MOCK CHOPPED LIVER

PAREVE | GLUTEN-FREE | PASSOVER | DO NOT FREEZE | MAKES
ABOUT 2 CUPS (500 ML)

2 cloves garlic

3 medium onions, quartered

1–2 Tbsp (15–30 mL) olive oil

1 pkg (8 oz/227 g) sliced
cremini mushrooms (about
2½ cups/625 mL)

¼ cup (60 mL) walnut pieces

3 hard-boiled eggs

Salt and freshly ground
black pepper

This is my favorite vegetarian version of chopped liver—it's perfect for Passover or all year round! It features an Omega-3 trio of olive oil, walnuts, and eggs. If you have a nut allergy, either omit the nuts or use pumpkin seeds (but not during Passover).

---

1. Drop garlic through the feed tube of a food processor fitted with the steel blade while the machine is running. Process until minced, about 10 seconds. Add onions and process with several quick on/off pulses, until coarsely chopped.

2. Heat olive oil in a large nonstick skillet on medium. Add onions and garlic (don't bother washing the food processor bowl). Sauté until golden, about 6–8 minutes. If the mixture begins to stick, add a little water.

3. Add mushrooms and sauté for 6–8 minutes, stirring occasionally, until browned. Remove pan from heat and cool slightly.

4. Process walnuts until coarsely ground, about 8–10 seconds. Add onion/mushroom mixture, eggs, salt, and pepper. Process with several quick on/off pulses, just until combined.

5. Transfer to a container, cover, and refrigerate until ready to serve. Serve chilled.

94 calories per ¼-cup (60 mL) serving, 6 g carbohydrates, 1 g fiber, 3 g sugar, 4 g protein, 6 g fat (1 g saturated), 27 mg sodium, 214 mg potassium

NORENE'S NOTES:

- **Legume lover's liver:** Replace mushrooms with 1½ cups (375 mL) canned chickpeas or lentils, rinsed and drained (preferably low-sodium or no-salt-added). Sauté onions and garlic for 8–10 minutes until well browned. (Note that legumes are not allowed for Ashkenazi Jews during Passover.)

- **Stuffed!** Serve in Bibb lettuce leaves, hollowed-out bell pepper halves, or large tomatoes. Alternately, stuff cherry tomatoes or mushroom caps with the mixture and serve as hors d'oeuvres.

DR. ED SAYS:

- **Cremini mushrooms,** a variety of the common white button mushroom, have more antioxidants than many vegetables including tomatoes, green peppers, and carrots. They are also a good source of protein, fiber, and potassium, as well as being low in carbs, sugar, sodium, and fat. At the same time, they provide vitamin B6, magnesium, folate, and some choline.

- **Eggs** are a welcome addition in a mainly vegetarian diet as they provide excellent quantities of high-quality protein, vitamin B12 (which is usually lacking in vegetarian diets), and choline. They are also a good source of vitamin B6, vitamin D, vitamin E, folate, and zinc. Simultaneously, they are also very low in carbs and sugar and are balanced in potassium and sodium.

> **DID YOU KNOW?** Choline is a precursor to the important neurotransmitter acetylcholine.

SARDINE SPREAD (MOCK CHOPPED HERRING)

PAREVE | GLUTEN-FREE OPTION | DO NOT FREEZE | MAKES ABOUT
3 CUPS (750 ML)

1 medium onion, cut into chunks

1 apple, peeled and cut
into chunks

2 cans (3¼ oz/106 g each)
sardines, well drained

1 slice flaxseed, whole wheat,
or rye bread

3 large hard-boiled eggs, halved

3 Tbsp (45 mL) white or cider
vinegar (or to taste)

Sweetener equivalent to
1 tsp (5 mL) sugar

This is an updated version of an old favorite. Sardines are high in
Omega-3 fatty acids and are a good source of protein and calcium.
Omega-3 eggs and flaxseed bread make this a heart-healthy spread.

1. In a food processor fitted with the steel blade, process onion, apple,
and sardines until finely minced, about 10 seconds.

2. Moisten bread by placing it briefly under running water; squeeze out
excess moisture and tear it into chunks. Add bread to the processor
along with eggs, vinegar, and sweetener; process for 8–10 seconds more,
or until combined.

3. Transfer to a serving bowl and cover well. Store in the refrigerator for
1–2 hours to blend flavors. Serve chilled.

157 calories per ½-cup (125 mL) serving, 10 g carbohydrates, 1 g fiber,
6 g sugar, 13 g protein, 7 g fat (2 g saturated), 386 mg sodium, 249 mg
potassium

NORENE'S NOTES:

· **Spread it around:** Serve a scoop on top of dark leafy greens or use
it to stuff hollowed-out tomatoes. Put it through a pastry bag and
pipe onto cucumber rounds or wholegrain crackers. This mixture also
makes a great filling for sandwiches or wraps. Your choice!

· **Eggs-actly!** Instead of 3 large eggs, use 2 hard-boiled eggs plus 2 egg
whites.

DR. ED SAYS:

· **Sardines** are one of the fish species with the highest concentrations
of Omega-3 fats. Norene's suggestion to serve this spread on top of
dark leafy greens is a great idea, because they enhance the impact
of the Omega-3 fats. Sardines are excellent sources of Omega-3 fats,
vitamin D, vitamin B12, and high-quality protein. They are also good
sources of magnesium, potassium, zinc, selenium, vitamins B6 and E,
and choline. All in all, a great brain nutrition source.

- **Overall,** this recipe is a welcome choice in a mostly vegetarian Mediterranean-type diet as it supplies much-needed high Omega-3 fats, vitamin D, vitamin B12, as well as protein. Sugar is slightly high due to the addition of an apple, but if you are concerned, then cut back on it. Potassium and sodium are nicely balanced.

DID YOU KNOW? Sardines are not only powerhouses for Omega-3 fats, but because they are a very small fish, they have much lower risk of carrying PCBs or other ocean-based toxins.

WINNIPEG HERRING SALAD

PAREVE | GLUTEN-FREE | PASSOVER | DO NOT FREEZE | MAKES
ABOUT 12 SERVINGS

1 jar (26 oz/600 g) herring fillets
in wine marinade

3 stalks celery, diced

1 yellow and/or orange bell
pepper, diced

3 or 4 firm, ripe tomatoes, diced

6 green onions, thinly sliced

2 Tbsp (30 mL) minced fresh dill

¼ cup (60 mL) vegetable oil

Sweetener equivalent to ¼ cup
(60 mL) brown sugar

This colorful, brain-boosting salad makes a great starter or appetizer. It feeds a large crowd or can be halved easily. I first heard about it from my friend Bev Binder of Winnipeg. She got the recipe from Lenore Kagan, who got it from Phyllis Spigelman. My friend Evelyn Schaefer also makes it, and now it's on my menu, too.

---

1. Drain herring and rinse well; discard onions from the marinade. Dice herring and place in a large bowl.

2. Add celery, peppers, tomatoes, green onions, dill, oil, and sweetener; mix well.

3. Cover and refrigerate overnight. Serve chilled.

187 calories per ½-cup (125 mL) serving, 8 g carbohydrates, 5 g sugar, 1 g fiber, 8 g protein, 14 g fat (2 g saturated), 446 mg sodium, 188 mg potassium

NORENE'S NOTES:

- **Oil right!** This recipe calls for vegetable oil, so it's suitable for Passover, but you can also use other neutral-flavored oils during the year (e.g., grapeseed, sunflower).

- **Variation:** Substitute pickled herring or any other type of jarred herring for a change in flavor. The choice is yours!

- **Add-ins:** Add 2 diced mini cucumbers. Instead of green onions, use 1 cup (250 mL) diced red onion. Pitted black olives add a colorful contrast.

DR. ED SAYS:

- **Herring,** another fish that I heartily recommend, is very high in Omega-3 fats and low in possible ocean toxins because of its small size. It is also an excellent source of vitamins D and B12 and high-quality protein. It has a similar profile of brain nutrients to that of sardines, which is discussed in Sardine Spread (p. 180).

- **Overall,** this recipe is similar in nutrients to the recipe for Sardine Spread, except that the vitamin C content is much higher due to the bell peppers and tomatoes.

DID YOU KNOW? It is very difficult to get vitamin D and vitamin B12 from vegetarian sources, so fatty fish is a great way to obtain these important brain nutrients. Vitamins D and B12 are especially important for older adults, who are the most at risk of memory loss and AD/dementia—as described in Chapter 7—Supplements they tend to have much lower blood levels of these nutrients as compared with the rest of the population.

DIY FROZEN GEFILTE FISH LOGS

PAREVE | GLUTEN-FREE OPTION | PASSOVER | FREEZES WELL |
MAKES 2 LOGS (16 SLICES)

FISH MIXTURE:

2 medium onions, cut into chunks

1 medium carrot, cut into chunks + extra slices for garnish

2 Tbsp (30 mL) dill

2 lb/1 kg ground fish (e.g., whitefish, pickerel, or pike, or even minced salmon)

4 large eggs

¼ cup (60 mL) ice cold water

¼ cup (60 mL) matzo meal (see Norene's Notes)

1½ tsp (7 mL) salt (use less if you're salt-sensitive)

½ tsp (2 mL) white pepper

1 tsp (5 mL) sugar

POACHING LIQUID:

2 medium onions, sliced

2 medium carrots, sliced

6 cups (1.5 L) water

1 tsp (5 mL) salt

1 tsp (5 mL) sugar

Looks complicated, cooks easy! It's easy to control the carb content when you make your own gefilte fish rather than buying the commercial variety. Use whatever fish is available locally—I've even used minced salmon. Thanks to my friend Rimma Tverskoy for asking me how to do it yourself!

1. **FISH MIXTURE:** Using a food processor fitted with the steel blade, process onions and carrot until finely minced, about 10 seconds. Add fish and process until smooth, about 30 seconds. Add the remaining ingredients and process 20–30 seconds longer, until very smooth and silky, scraping down the sides of the bowl as necessary. (If using a small processor, prepare fish mixture in 2 batches.)

2. Moisten 2 sheets of parchment paper under running water. Squeeze gently to remove excess moisture and make them flexible.

3. Moisten your hands and shape fish mixture into 2 logs. Wrap each log in moistened parchment paper, twisting the ends to seal tightly. Place logs in a resealable freezer bag (or bags) and freeze until needed.

4. **POACHING LIQUID:** Combine onions, carrots, water, salt, and sugar in a large, wide pot and bring to a boil. Carefully add frozen logs to the liquid and bring back to a boil. If needed, add more water so fish is completely covered.

5. Simmer, partially covered, for 2 hours.

6. Let logs cool in liquid. Carefully remove them from liquid using a wide slotted spatula. Chill until serving time.

7. Unwrap logs and transfer to a serving platter. Slice, garnishing each piece with a carrot slice. Delicious with horseradish.

140 calories per 1-inch (2.5 cm) slice, 6 g carbohydrates, 1 g fiber, 2 g sugar, 16 g protein, 6 g fat (1 g saturated), 431 mg sodium, 325 mg potassium

NORENE'S NOTES:

- **Gluten-free/passover variation:** Either substitute ground almonds for matzo meal or use gluten-free matzo meal.

- **Oven-poached variation:** Instead of simmering frozen logs and vegetables on the stovetop, place in a deep pan. Add boiling water to cover completely. Cover tightly and cook at 350°F (175°C) for 2 hours. Once cooled, remove from liquid and chill.

- **Loaf-ing around!** Place unwrapped frozen log(s) in a greased loaf pan (or pans). Top each one with 1 cup (250 mL) Simple Salsa (p. 170) or tomato sauce. Bake, uncovered, for 75–90 minutes at 350°F (175°C).

- **Gefilte fish balls:** Prepare fish mixture as directed in Step 1. Omit Steps 2–3. Shape mixture into balls, moistening your hands with cold water for easier handling. Carefully add to Poaching Liquid. Simmer, partially covered, for 2 hours.

- **Freeze with ease:** If frozen, cooked gefilte fish will become watery. Simmer thawed fish balls for about 15 minutes in water to cover, then drain well. Fish will taste freshly cooked!

- **Miniatures:** At the end of Step 1, shape fish mixture into tiny balls (you should get 4–5 dozen, depending on size). Simmer in Poaching Liquid for 1 hour. Perfect for a party!

DR. ED SAYS:

- **Fish:** Keep in mind that pike and pickerel, being non-fatty fish, tend to be lower in Omega-3 content. So, if you want to maximize this nutrient, use whitefish or minced salmon. Fish provides the important vitamin D and vitamin B12 nutrients, excellent high-quality protein, and other brain nutrients previously mentioned. However, because of dilution with matzo meal and other ingredients, the content of these nutrients will not be as high as in the previous recipes mentioned.

- **Eggs,** as described in Mock Chopped Liver (p. 178), will also provide important nutrients that come primarily from animal-based sources.

> **DID YOU KNOW?** Mincing fish tends to emulsify the fish oil, and there is some evidence that emulsified fish oil will be better absorbed.

MINI VEGGIE LATKES WITH SMOKED SALMON

DAIRY | PAREVE OPTION | GLUTEN-FREE OPTION | PASSOVER |
REHEATS AND/OR FREEZES WELL | MAKES 48 MINI LATKES

1 medium onion, cut into chunks

1 Idaho (russet) potato,
cut into chunks

1 medium sweet potato,
cut into chunks

1 medium carrot, cut into chunks

1 medium zucchini,
cut into chunks

1 red bell pepper, cut into chunks

2 Tbsp (30 mL) fresh dill
+ extra for garnish

2 large eggs

⅓ cup (80 mL) matzo meal
(preferably whole wheat)

½ tsp (2 mL) salt

Freshly ground black pepper

3 Tbsp (45 mL) olive oil, for frying
(add more as needed)

1 cup (250 mL) plain Greek yogurt
(skim or 1%)

¼ lb/125 g smoked salmon, cut
into bite-sized pieces

Dill-icious! Whenever I make these, everyone devours them! You can peel the potato and sweet potato if you prefer, but I just scrub them well. That's more a-peeling!

1. In a food processor fitted with the steel blade, process vegetables and dill in batches until finely minced, about 8–10 seconds per batch.

2. Transfer minced vegetables to a large mixing bowl and add eggs, matzo meal, salt, and pepper; mix well.

3. Spray a large nonstick skillet with nonstick cooking spray. Add 1 Tbsp (15 mL) oil and heat over medium-high. Drop mixture from a teaspoon into hot oil to form pancakes (latkes). Flatten them slightly with the back of the spoon. Reduce heat to medium and brown well, about 2 minutes per side. Remove latkes from the skillet and drain on paper towels. Add additional oil to the skillet as needed and stir batter before cooking each new batch of latkes. (Can be made in advance and kept warm in a 250°F/120°C oven.)

4. When ready to serve, arrange latkes on a platter and top each with a dollop of Greek yogurt, smoked salmon, and a sprig of dill.

29 calories per latke, 3 g carbohydrates, trace fiber, <1 g sugar, 2 g protein, 1 g fat (0 g saturated), 32 mg sodium, 62 mg potassium

NORENE'S NOTES:

- **Grate tip!** Grate onion and potato together to prevent potato from turning dark. Idaho (russet) potatoes are higher in starch and less watery than most other potatoes when grated.

- **Green cuisine!** Instead of zucchini, use 1 pkg (10 oz/300 g) frozen spinach, thawed and squeezed dry.

- **Gluten-free option:** Use gluten-free matzo meal or panko crumbs.

- **Pareve option:** Instead of Greek yogurt, use either coconut yogurt or non-dairy sour cream.

DR. ED SAYS:

- **Potatoes** add great taste and texture. Keep in mind, however, that they are mostly starch and convert easily to sugars. The nutritional analysis shown for carbs is deceptive because it is for only one mini latke—and you can never eat just one! So, try to limit the number of latkes you eat.

- **Greek yogurt and smoked salmon** add vitamins D and B12, Omega-3, and a high-quality protein to the recipe, as well as active cultures from the yogurt, which may promote brain health.

> DID YOU KNOW? Current research, which is still in its infancy, is studying the gut/brain axis, and it is thought that the ability of active cultures in yogurt to control inflammation could have benefits for brain maintenance.

MEDITERRANEAN STUFFED MUSHROOMS

DAIRY | PAREVE OPTION | GLUTEN-FREE | PASSOVER | REHEATS
AND/OR FREEZES WELL | MAKES 24 STUFFED MUSHROOMS

24 large cremini mushrooms

1 Tbsp (15 mL) olive oil

1 medium onion, chopped

2 cloves garlic (about 1 tsp/ 5 mL minced)

½ cup (125 mL) roasted red bell peppers, drained and chopped (see Norene's Notes)

⅓ cup (80 mL) chopped sun-dried tomatoes (optional)

1 pkg (10 oz/300 g) frozen chopped spinach, thawed and squeezed dry

2 Tbsp (30 mL) chopped fresh basil (or 1 tsp/5 mL dried)

Salt and freshly ground black pepper

½ cup (125 mL) grated low-fat mozzarella or Parmesan cheese

These are excellent as either an appetizer or a low-carb side dish. A food processor makes quick work of preparing the stuffing. For a dairy-free version, see Norene's Notes.

1. Wash mushrooms quickly and pat dry with paper towels. Remove stems and chop coarsely, reserving mushroom caps.

2. In a large nonstick skillet, heat oil on medium. Add onion, garlic, and chopped stems. Sauté about 5 minutes, or until tender. Stir in roasted bell peppers, sun-dried tomatoes (if using), and spinach. Cook until most of the moisture has disappeared, about 3–4 minutes, stirring occasionally. If the mixture begins to stick, add a little water. Season with basil, salt, and pepper; let cool.

3. Stuff mushroom caps with the onion/garlic mixture, using a tea-spoon to mound the filling slightly. Arrange stuffed mushrooms in an oblong baking dish sprayed with nonstick cooking spray. Sprinkle with Parmesan. (Can be prepared in advance and refrigerated, covered, overnight.)

4. Bake, uncovered, in a preheated 350°F (175°C) oven for 15 minutes, until golden.

24 calories per stuffed mushroom, 2 g carbohydrates, 1 g fiber, 1 g sugar, 2 g protein, 1 g fat (0 g saturated), 29 mg sodium, 151 mg potassium

NORENE'S NOTES:

• **Roasted red peppers:** Preheat broiler or BBQ. Broil or grill red bell peppers until skins are blackened and blistered, about 12–15 minutes, turning them occasionally. Immediately place hot peppers in a bowl, cover, and let cool. Scrape off skins, using a paring knife. Rinse quickly under cold water to remove any bits of charred skin. Cut peppers in half and discard stems, cores, and seeds. Cut peppers into long, narrow strips. Refrigerate or freeze.

RECIPE CONTINUED . . .

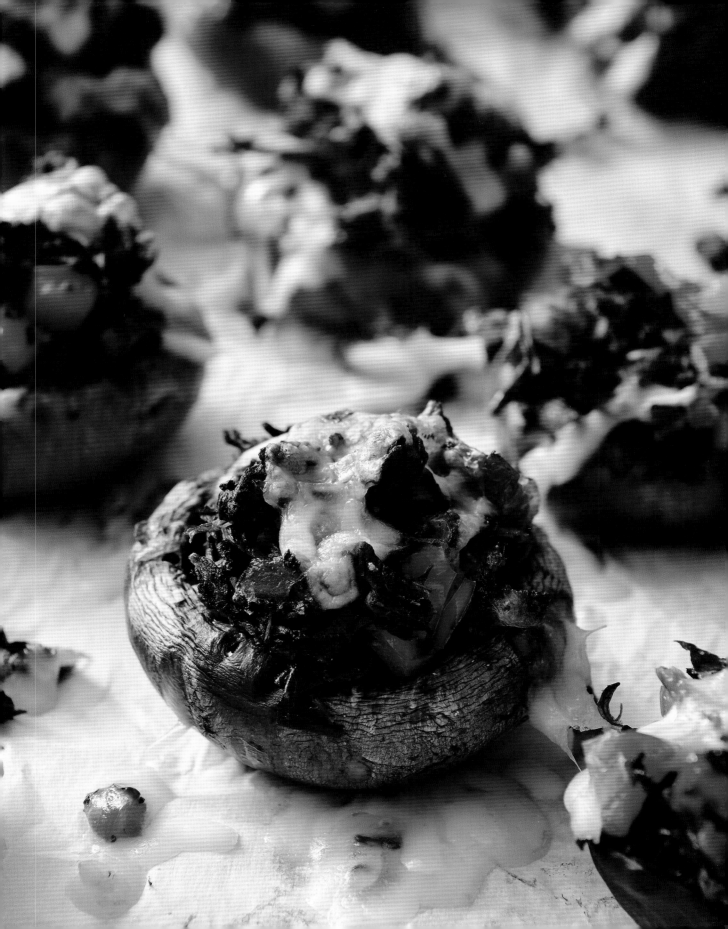

- **Variation:** Instead of roasted red peppers and sun-dried tomatoes, use ½ cup (125 mL) chopped red bell pepper and 1 stalk chopped celery. Instead of basil, use ½ tsp (2 mL) dried thyme.

- **Switch it up:** For a different twist, use the filling from Spanakopita Roll-Ups (p. 195).

- **Pareve option:** Omit cheese and sprinkle mushrooms with chopped almonds.

DR. ED SAYS:

- **Cremini mushrooms:** I always like to see mushrooms in a recipe because of their high and unique antioxidant content, their fiber and protein contribution, and the fact that they provide good amounts of important brain vitamins and minerals. They are also very low in sugar and digestible carbs. For more information, see Mushroom Mock Chopped Liver (p. 178).

- **Spinach** is used extensively in this book because it has been highlighted as especially beneficial for brain health. This is attributed to its high content of carotenoid antioxidants, especially lutein and zeaxanthin, as well as its high content of the brain-related nutrients, vitamin E, folate, vitamin C, magnesium, and manganese.

- **Overall,** the nutrient content for each stuffed mushroom will be relatively small because of its small size. However, if you consume several, you will get substantial levels of protein, fiber, antioxidants, vitamin C (primarily from the bell peppers and spinach), vitamin B12, folate, magnesium, and zinc.

> DID YOU KNOW? Lutein and zeaxanthin have been found to be important to prevent macular degeneration in the eyes, because the eyes are linked to the brain. This has led to research and discovery of their benefits for the brain.

CRISPY CRUNCHY CHICKPEAS

DAIRY-FREE | GLUTEN-FREE | DO NOT FREEZE | MAKES ABOUT
1¼ CUPS (310 ML)

These are totally addictive! They make a super snack on their own, as a crunchy addition to salads and casseroles, or instead of croutons in soup.

1 can (19 oz/540 g) chickpeas (preferably low-sodium or no-salt-added)

1 Tbsp (15 mL) olive oil

½ tsp (2 mL) salt

¼ tsp (1 mL) freshly ground black pepper

½ tsp (2 mL) garlic powder

¼ tsp (1 mL) oregano

1. Preheat oven to 350°F (175°C). Line a large, rimmed baking sheet with parchment paper.

2. Place chickpeas in a strainer over a bowl and drain well. If desired, reserve chickpea liquid (see Norene's Notes).

3. Rinse chickpeas under cold running water; pat dry with paper towels.

4. Transfer chickpeas to a large bowl, drizzle with olive oil, and sprinkle with seasonings. Mix well.

5. Spread in a single layer on the prepared baking sheet. Roast, uncovered, for 50–60 minutes, or until crisp and golden, stirring every 15 minutes.

6. Remove from oven and let cool. Store in a loosely covered bowl or container at room temperature. Serve at room temperature.

144 calories per ¼-cup (60 mL) serving, 20 g carbohydrates, 5 g fiber, 1 g sugar, 7 g protein, 4 g fat (0 g saturated fat), 220 mg sodium, 206 mg potassium

NORENE'S NOTES:

- **Aquafaba:** The leftover liquid from canned chickpeas is known as aquafaba. It can be used to replace egg whites and whole eggs in many sweet and savory recipes. Substitute 3 Tbsp (45 mL) chickpea liquid for 1 egg; substitute 2 Tbsp (30 mL) for 1 egg white. Don't replace more than 3 eggs in a recipe.

- **Spice it up!** Chili powder, cayenne, cumin, turmeric, or curry powder will add a spicy kick to these crunchy nibbles. Or sprinkle with your favorite mix of herbs and spices. Always different, always delicious!

RECIPE CONTINUED . . .

CRISPY CRUNCHY CHICKPEAS (continued)

DR. ED SAYS:

- **Chickpeas** (garbanzo beans) are seeds in the legume family, which also includes kidney beans, black beans, and peanuts. They have a relatively low moisture content and are therefore nutrient-dense. They are very rich in fiber and protein, B vitamins B6 and folate, and contain good amounts of magnesium, manganese, and zinc. Although they have a high carb content, their glycemic index is very low for two reasons: firstly, because of the fiber, and secondly, because their starch content is high in the resistant starch amylose, which acts in many ways like fiber. Part of chickpeas' fiber content is a soluble fiber called raffinose, which acts as a food source for beneficial bacteria in the gut.

> DID YOU KNOW? Chickpeas, which first appeared in Turkey in 3500 BCE, are the main ingredient in hummus and falafel. India produces the most chickpeas worldwide.

KALE CHIPS

PAREVE | GLUTEN-FREE | PASSOVER | DO NOT FREEZE | MAKES
2 SERVINGS

Chip, chip, hooray! You'll flip over these scrumptious baked kale chips—they're much healthier than potato chips. I often devour these straight from the pan while waiting for them to cool! You can also make spinach chips (see Norene's Notes).

½ bunch kale
(see Norene's Notes)

2 tsp (10 mL) extra virgin olive oil

¼ tsp (1 mL) salt (or to taste)

½ tsp (2 mL) garlic powder

¼ tsp (1 mL) onion powder

¼ tsp (1 mL) chili powder
or flakes

1. Preheat oven to 300°F (150°C). Line a large, rimmed baking sheet with parchment paper.

2. Remove and discard kale stems. Tear leaves into large pieces—you should have 4–5 cups (1–1.25 L).

3. Wash and dry leaves thoroughly—either use a lettuce spinner or wrap in towels.

4. Place kale on the prepared baking sheet. Drizzle evenly with oil, massaging it into the leaves to coat the small nooks and crannies. Sprinkle evenly with seasonings. Spread out kale leaves in a single layer, not overlapping, to ensure crispness.

5. Bake uncovered for 10 minutes. Rotate pan front to back for even browning. Bake 15 minutes longer, until dry and crisp. Watch carefully to prevent burning. (Note: Kale will shrink a lot.)

6. Let cool on pan for 5 minutes to let kale leaves crisp up. Enjoy!

82 calories per 85-g serving, 8 g carbohydrates, 3 g fiber, 3 g sugar, 4 g protein, 5 g fat (<1 g saturated fat), 331 mg sodium, 395 mg potassium

NORENE'S NOTES:

- **Spinach chips:** Substitute baby spinach for kale. There's no need to remove the stems and if it's prewashed then you don't need to wash or dry the leaves—so easy!

- **Size matters!** Kale and spinach are sold as bunches, or in a bag or container. A common container size is 11 oz (312 g), so use half the amount for this recipe (5½ oz/156 g), almost 4 cups (1 L). The weight of 2 cups (500 mL) kale or spinach is about 3 oz (85 g).

RECIPE CONTINUED . . .

KALE CHIPS (continued)

- **Low and slow!** Most recipes recommend baking kale/spinach chips at 350°F (175°C) for 10–12 minutes. However, using a lower baking temperature and longer baking time results in perfectly crisp chips.

- **Crispy chips:** Dry kale/spinach leaves thoroughly before baking, then spread out in a single layer after seasoning. They are best when eaten immediately as they get soggy. Store loosely covered at room temperature for a day or two. Re-crisp for 5–10 minutes at 300°F (150°C).

- **Parmesan kale chips:** At the end of Step 4, sprinkle leaves with ¼ cup (60 mL) grated Parmesan cheese (vegans can use nutritional yeast). Bake as directed. These are super as a salad topping or in omelets.

DR. ED SAYS:

- **Kale,** the predominant ingredient in this recipe, supplies most of the brain-healthy nutrients. This dark leafy green is packed with antioxidants that can act both to counter the harmful effects of oxygen and as anti-inflammatories. Kale is a good source of fiber, vitamin B6, folate, and magnesium. When possible use organic kale since leafy greens tend to have more residual pesticides than many other foods.

- **Spinach** is another leafy green that helps boosts brain health. It is very low in fat and available carbs, plus it is an excellent source of fiber, vitamin C, folate, magnesium, and potassium. It is also a good source of vitamin E and B6.

- **Overall,** this addictive, brain-boosting snack is an excellent source of complex antioxidants, vitamin C, and plant-based Omega-3 fats. Although kale is a good source of fiber, folate, and magnesium, spinach is a great replacement as it provides an excellent source of these nutrients. As an additional bonus, spinach contains a component called phytate, which protects you from the brain-damaging effects of iron.

SPANAKOPITA ROLL-UPS

DAIRY | REHEATS AND/OR FREEZES WELL | MAKES 60 ROLL-UPS

These eye-catching hors d'oeuvres are truly a sight for sore eyes! Health experts believe that eating lutein-rich, brain-boosting vegetables like spinach and broccoli at least twice a week may lower your risk of cataracts and/or macular degeneration.

---

1. Preheat oven to 375°F (190°C). Line a rimmed baking sheet with parchment paper.

2. **FILLING:** Heat oil on medium-high. Add onion, bell pepper, and garlic and sauté for 3–4 minutes, until softened. (Alternately, microwave in a glass bowl on high for 3–4 minutes.)

3. In a food processor fitted with the steel blade, process spinach until finely chopped. Add cheese, egg, pepper, and dill. Process just until combined. Add onion mixture and pulse briefly to combine.

4. **DOUGH:** Place one sheet of phyllo dough on a dry work surface, with the long side facing you. Brush lightly with oil. Top with a second sheet of dough and brush lightly with oil. (Keep the remaining dough covered with plastic wrap to prevent it from drying out.)

5. **ASSEMBLY:** Spoon a quarter of the spinach filling in a narrow band along the bottom edge of the phyllo, leaving a 1-inch (2.5 cm) border on the bottom edge and on both sides. Fold both sides inwards then roll up dough into a long, narrow cylinder, starting from the edge closest to you. Place seam side down on the prepared baking sheet. Repeat with the remaining dough and filling, forming 4 rolls.

6. Lightly brush tops of each roll with oil. Using a sharp knife, mark 1-inch (2.5 cm) slices along the top of each roll, cutting partially through the dough, but not through the filling. You will get about 15 slices from each roll. (Rolls may be frozen at this point. No need to thaw before baking or reheating—just add 2–3 minutes to baking time.)

7. Bake for 20 minutes, until golden. Slice and serve. To reheat, bake uncovered at 325°F (160°C) for 10 minutes.

RECIPE CONTINUED . . .

FILLING:

1 Tbsp (15 mL) olive oil

1 medium onion, chopped

½ red bell pepper, chopped

2–3 cloves garlic (about 2 tsp/ 10 mL minced)

2 pkgs (10 oz/300 g each) frozen or fresh spinach, cooked and squeezed dry

1 cup (250 mL) crumbled feta or goat cheese

1 large egg

Freshly ground black pepper

2 Tbsp (30 mL) minced fresh dill (or 2 tsp/10 mL dried)

DOUGH:

8 sheets phyllo dough, thawed (see Norene's Notes)

¼ cup (60 mL) olive oil

29 calories per roll-up, 2 g carbohydrates, 0 g fiber, 0 g sugar, 1 g protein, 2 g fat (1 g saturated fat), 44 mg sodium, 41 mg potassium

NORENE'S NOTES:

- **Dairy good!** Instead of feta or goat cheese, substitute 1 cup (250 mL) light ricotta cheese. Alternately, combine ½ cup (125 mL) light ricotta, ½ cup (125 mL) light feta, and ¼ cup (60 mL) grated Parmesan cheese.

- **Variation:** Use broccoli instead of spinach. If desired, add ½ cup (125 mL) minced sun-dried tomatoes, rinsed and drained, to the filling.

- **Leftover filling?** Stuff large mushroom caps with filling and sprinkle with sesame seeds. Bake, uncovered, at 350°F (175°C), for 15 minutes.

- **Easy doughs it!** One 1-lb (500 g) package of phyllo dough contains 20–24 sheets. Phyllo dough can be found in the supermarket freezer. To thaw, place package in the refrigerator overnight. Defrosted dough will keep 3–4 weeks in the refrigerator. Don't refreeze dough that has been thawed.

- **Cover up!** When working with phyllo, keep it well covered with plastic wrap to prevent it from drying out. If you cover it with a damp cloth and it is too wet the dough will be soggy.

- **Tear-iffic tip!** If phyllo dough tears, don't cry—patch it together with a little oil.

DR. ED SAYS:

- **Spinach,** one of the two major ingredients, is an abundant source of brain-healthy nutrients, as described in Mediterranean Stuffed Mushrooms (p. 188).

- **Feta and goat cheeses** are both rich sources of protein and important B vitamins, as well as very low in sugars and carbs. They are also excellent sources of calcium, which will not be complexed with the oxalate in the spinach. So, the combination of cheese and spinach in this recipe is appropriate. The one drawback of feta is its high sodium content at over 1000 mg per 100 g. Goat cheese would be a better choice for those who are sodium-sensitive, as its sodium level is less than half that of feta, even though its calcium level is slightly lower too.

- **Overall,** because of the small weight per roll-up, the nutritional profile is non-remarkable. However, as you will probably consume several, it becomes quite acceptable.

DID YOU KNOW? Spinach contains high amounts of the antinutrient oxalate, which can interfere with calcium absorption from plant sources or supplements. There are several ways to get around it: (1) Eat dairy products to ensure the calcium you get does not complex with the oxalate. This is because dairy products contain high levels of calcium, and because the calcium is already bound to dairy protein and available for use by the body. (2) Consume your calcium-rich foods and supplements at a time when you do not consume spinach. 3) Boil the spinach, so that the oxalate dissolves into the water.

SALMON RICE PAPER ROLLS

PAREVE | GLUTEN-FREE OPTION | DO NOT FREEZE | MAKES 12 ROLLS

1 cup (250 mL) sushi rice

½ lb (250 g) boneless, skinless salmon fillet

1–2 Tbsp (15–30 mL) extra virgin olive oil

½ tsp (2 mL) paprika

½ tsp (2 mL) garlic powder

Salt and freshly ground black pepper to taste

1 cup (250 mL) shredded carrots

3 green onions, julienned (reserve some as a garnish)

1 large cucumber, julienned (do not peel)

½ large red pepper, julienned

½ cup (125 mL) shredded purple cabbage

12 rice paper spring roll wrappers

DIPPING SAUCE:

2–3 Tbsp (30–45 mL) honey

1 Tbsp (15 mL) lime juice

¼ cup (60 mL) soy sauce or tamari

2 Tbsp (30 mL) rice vinegar

1 tsp (5 mL) Sriracha

Salt and freshly ground black pepper to taste

Cookbook author Amy Stopnicki always keeps rice paper spring roll wrappers in her pantry. The filling can be changed easily—either add an ingredient or take one out, the sky is the limit to what you can create! I've modified Amy's recipe from *Kosher Taste,* adding cucumber, red bell pepper, and purple cabbage to boost the nutrient content. Just assemble everything in advance, then get ready to roll! To switch it up, serve with Peanut Sauce (see Norene's Notes).

1. Prepare sushi rice according to package instructions.

2. Preheat oven to 400°F (200°C). Coat salmon with oil, paprika, garlic powder, salt, and pepper.

3. Bake, uncovered, for 10–12 minutes. When done, salmon will flake when lightly pressed. Once cooled, break it into small chunks.

4. Place salmon, carrots, green onions, cucumber, red pepper, and cabbage in separate piles on a large tray.

5. Pour warm water into a pie plate or large bowl. Working with one sheet at a time, dip rice paper wrapper in warm water for 15 seconds, just until softened and translucent. Immediately remove from water and place on a flat work surface.

6. **ASSEMBLY:** Place a tablespoon each of cooked rice and salmon with some carrots, green onion, cucumber, bell pepper, and cabbage in the center of a wrapper. Fold in sides, then roll up tightly like a jelly roll. Repeat with the remaining rolls.

7. **DIPPING SAUCE:** Combine all sauce ingredients in a mixing bowl.

8. **TO SERVE:** Slice each roll in half diagonally. Arrange on individual plates, with one half on top of the second half. Place a small cup of dipping sauce on each plate. Garnish with reserved green onions.

157 calories per roll, 26 g carbohydrates, 1 g fiber, 5 g sugar, 7 g protein, 2 g fat (0 g saturated), 306 mg sodium, 168 mg potassium

- **Switch it up:** Either serve with Peanut Sauce (see recipe for Chicken Satay, p. 295), or Peanut Dressing/Marinade (p. 427). Scrumptious!

- **Lower-sodium option:** Reduce the sodium content by using low-sodium soy or tamari sauce. Alternatively, use half soy sauce, half water.

DR. ED SAYS:

- **Rice** is loaded with starch, which converts easily to sugars, so the combination of digestible carbs and sugar is fairly high. Although the other ingredients are quite nutritious, this is one recipe not to over-indulge in. There is a type of rice called black rice that retains the outer bran layer and is rich in fiber, important anthocyanin brain anti-oxidants, and vitamin E. I heartily recommend it over white or even brown rice.

- **Salmon** is an excellent counterpoint to the poor nutrition of the rice. It is high in Omega-3 fats as well as vitamins D and B12. It is also a good source of magnesium, potassium, zinc, selenium, vitamins B6 and E, and choline.

- **Overall,** this recipe provides significant amounts of vitamin E, vitamin D, vitamin B6, and vitamin B12, as well as some Omega-3 fats and minerals. These nutrients are primarily provided by the salmon. The carb/sugar combination is high, due primarily to the white rice, so enjoy in moderation.

DID YOU KNOW? Black rice is sometimes called forbidden rice because it was once reserved exclusively for the health of the Chinese emperor and forbidden to everyone else.

TORTILLA PINWHEELS

PAREVE | GLUTEN-FREE OPTION | DO NOT FREEZE | MAKES ABOUT
24 PINWHEELS

1⅓ cups (330 mL) homemade
or store-bought hummus
(e.g., Garden Vegetable
Hummus, p. 167)

Four 10-inch (25 cm) whole wheat
flour, corn, or gluten-free tortillas

6 oz (150 g) baby spinach leaves
+ extra for garnish

½ cup (125 mL) roasted red
peppers (from a jar or homemade,
p. 188), cut into narrow strips

½ cup (125 mL) matchstick
carrots

These pinwheels are so pretty when you use different-colored tortillas. They come in a variety of colors, such as red, green, and yellow, and
are available in whole wheat, sun-dried tomato, pesto, and spinach.
Experiment with different fillings and combinations (see Norene's Notes).

1. Spread a thin layer of hummus on each tortilla, leaving a ½-inch
(1 cm) border around the outer edge. Place a row of spinach leaves across
the middle of each tortilla. Top with roasted pepper strips and carrots.

2. Roll tortillas up tightly and cover with plastic wrap. Refrigerate for
1 hour or up to 24 hours.

3. Shortly before serving, remove plastic wrap and trim ends. Slice each
roll on the bias into 6 pieces. Arrange on a large platter lined with spinach leaves and serve chilled. (Can be prepared up to a day in advance.
Cover tightly when storing in the refrigerator so they don't dry out.)

60 calories per pinwheel, 8 g carbohydrates, 4 g fiber, 0 g sugar, 2 g
protein, 2 g fat (0 g saturated), 103 mg sodium, 43 mg potassium

NORENE'S NOTES:

- **Variations:** Instead of roasted peppers, use roasted or steamed
  asparagus spears. Different-colored bell peppers add flavor and
  visual appeal. Use Bibb lettuce, mixed salad greens, kale, or radicchio
  leaves instead of spinach. Other fillings could include egg, tuna, or
  salmon salad, or grilled veggies. Use your imagination!

- **Lox de-light!** Spread tortillas with light cream cheese (use plain or
  herb-flavored, or dairy-free cream cheese substitute), then top with
  strips of lox and baby spinach leaves.

- **Hummus** is a focus of this recipe. Since its main component is chickpeas, hummus provides a rich source of brain-friendly nutrients, as described in Crispy Crunchy Chickpeas (p. 191).

- **Spinach** provides a solid nutritional base for the brain and its benefits have been described repeatedly wherever it has been used in this book.

- **Overall,** due primarily to the spinach and hummus, we have a good source of vitamin C and fiber, and reasonable amounts of folate, magnesium, zinc, and vitamin E. We also have a good mix of fat-soluble carotenoid antioxidants, including lutein and zeaxanthin, in both the spinach and carrots, and water-soluble flavonoid polyphenols in the bell peppers.

> **DID YOU KNOW?** The word hummus is Arabic, meaning chickpeas. The complete dish is called hummus bi tahini, or hummus with tahini.

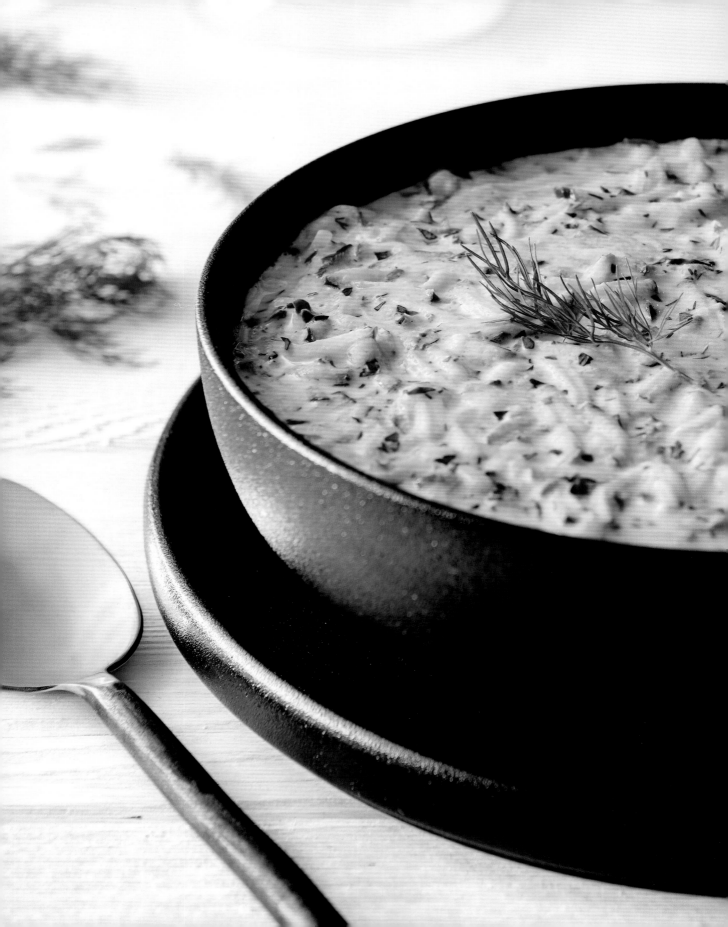

SUPER SOUPS

FILL UP WITH SOUP: Did you know that if you eat a bowl of vegetable soup you will feel full for a longer period of time than if you drink a glass of water and eat the vegetables separately? Your body and brain actually recognize water differently when it's combined with food. So, get smart and eat soup often to help control your appetite.

"EAU" SO GOOD! The water content in soups ranges from 80% to 95%. The recipes in this book are packed with water-rich vegetables so you can enjoy a large portion of soup that's low in calories and nutrition-packed. These soups also contain low-to-medium GI ingredients, are low in fat, and contain dietary fiber to help prevent rebound hunger.

SLOW DOWN, YOU EAT TOO FAST! It takes 20 minutes for your brain to know that your stomach is full. So, starting a meal with soup helps fill you up and takes the edge off your hunger. Chunky soups take longer to eat and are more satisfying than clear, thin broths.

HOMEMADE IS BEST: You're in control when you make homemade soups. They're quick to make and less expensive than commercial soups, which are usually loaded with sodium, fat, and calories.

MULTIVITAMIN IN A BOWL: Soups with vegetables, grains, and legumes are a wonderful way to incorporate more protein, fiber, vitamins, minerals, and phytonutrients (nutrients and antioxidants found in plants that help maintain health and control inflammation) into your diet.

BOWL THEM OVER! To make soup, all you need are vegetables (fresh or frozen), lean protein (beans, lentils, chicken, or tofu), whole grains (brown rice, barley, or quinoa), chicken or vegetable broth (or water) and herbs and spices.

CUT THE FAT! One tablespoon of olive or canola oil is enough to sauté 3–4 cups (750–1000 mL) of vegetables. Use nonstick cookware or spray the inside of your pot with nonstick cooking spray before adding veggies. If veggies start to stick, add a little water or broth instead of oil. You can also sauté vegetables in chicken or vegetable broth instead of fat. Another option is to roast the veggies at 400°F (200°C), drizzled with just a little oil. However, you don't have to worry too much about fat as long as it is not saturated fat. In fact, recent research attributes longer life and lower incidence of disease with higher amounts of unsaturated fat, which replaces digestible carbs.

COOK IT SLOW: A slow cooker is excellent for making large quantities of soup for people on the go. If your recipe calls for 15–30 minutes of cooking, slow-cook it for 4–8 hours on low, or 1½–2 hours on high. If your recipe calls for 30–60 minutes of cooking, slow-cook it for 6–8 hours on low, or 3–4 hours on high. There is little evaporation in a slow cooker, so adjust the seasonings accordingly.

MICROWAVE MAGIC! Use a microwave oven for smaller, quick-cooking soups. An 8-cup (2 L) glass batter bowl is a perfect size. Cooking time is similar to cooking soups on the stove top. Microwave soups, covered, on high power. Soups cooked in the microwave don't stick, so you don't need to add much fat and cleanup is easy.

IN THE THICK OF IT! If your soup is too watery, simmer it, uncovered, to reduce some of the liquid. If it's still too thin, purée part of the cooked vegetables in a food processor, then stir them back into the soup—the puréed vegetables will give it a thicker consistency. Alternatively, use an immersion blender right in the pot and purée until the desired texture is reached.

BEAN CUISINE! Puréed canned white beans are a sneaky way to thicken your soup and add some fiber! Just 1 cup (250 ml) puréed vegetables or legumes will thicken 3–4 cups (750–1000 mL) broth.

THIN IS IN: If your soup is too thick, thin it with a little water or vegetable or chicken broth, and adjust seasonings as needed.

YOUR CHOICE: If you don't have homemade broth on hand, use canned, bottled, or packaged broth (see "Broth in a Box," below). You can also use bouillon cubes or instant powdered soup mix, but they are often high in sodium.

BROTH IN A BOX: Good-quality brands of vegetable and chicken broth are now available in Tetra paks, like the kinds used for soy milk. One box contains about 4 cups (1 L) (35 oz/1 L) and doesn't require refrigeration until opened. Perfect in a pinch!

LOWER-SODIUM OPTION: Just 1 cup (250 mL) canned vegetable or chicken broth contains about 1000 mg of sodium, almost ½ tsp (2 mL) salt, and bouillon cubes and instant soup mix are usually loaded with sodium. A quick trick to reduce the sodium is to add double the amount of water. Beware—some brands contain MSG and partially hydrogenated fats.

COLD FACTS: Make sure soups (or any cooked foods) are completely cooled before you transfer them to freezer-safe containers. Store soup in 1- or 2-cup (250 or 500 mL) containers, leaving 2 inches (5 cm) at the top to allow for expansion. Cover and freeze. Square containers take up less space than round ones.

SOUP CUBES: Freeze small quantities of chicken or vegetable broth in ice cube trays. One cube equals 2 Tbsp (30 mL) soup—so handy for adding to recipes when a small amount is needed.

HOT STOCK TIP: To reheat soup in the microwave, allow 2 minutes per 1 cup (250 mL) on high power, stirring once or twice during heating. If soup is frozen there's no need to defrost it first. To defrost 1 cup (250 mL) of soup takes 3–4 minutes on high power, then another 2–3 minutes on high to heat up.

MEAL IN A BOWL: Add diced cooked poultry, lean beef, or extra-firm tofu cubes to your favorite soup(s) to boost the protein content.

DR. ED SAYS: Keep in mind that because most soups are heavily diluted with water, the nutritional content per serving will not be as high as the equivalent solid food. Nevertheless, soups are part and parcel of any good diet plan.

VEGETABLE BROTH (ALMOST CHICKEN SOUP)

PAREVE | MEAT OPTION | GLUTEN-FREE | PASSOVER | REHEATS
AND/OR FREEZES WELL | MAKES ABOUT 8 CUPS (2 L)

This could be called "chicken soup without the chicken"! Serve this low-sodium broth on its own or use it in recipes calling for vegetable broth. Perfect for the vegetarians at your table!

---

1. Place all ingredients into a large soup pot (or see Norene's Notes). Water should cover vegetables by no more than 1 inch (2.5 cm). Bring to a boil over high heat. Reduce heat to low and simmer, partially covered, for 35–40 minutes.

2. Remove from heat and cool completely.

3. Using a colander, strain liquid into a large bowl. Reserve cooked vegetables (can be puréed, see Norene's Notes).

4. Ladle cooled broth into containers and cover tightly. Refrigerate or freeze until ready to use.

24 calories per 1-cup (250 mL) serving, 5 g carbohydrates, 2 g fiber, 3 g sugar, 1 g protein, 0 g fat (0 g saturated fat), 33 mg sodium, 180 mg potassium

NORENE'S NOTES:

- **Soup socks rock!** In Step 1, place vegetables in a cheesecloth bag and make a knot; cook soup as directed. Remove bag of vegetables from the cooled soup—no need to strain the soup or yourself!

- **Veggie power:** Onion skins add a rich, golden color to the broth—just be sure to wash the onions well. Add a cup or two of chopped leeks, tomatoes, turnips, squash, zucchini, and/or celery tops. Don't add strong-flavored vegetables (e.g., cabbage, broccoli, or cauliflower) because their flavor will overwhelm the broth. Starchy vegetables (e.g., potatoes and sweet potatoes) will make the broth cloudy.

RECIPE CONTINUED . . .

2 large onions, cut into large chunks (peeling is optional)

7 or 8 medium carrots, cut into large chunks

4 stalks celery, cut into large chunks

1 red bell pepper, cut into large chunks

1 cup (250 mL) mushrooms (optional)

9 cups (2.25 L) cold water

Salt (optional)

Freshly ground black pepper

3–4 cloves garlic

½ cup (125 mL) fresh dill

- **Mushroom magic!** For a full, rich flavor, add a handful of reconstituted dried mushrooms that have been soaked in hot water for 20 minutes. Also add their soaking liquid to the broth; cook as directed.

- **Sodi-yum?** Nutrients are calculated without salt. Many chefs leave broth unsalted until they are ready to use it.

- **Purée power:** Discard onion skins. Purée cooked vegetables from broth in a food processor or blender, then return them to the broth. Cooked vegetables contain valuable nutrients and flavor. Kids love this soup—it's a smart way to sneak veggies into their tummies.

- **Chicken soup for the bowl:** Add 3 lb (1.4 kg) cut-up chicken pieces in Step 1 (use a separate soup sock for the chicken). Bring to a boil; skim off the foam that rises to soup's surface. Increase cooking time to 1½–2 hours.

DR. ED SAYS:

- **Nutrition note:** Since the vegetables are discarded after boiling, the main nutrition comes from the vegetable extracts. Simmering the soup after bringing it to a boil will help preserve some of the nutrients as opposed to continued boiling.

- **Celery,** at first glance, is not a very nutritious ingredient except for its high fiber content, which represents about a third of its dry weight. The lack of nutrient density is due to its high water content at 95% by weight. However, celery has a variety of phytochemicals and antioxidants that are advantageous for a number of health issues.

- **Overall,** this recipe is very low in calories, high in fiber, and has a reasonable source of vitamin E, vitamin C, vitamin B6, and folate. It is also low in sodium, unlike commercial soups.

DID YOU KNOW? A ⅔-cup (160 mL) serving of commercial vegetable broth contains upwards of 500 mg of sodium.

DID YOU KNOW? Celery is a double-edged sword (or stalk). On the one hand, its antioxidants and phytonutrients have been recommended to control inflammation, blood pressure, and even the risk of certain cancers. One of its anti-inflammatory compounds, called apigenin, has been shown to improve learning and memory in mice. On the other hand, if eaten in quantity, celery contains compounds to which people may be allergic and which can cause dermatitis and sensitivity to UV rays.

MINIATURE "NOTSA" BALLS (CHICKEN KNEIDLACH)

MEAT | GLUTEN-FREE OPTION | PASSOVER | REHEATS AND/OR
FREEZES WELL | MAKES 24 MINIS

1 medium onion, cut into chunks

1 stalk celery, cut into chunks

2 Tbsp (30 mL) fresh dill

1 lb (500 g) lean ground
chicken or turkey

1 large egg

1 Tbsp (15 mL) vegetable
or olive oil

3 Tbsp (45 mL) matzo meal
(whole wheat or gluten-free)
or almond meal

½ tsp (2 mL) salt

Freshly ground black pepper

2 Tbsp (30 mL) club soda
or cold water

10 cups (2.5 L) lightly
salted water

These low-carb chicken kneidlach (matzo balls) are a luscious alternative to regular matzo balls. For people who aren't able to use matzo meal, these can be made with ground almonds, making them gluten-free.

1. In a food processor fitted with the steel blade, process onion, celery, and dill until minced, about 10 seconds. Add ground chicken, egg, oil, matzo meal, salt, pepper, and club soda; process just until mixed. Transfer to a bowl, cover, and chill for 20–30 minutes.

2. Bring salted water to a boil in a large pot. Wet your hands and shape mixture into walnut-sized balls. Drop into boiling water, cover tightly, and simmer for 20–25 minutes, or until cooked through.

3. Using a slotted spoon, carefully remove balls from water and transfer to bowls of hot Vegetable Broth (p. 207) or chicken soup.

41 calories per mini, 1 g carbohydrates, 0 g fiber, trace sugar, 5 g protein, 2 g fat (trace saturated fat), 70 mg sodium, 14 mg potassium

NORENE'S NOTES:

- **Freeze with ease:** Arrange cooked matzo balls in a single layer on a rimmed baking sheet lined with wax paper. When frozen, transfer to a resealable freezer bag. To reheat, add frozen "Notsa" Balls to simmering soup. They will take about 10 minutes to defrost and heat through.

- **Grind it right:** Ground chicken usually contains dark meat, increasing the fat content. You can grind chicken breasts yourself in a food processor. Cut 1 lb (500 g) chilled boneless, skinless chicken breasts into 1-inch (2.5 cm) chunks and process 15–20 seconds, until minced.

DR. ED SAYS:

- **Matzo meal or almond flour** is the basis for the "Notsa" Balls. If you don't have a strong preference for the taste of matzo meal, always go for the almond flour because it is nutrient-dense with important brain-healthy components, including fiber, vitamin E, folate, choline, and an important class of polyphenol antioxidants called proanthocyanidins. Almonds are also very low in digestible carbs and sugars and, as a result, have a low glycemic index. In addition, they are gluten-free.

- **Lean chicken and turkey** are excellent sources of high-quality protein, and if you stick with lean white meat the protein content can represent more than 85% of the dry weight of the poultry. Even with its water content, you are getting about 22 g per serving (a third of the daily recommended amount). In addition, lean poultry provides good amounts of vitamin B6, vitamin D, and vitamin B12.

- **Overall,** the carbs, saturated fat, and calories are quite low for each miniature ball and the protein quite high—but can anyone eat just one?

> DID YOU KNOW? High-quality protein means that the protein contains all the amino acids that the body needs in efficiently usable amounts. This means that, gram for gram, you are getting much better utilization than poor-quality proteins. High-quality proteins are eggs, dairy, and meat, medium-quality are vegetable proteins, and zero-quality is collagen (skin) or gelatin.

AUTUMN VEGETABLE SOUP

PAREVE | GLUTEN-FREE | PASSOVER | REHEATS AND/OR FREEZES
WELL | MAKES ABOUT 15 CUPS (3.75 L)

2 Tbsp (30 mL) olive oil

1 large or 2 medium onions,
chopped

2–3 stalks celery, chopped

6 medium carrots, chopped

3 medium sweet potatoes, cut
into chunks

1 medium butternut or acorn
squash, peeled and cut into
chunks (about 5 cups/1.25 L)

1 cup (250 mL) sliced mushrooms

2 medium zucchinis,
cut into chunks

10 cups (2.5 L) water

4–6 bay leaves

2 tsp (10 mL) salt (or to taste)

½ tsp (2 mL) freshly ground
black pepper

2 Tbsp (30 mL) finely
chopped fresh dill

2 Tbsp (30 mL) finely chopped
fresh parsley

2 cloves garlic, crushed
(or ½ tsp/2 mL garlic powder)

Thanks to Valerie Kanter of Chicago, editor of the Kosher cookbook *Crowning Elegance*, for sharing her scrumptious low-carb autumn vegetable soup—it's wonderful all year round. She often serves it from her slow cooker for the Sabbath lunch. It's a winner!

---

1. Heat oil in a large soup pot over medium heat. Sauté onions, celery, and carrots for 5 minutes, until tender, stirring occasionally. Add sweet potatoes, squash, mushrooms, and zucchini; mix well.

2. Add water, bay leaves, salt, and pepper; bring to a boil. Reduce heat to low and simmer, partially covered, for 2 hours, stirring occasionally. If soup becomes too thick, add a little more water. Remove bay leaves and discard.

3. Using a potato masher, coarsely mash vegetables in the pot—soup will be somewhat chunky. Stir in dill, parsley, and garlic; adjust seasonings to taste.

81 calories per 1-cup (250 mL) serving, 15 g carbohydrates, 3 g fiber, 4 g sugar, 2 g protein, 2 g fat (0 g saturated fat), 357 mg sodium, 455 mg potassium

NORENE'S NOTES:

- **Short cuts:** To make it easier to cut a squash, slash tough outer skin in several places with a sharp knife. Microwave, uncovered, on high power for 4-5 minutes. Cool for 5 minutes, then cut in half or into large pieces. Remove seeds and stringy fibers—an ice-cream scoop or large spoon works perfectly.

- **Love me tender!** Summer squash varieties include yellow and green zucchini, crookneck, vegetable marrow, and pattypan/scallop squash—all have thin, edible skins and soft seeds. Summer squash cooks quickly because of its high water content.

- **Bay watch!** Always remove and discard bay leaves after cooking. A bay leaf won't rehydrate even after boiling, so if left in the soup someone could choke on it. Count how many you put in and how many you take out. Or, better yet, tie them up in a square of cheesecloth for easy removal after cooking.

- **Slow cooker method:** At the end of Step 1, combine sautéed vegetables with water and seasonings in the insert of your slow cooker. Cook, covered, for 6–8 hours on low or 3–4 hours on high. No peeking!

DR. ED SAYS:

- **Bay leaves,** also known as laurel leaves, actually contain good levels of vitamins A, C, B6, and folate, as well as magnesium and excellent levels of fiber. The problem is that because they are used primarily as a spice, the quantity used is too small to make a difference. So, their main use, aside from flavoring, is in alternative medicines for minor health problems.

- **Squash and carrots** are good sources of fiber and carotenoid antioxidants, which are fat soluble. Sautéing in oil will help release these antioxidants into the soup and make them available to the body. They are also high in potassium and low in sodium, and squash is a good source of vitamins C and E and some B vitamins, as well as magnesium and manganese.

- **Overall,** this recipe provides good amounts of vitamins E, C, B6, and folate, as well as magnesium and fiber.

> **DID YOU KNOW?** Bay leaves were used to crown victorious athletes in ancient Greece. They were also considered a sacred herb in both Greece and Rome because they were used for so many maladies. When bay leaves are burned they release essential oils that provide a relaxing and calming atmosphere.

SLOW COOKER VEGETABLE SOUP

PAREVE | MEAT OPTION | REHEATS AND/OR FREEZES WELL |
MAKES ABOUT 18 CUPS (4.5 L)

2 medium onions, cut into
chunks

1 medium sweet potato, peeled
and cut into chunks

3 stalks celery, cut into chunks

3 large carrots, cut into chunks

1 red bell pepper, cut into chunks

¼ cup (60 mL) minced fresh dill
(or 1 Tbsp /15 mL dried)

¾ cup (185 mL) pearl or pot
barley, rinsed and drained

1 cup (250 mL) dried red lentils,
rinsed and drained

12 cups (3 L) vegetable broth or
water (preferably low-sodium or
no-salt-added)

Salt and freshly ground
black pepper

Quick prep, slow cook! Chop the vegetables in a food processor, then put everything into the slow cooker and let this carefree soup cook all day while you are away at work or out doing errands. It's packed with fiber, phytochemicals, and flavor—and it's virtually fat-free! It makes a big batch, so get ready to freeze some for future meals.

---

1. In a food processor fitted with the steel blade, process vegetables in batches, using quick on/off pulses, until finely chopped.

2. Transfer chopped vegetables to a slow cooker, along with dill, barley, lentils, broth, salt, and pepper. Cover and cook on low for 8–10 hours (or on high for 4–6 hours), until vegetables are tender. (The extra 2 hours of cooking time won't affect the finished dish if dinner is delayed.)

99 calories per 1-cup (250 mL) serving, 20 g carbohydrates, 4 g fiber, 3 g sugar, 5 g protein, 0 g fat (0 g saturated fat), 112 mg sodium, 202 mg potassium

NORENE'S NOTES:

• **Everything but the kitchen sink soup:** Vary this soup depending on what you have on hand. Try it with chopped mushrooms, zucchini, or tomatoes. Instead of sweet potato, use regular potato, turnip, or squash. Instead of lentils, use green or yellow split peas. Canned drained kidney beans are also a good addition. As a guideline, fill the pot halfway with vegetables. Add barley and legumes, then add enough vegetable broth or water to fill the pot to within 1 inch (2.5 cm) from the top. Sometimes I add a cup of leftover tomato sauce. Always different, always delicious!

• **Size counts:** I have a 6-quart slow cooker, but if yours is smaller, use less vegetables, seasonings, and liquid. As a guideline, fill the pot halfway with vegetables. Add ½ cup (125 mL) barley and ¾ cup (185 mL) lentils, then add enough vegetable broth or water to fill the pot to within 1 inch (2.5 cm) from the top.

- **Quick tip:** This soup will cook faster if you add boiling water instead of tap water. Cook on high for 4-6 hours.

- **Meat option:** For a meatier flavor, add a few soup bones or lean stewing beef. Cooking time will be the same.

- **No slow cooker?** You can also cook this soup on the stovetop. Combine all the ingredients in a large soup pot that has been sprayed with nonstick cooking spray. Bring to a boil, then cover partially and simmer for 2–2½ hours, stirring occasionally.

DR. ED SAYS:

- **Lentils** belong to the legume family and, as with most legumes, they have a very high fiber content, as well as a very low GI to control blood sugar. They also have the highest protein concentration of beans outside soya, and are rich in vitamin B6, folate, magnesium, zinc, potassium, and manganese, while being low in fat and sodium. Lentils also contain relatively large and varied amounts of polyphenol antioxidants, which are extracted easily into soup.

- **Barley** is a grain but has a nutritional profile similar to lentils and other legumes. Although its carb content is higher than lentils, its high fiber content helps to make it the grain with the lowest GI, which is good for controlling blood glucose. See Barley Basics, p. 406.

- **Overall,** the recipe provides reasonable levels of vitamins C, B6, and folate, and magnesium. It also contains a variety of polyphenol antioxidants, which are readily extracted into the soup.

> **DID YOU KNOW?** Lentils, like many dried beans, contain significant amounts of purines, which break down to uric acid and can cause gout and kidney stress. So, if you have high uric acid levels or kidney disease, you should not overindulge in beans. High purines also occur in organ meats and some fish.

MIGHTY MINESTRONE

DAIRY OPTION | PAREVE | GLUTEN-FREE | REHEATS AND/OR
FREEZES WELL | MAKES ABOUT 10 CUPS (2.5 L)

2 Tbsp (30 mL) olive oil

2–3 cloves garlic (about
1 Tbsp/15 mL minced)

2 stalks celery, chopped

2 medium carrots, chopped

1 medium onion, chopped

1 can (28 oz/796 g) whole
tomatoes, including liquid

1 can (19 oz/540 g) red kidney
beans, drained and rinsed

3 medium zucchinis, chopped

2 cups (500 mL) vegetable or
chicken broth (preferably low-
sodium or no-salt-added)

1 tsp (5 mL) dried oregano

Salt and freshly ground
black pepper

Chopped fresh basil
(for garnish)

This quick and easy fiber-filled soup comes from my late cousin, Elsie
Gorewich. It was a favorite of her late daughter Nancy, who included
the recipe in her cookbook, *Souperb!* Every year Nancy compiled a small
cookbook that she sent to family and friends. I'm so glad I have my own
copy, which is part of my treasured cookbook collection.

1. Heat oil in a large soup pot on medium. Add garlic, celery, carrots,
and onion; sauté until tender, about 5–7 minutes. Add tomatoes, kidney
beans, zucchini, broth, and oregano; bring to a boil.

2. Reduce heat and simmer, partially covered, for 25–30 minutes. Stir
occasionally. If soup becomes too thick, thin with a little broth or water.

3. Season with salt and pepper. If necessary, add a pinch of sugar or
sweetener (some brands of canned tomatoes are more acidic than others; the sweetness helps counter that acidity). Garnish with fresh basil
and serve.

106 calories per 1-cup (250 mL) serving, 16 g carbohydrates, 6 g fiber,
5 g sugar, 5 g protein, 3 g fat (1 g saturated fat), 96 mg sodium, 525 mg
potassium

NORENE'S NOTES:

- **Variation:** Replace zucchini with trimmed green or yellow beans, cut
into 1-inch (2.5 cm) pieces.

- **Machine cuisine**: Speed up preparation by chopping the vegetables
in batches in the food processor, using quick on/off pulses.

- **Microwave magic!** Combine oil, garlic, celery, carrots, and onion in a
3-quart microwaveable bowl. Microwave, covered, on high power for
5 minutes. Add the remaining ingredients and microwave, covered, on
high for 20 minutes, stirring once or twice.

- **Dairy option:** For a calcium boost, add a sprinkling of grated Parmesan cheese at serving time.

DR. ED SAYS:

- **Tomatoes** are known for their high carotenoid antioxidant content, especially lycopene, a powerful antioxidant and anti-inflammatory (which makes it important for the brain). Lycopene is believed to contribute positively to lower cardiovascular disease and cancer prevention. Because carotenoids are fat-soluble, and because lycopene needs heat and maceration to be released from the tomato, this recipe, which involves sautéing and heating, is an ideal vehicle for the provision of carotenoids to the diet. For example, raw tomatoes provide about 5 mg of lycopene/cup while tomato paste provides 75 mg per cup.

- **Zucchini** is considered part of the squash family. Because it is mostly water at 95% moisture, it does not provide great amounts of brain-healthy vitamins and minerals, but does have reasonable levels of fiber, vitamins B6, C, and folate, magnesium, and potassium. It is also low in fat and sodium. Zucchini also contains some plant polyphenol antioxidants. On a dry weight basis, its sugar content is about 50%, but because of its high moisture content, this translates to a reasonable 3 g per cup of chopped zucchini.

- **Overall,** this recipe is a good source of vitamins E, C, B6, and folate, as well as magnesium and zinc. It even has a respectable 5 g of protein per serving in a soup that is low in sodium, high in potassium, and high in fiber.

> DID YOU KNOW? Slowly simmered soups are a great way to get powerful plant antioxidants in your diet. Low heat and stirring help liberate the fat-soluble antioxidants, while slow simmering also helps extract the water-soluble polyphenol antioxidants without too much heat degradation.

BLACK BEAN, BARLEY, AND VEGETABLE SOUP

PAREVE | REHEATS AND/OR FREEZES WELL | MAKES ABOUT
15 CUPS (3.75 L)

1–2 Tbsp (15–30 mL) olive oil

3 cloves garlic (about 1 Tbsp/
15 mL minced)

2 medium onions, chopped

2 stalks celery, chopped

10 cups (2.5 L) water or vegetable
or chicken broth (preferably
low-sodium or no-salt-added)

3 medium carrots, chopped
(or 12 baby carrots)

1½ cups (375 mL) mushrooms,
chopped

1 medium sweet potato
(or 2 medium potatoes), peeled
and chopped

½ cup (125 mL) pearl barley,
rinsed and drained

1 cup (250 mL) dried red lentils,
rinsed and drained

1 can (19 oz/540 g) black beans,
drained and rinsed

2 tsp (10 mL) salt (or to taste)

1 tsp (5 mL) freshly ground black
pepper (or to taste)

¼ cup (60 mL) minced fresh dill
and/or finely chopped fresh basil

¼ cup (60 mL) minced
fresh parsley

Black beans are easier to digest than other beans, are very high in antioxidants, and are a good source of protein. This high-fiber soup is enhanced with fresh herbs—it's "soup-herb"! Don't let the long list of ingredients deter you. To save prep time, use a food processor to chop the vegetables.

1. Heat oil in a large soup pot over medium heat. Add garlic, onions, and celery; sauté for 5–7 minutes, until golden. If vegetables start to stick, add a little water.

2. Add water, carrots, mushrooms, sweet potato, barley, lentils, black beans, salt, and pepper; bring to a boil.

3. Reduce heat and simmer, partially covered, for 1 hour, until vegetables are tender, stirring occasionally. If soup becomes too thick, add a little water.

4. Add dill and parsley, and adjust seasonings to taste before serving.

130 calories per 1-cup (250 mL) serving, 23 g carbohydrates, 5 g fiber, 2 g sugar, 6 g protein, 2 g fat (0 g saturated fat), 341 mg sodium, 329 mg potassium

NORENE'S NOTES:

- **GI go!** Black beans, barley, and lentils all have a low glycemic index, making this soup an excellent choice for diabetics or those who are insulin-resistant.

- **Lower-sodium option:** Although canned black beans are more convenient than dried because they don't need soaking and cooking, they are higher in sodium. Instead, either choose organic brands of canned black beans, which contain a fraction of the sodium of regular canned beans, or buy low-sodium or no-salt-added beans.

- **Black beans** are in the legume family. They are low in moisture, thus making them very nutrient-dense. Even though black beans have a very high carb content, they also have a very high fiber content, which to a great degree compensates for the high carbs and results in a low glycemic index. They are very rich in brain nutrients, being excellent sources of fiber, protein, zinc, magnesium, manganese, choline, and folate. As a bonus, black beans—and beans in general—are quite high in antioxidants. One caution is that they do contain significant amounts of oxalates, which can cause kidney stones if you are susceptible.

- **Overall,** a serving contains excellent fiber content, good protein, folate, magnesium, vitamin C, and zinc, and is a great source of antioxidants.

DID YOU KNOW? In a study carried out by the USDA, beans occupied three out of four of the top spots in antioxidant content of 100 common foods. These were red beans, red kidney beans, and pinto beans. Black beans came in at about half the levels of the beans just mentioned, but this is still considered high.

LENTIL BARLEY SOUP

PAREVE | REHEATS AND/OR FREEZES WELL | MAKES ABOUT
9 CUPS (2.25 L)

1 large onion, chopped

1–2 stalks celery, chopped

2 medium carrots, chopped

2 cloves garlic (about 1 tsp/
5 mL minced)

¾–1 cup (185–250 mL) chopped
mushrooms

¾ cup (185 mL) dried red lentils,
rinsed and drained

½ cup (125 mL) pearl barley,
rinsed and drained

8 cups (2 L) vegetable broth or
water (preferably low-sodium or
no-salt-added)

1 bay leaf (optional)

1 tsp (5 mL) salt (or to taste)

½ tsp (2 mL) freshly ground
black pepper

2 Tbsp (30 mL) minced fresh dill

2 Tbsp (30 mL) fresh parsley

This simply delicious soup is high in soluble fiber, which helps stabilize blood sugar. My late mother's original version contained more starch, but I modified it and added lentils, a bay leaf, and parsley. Mom's mantra was, "Eat some soup. It will fill you up!" Double up the recipe for a large crowd.

---

1. Combine all ingredients except dill and parsley in a large soup pot and bring to a boil. Reduce heat and simmer, partially covered, for 1 hour, or until the lentils are soft. Stir occasionally.

2. Stir in dill and parsley and simmer 5–10 minutes longer. Discard bay leaf and adjust seasonings to taste. If soup becomes too thick, add a little water.

130 calories per 1-cup (250 mL) serving, 26 g carbohydrates, 5 g fiber, 3 g sugar, 6 g protein, 1 g fat (0 g saturated fat), 297 mg sodium, 250 mg potassium

NORENE'S NOTES:

- **Hidden treasures:** Red lentils melt into the soup and virtually disappear, making it an excellent way to sneak some fiber into your family's diet.

- **Lima bean and barley soup:** Instead of lentils, use ¾ cup (185 mL) lima beans that have been presoaked overnight in triple their volume of cold water, then drained and rinsed (see "Overnight Soak Method," p. 345). Increase cooking time in Step 1 to 1½–2 hours.

DR. ED SAYS:

- **Lentils and barley** have already been discussed in detail in the Slow Cooker Vegetable Soup recipe (p. 215), but these two ingredients, the main components of the current recipe, are two of the best choices for a soup because of their high fiber, low glycemic index, and high nutrient density, as well as their significant quantities of antioxidants.

- **Mushrooms** have also been discussed in detail in earlier recipes, and are welcome in any recipe because of their unique contribution of antioxidants, their ability to produce vitamin D, their protein content, their B vitamin contribution, their fiber content, and their low fat and carb contents.

DID YOU KNOW? One of the side effects of a high-fiber diet, especially soluble fiber, is that you become prone to passing gas, which is produced when bacteria in the gut break down the fiber. However, there are enzymes on the market that you can consume in pill form that will break down the soluble fiber before it reaches the gut and thus prevent excess gas formation. Unfortunately, by using these pills, you are also reducing the amount of fiber in the food and its beneficial effects. The average person passes gas 14 times a day, so there's no reason to try and prevent this normal process.

LOVE THAT LENTIL SOUP!

PAREVE | GLUTEN-FREE | REHEATS AND/OR FREEZES WELL | MAKES ABOUT 14 CUPS (3.5 L)

2 cups (500 mL) dried red lentils

⅔ cup (160 mL) brown rice

2 Tbsp (30 mL) olive oil

2 large onions, chopped

2 cloves garlic (about 2 tsp/ 10 mL minced)

8 cups (2 L) vegetable broth (preferably low-sodium or no-salt-added)

6 cups (1.5 L) water

1 Tbsp (15 mL) ground cumin

1 tsp (5 mL) salt (or to taste)

½ tsp (2 mL) freshly ground black pepper

1 Tbsp (15 mL) lemon juice (preferably fresh)

¼ cup (60 mL) minced fresh parsley (or 1 Tbsp/15 mL dried)

This soup really lives up to its name—everyone who tastes it loves it! It reminds people of the popular soup you might find at a Middle Eastern restaurant in Toronto. This recipe makes a huge batch but it won't last long! You can easily make half the recipe for a small family.

1. Rinse lentils and rice thoroughly in a strainer. Drain well and set aside.

2. Heat oil in a large soup pot on medium. Add onions and garlic; sauté until golden, about 5–7 minutes. Add broth, water, cumin, lentils, and rice. Bring to a boil.

3. Reduce heat, cover partially, and simmer for 35–40 minutes, stirring occasionally. Add salt, pepper, lemon juice, and parsley. If too thick, thin with a little water.

171 calories per 1-cup (250 mL) serving, 29 g carbohydrates, 4 g fiber, 2 g sugar, 8 g protein, 3 g fat (trace saturated fat), 189 mg sodium, 247 mg potassium

NORENE'S NOTES:

• **Red to green!** Although this soup is made with red lentils, the color becomes yellowish green when cooked.

• **Freeze with ease!** If you freeze the soup, it will separate when thawed. Not to worry though—just stir it when reheating and it will be the same as if you had just made it.

DR. ED SAYS:

• **Vegetable broth** is only 2% solids and, as a result, the nutrient contribution is minimal beyond the extracted antioxidants. However, because it is an aqueous extract of vegetables, it can contain significant levels of sugars and available carbs and potentially high sodium levels. Therefore, when purchasing, look for low level of sugar and sodium. Another option would be to make your own Vegetable Broth (p. 207).

- **Brown rice** is very high in carbs at 87% of its dry weight, whereas fiber is only about 7% of its dry weight. As a result, its glycemic index is relatively high at 68. Therefore, even though it does contain more nutrients than white rice, including magnesium and B vitamins, it should be consumed in moderation.

- **Overall,** this recipe is a good source of vitamin C, vitamin B6, folate, magnesium, and zinc. It is also an excellent source of antioxidants, fiber, and protein, primarily due to the lentils.

DID YOU KNOW? There are two types of fiber. One is called soluble fiber, and is found in fruits, legumes, nuts, and some cereals such as oats. This type of fiber is good for slowing sugar absorption and cholesterol. The other type of fiber is called insoluble fiber, and is found primarily in whole grains, seeds, and the skins of fruits and vegetables. This type of fiber is a bulking agent and is good for keeping you regular and avoiding constipation. Most fruits and vegetables will contain both types in differing quantities.

CABBAGE LENTIL BORSCHT

PAREVE | REHEATS AND/OR FREEZES WELL | MAKES ABOUT
16 CUPS (4 L)

2 Tbsp (30 mL) olive or canola oil

3 medium onions, chopped

1 pkg (16 oz/500 g) coleslaw mix

3 cloves garlic (about 1 Tbsp/
15 mL minced)

8 cups (2 L) water, vegetable, or
chicken broth (preferably low-
sodium or no-salt-added)

1 cup (250 mL) tomato juice
(preferably low-sodium)

1 can (28 oz/796 mL) diced
or whole tomatoes, including
liquid (preferably low-sodium or
no-salt-added)

1 can (5½ oz/156 g) tomato paste
(preferably low-sodium)

1 cup (250 g) dried green,
brown, or red lentils, rinsed
and drained

Sweetener equivalent to ¼ cup
(60 mL) brown sugar (or to taste)

½ tsp (2 mL) freshly ground
black pepper

1 bay leaf

2 tsp (10 mL) salt (or to taste)

2 Tbsp (30 mL) lemon juice
(preferably fresh)

2 Tbsp (30 mL) minced fresh dill

Big soup, little effort! Bagged coleslaw mix speeds up preparation for this scrumptious soup and lentils boost the fiber content. Most of the ingredients are probably in your kitchen.

1. Heat oil in a large soup pot over medium heat. Add onions and sauté for 5 minutes, until tender. Add coleslaw mix and garlic and cook 5–7 minutes longer, until tender, stirring occasionally.

2. Stir in water, tomato juice, tomatoes, tomato paste, lentils, sweetener, pepper, and bay leaf; bring to a boil. Reduce heat and simmer, partially covered, for 1½ hours, until lentils are tender. If soup gets too thick, add a little water or broth.

3. Stir in salt, lemon juice, and dill; simmer 5 minutes longer to blend the flavors. Remove and discard bay leaf before serving.

83 calories per 1-cup (250 mL) serving, 14 g carbohydrates, 3 g fiber, 5 g sugar, 3 g protein, 2 g fat (0 g saturated fat), 323 mg sodium, 229 mg potassium

NORENE'S NOTES:

· **Grate idea!** Instead of coleslaw mix, use 6 cups (1.5 L) grated cabbage and 1 grated carrot. If you want to include more vegetables, add 2 stalks chopped celery and 1 chopped zucchini.

· **Color your world!** Green or brown dried lentils will retain their shape, whereas red dried lentils will disintegrate during cooking and disappear into the soup.

· **Cooking tip:** Always add salt and lemon juice at the end of the cooking time to soups or stews that contain beans or lentils. If you add them at the start of the cooking process, the lentils won't soften completely. The only exception is lima beans—salt is added at the start of cooking.

- **Cabbage,** part of the cruciferous vegetable family, is provided in the form of coleslaw mix in this recipe. It is high in magnesium, vitamin C, and fiber. It is also a good source of zinc and folate and is reasonably low in available carbs and sugar, which results in a low glycemic index. Cabbage is also a good source of phenolic antioxidants. To maximize the antioxidant content, consider using red cabbage, which has significantly higher water-soluble phenolic antioxidants, as well as fat-soluble carotenoid antioxidants such as lutein and zeaxanthin.

- **Overall,** this recipe is a good source of fiber and vitamin C, and is a reasonable source of vitamin E and vitamin B6. It is somewhat high in sugar at 5 g per serving, primarily due to the tomatoes and tomato juice.

DID YOU KNOW? The cruciferous vegetable family (e.g., cabbage, broccoli, Brussels sprouts, etc.), has sulfur-containing compounds. These will cause gas released in the gut from the fiber to have an odor similar to rotting eggs or vegetables.

BROCCOLI & RED PEPPER SOUP

DAIRY OPTION | PAREVE | GLUTEN-FREE | PASSOVER | REHEATS
AND/OR FREEZES WELL | MAKES ABOUT 8 CUPS (2 L)

1 Tbsp (15 mL) olive oil

1 medium onion, chopped

1 red bell pepper, chopped

2 cloves garlic (about 2 tsp/
10 mL minced)

2 carrots, coarsely chopped
(or 12 baby carrots)

1 bunch broccoli, trimmed
and coarsely chopped (about
4 cups/1 L)

6 cups (1.5 L) vegetable broth
(preferably low-sodium or
no-salt-added)

1–2 tsp (5–10 mL) salt (or to taste)

½ tsp (2 mL) freshly ground black
pepper

1 Tbsp (15 mL) chopped
fresh basil

3 Tbsp (45 mL) chopped fresh dill

Broccoli rocks in this stalk-filled soup! This low-cal, low-carb soup is a light "weigh" to start a meal and curb your appetite.

1. Heat oil in a large saucepan over medium heat. Add onion, red pepper, and garlic; sauté 3–4 minutes, until vegetables are tender. Stir in carrots and broccoli and mix well.

2. Add broth, salt, and pepper, and bring to a boil. Reduce heat and simmer, partially covered, for 20 minutes, until broccoli is tender. Stir in basil and dill. Remove from heat and cool slightly.

3. Using an immersion blender, purée soup right in the pot, or purée in batches in a blender or food processor. Adjust seasonings to taste.

58 calories per 1-cup (250 mL) serving, 9 g carbohydrates, 3 g fiber, 4 g sugar, 2 g protein, 2 g fat (0 g saturated fat), 331 mg sodium, 223 mg potassium

NORENE'S NOTES:

- **Fresh or frozen?** Frozen broccoli, which is mostly florets, may actually contain more beta carotene than fresh broccoli. Add either fresh or frozen broccoli florets to this nutritious soup. The stems from fresh broccoli can be grated and used instead of cabbage when making stir-fries or coleslaw.

- **Fresh or dried?** When using fresh herbs, add them at the end of cooking. If using dried herbs, add them at the beginning of cooking.

- **Dairy option:** Serve soup with a dollop of light sour cream or plain yogurt, or stir in a little milk (skim or 1%).

- **Broccoli** is part of the cruciferous vegetable family. It is actually higher in nutritional value than cabbage, with high quantities of vitamin C, and good quantities of fiber, vitamin B6, folate, magnesium, and zinc. It is also a star when it comes to antioxidants that are important to the brain, and is high both in carotenoids, including high amounts of lutein and zeaxanthin, and in phenolic flavonoid antioxidants, with excellent amounts of kaempferol (which was shown to be important in research into the MIND Diet).

- **Overall,** this recipe is an excellent source of vitamin C and other phytoantioxidants, and a good source of vitamin B6, folate, and fiber. It is, however, one of the few soup recipes in this book where the sodium is higher than the potassium—though not by much.

> **DID YOU KNOW?** Quercetin is another flavonoid antioxidant found in broccoli, as well as in the onions and peppers included in this recipe. It is both an antioxidant and anti-inflammatory, and is thought to reduce deaths related to heart disease, especially in older-age adults. Its anti-inflammatory properties make it useful for preserving brain function.

BROCCOLI, SQUASH, AND SWEET POTATO SOUP

PAREVE | GLUTEN-FREE | PASSOVER | REHEATS AND/OR FREEZES
WELL | MAKES ABOUT 12 CUPS (3 L)

1 acorn or butternut squash
(2 lb/1 kg)

1 Tbsp (15 mL) olive or
grapeseed oil

2 large onions, coarsely chopped

2 cloves garlic (about 2 tsp/
10 mL minced)

1 bunch broccoli, cut into chunks
(about 4 cups/1 L)

2 medium sweet potatoes, peeled
and cut into chunks

2 medium carrots, peeled and cut
into chunks (or 8 baby carrots)

8 cups (2 L) vegetable or chicken
broth (preferably low-sodium
or no-salt-added)

¼ cup (60 mL) chopped fresh dill

1–2 tsp (5–10 mL) salt (or to taste)

Freshly ground black pepper

This scrumptious soup is packed with beta carotene and is very nourishing—it's like a multivitamin in a bowl!

1. Pierce squash in several places with a sharp knife. Microwave, uncovered, on high power for 6–8 minutes, turning squash over halfway through cooking. Squash should be three-quarters cooked. Once cool enough to handle, cut in half and discard seeds. Scoop out flesh and cut into chunks. (An ice-cream scoop does a great job!) You should have 4–5 cups (1–1.25 L).

2. Heat oil in a large soup pot on medium. Add onions and garlic; sauté for 5–7 minutes, until golden. Add broccoli, sweet potatoes, carrots, and squash; mix well.

3. Stir in broth, dill, salt, and pepper; bring to a boil. Reduce heat to low and simmer, partially covered, for 30 minutes, stirring occasionally, until vegetables are tender. Remove from heat and cool slightly.

4. Using an immersion blender, purée soup right in the pot, or purée in batches in a blender or food processor. If soup is too thick, add a little water or broth.

94 calories per 1-cup (250 mL) serving, 20 g carbohydrates, 4 g fiber, 4 g sugar, 3 g protein, 1 g fat (0 g saturated fat), 239 mg sodium, 485 mg potassium

NORENE'S NOTES:

- **Squash anyone?** Winter varieties of squash include acorn, butternut, buttercup, Hubbard, and spaghetti. All have deep yellow-to-orange flesh, seeds, and hard, thick skins. Choose squash that is heavy for its size, with a hard, outer skin that is free of moldy spots or blemishes. Most squash is interchangeable in recipes.

- **Store it right!** Store squash and sweet potatoes in a cool, dark place. Squash will keep for 1–2 months and sweet potatoes will keep up to a month.

- **Sweet news!** Did you know that sweet potatoes are packed with more beta carotene than carrots or winter squash?

- **Variation:** Replace broccoli with cauliflower florets.

DR. ED SAYS:

- **Sweet potatoes** are not only a better choice for taste, but also contain more nutrients than white potatoes, especially antioxidants. Sweet potatoes are a rich source of beta carotene and vitamin A antioxidants compared with white potatoes, which do not have significant quantities of antioxidants. Nevertheless, even though sweet potatoes have a higher fiber content than white potatoes, they also have a higher carb content, which makes for a rather high glycemic index.

- **Overall,** this recipe is an excellent source of vitamin C and fiber, and a good source of vitamin B6, folate, magnesium, and potassium. As well, it is an excellent source of carotenoid antioxidants from the sweet potatoes, carrots, squash, and broccoli.

> **DID YOU KNOW?** Even though many starchy foods have reasonable fiber content, their available carb content tends to overwhelm the fiber, resulting in poor glycemic index scores. These foods—primarily grains and root tubers—should be eaten in moderation.

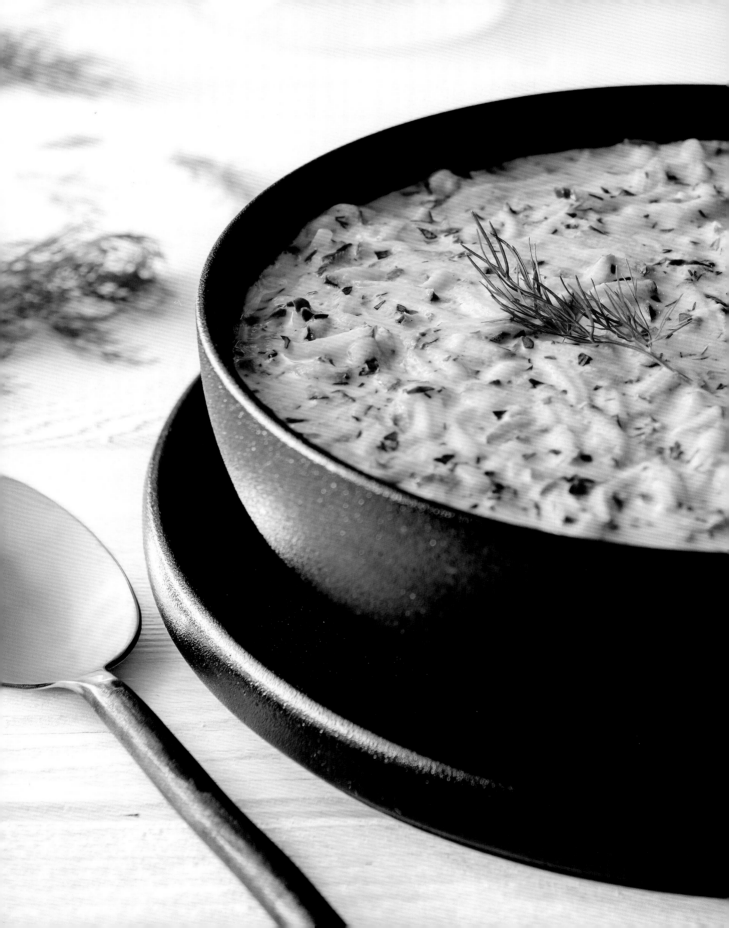

COOL AS A CUCUMBER SOUP

DAIRY-FREE OPTION | GLUTEN-FREE | PASSOVER | DO NOT FREEZE |
MAKES ABOUT 6 CUPS (1.5 L)

No cooking required for this low-cal, low-carb, calcium-packed summer cooler; it's really refreshing and perfect for Passover. When my late mother tasted it she said, "Your grandmother would have been here first thing in the morning for lunch if she knew you had this in your refrigerator!"

1½ cups (375 mL) grated unpeeled cucumber (English or minis)

2 green onions, chopped

3 cloves garlic (about 1 Tbsp/ 15 mL minced)

2 cups (500 mL) plain yogurt (skim or 1%)

2 cups (500 mL) milk (skim or 1%)

Salt and freshly ground black pepper

½ cup (125 mL) minced fresh parsley + extra for garnish (optional)

3–4 Tbsp (45–60 mL) minced fresh dill + extra for garnish (optional)

1. Combine all ingredients in a large bowl and mix well.

2. Cover and chill for several hours or overnight. Garnish with additional minced fresh parsley or dill and serve chilled.

83 calories per 1-cup (250 mL) serving, 13 g carbohydrates, <1 g fiber, 11 g sugar, 8 g protein, 0 g fat (0 g saturated fat), 102 mg sodium, 424 mg potassium

NORENE'S NOTES:

- **Variation:** Use Greek yogurt (skim or 1%), which is higher in protein and lower in carbs, instead of regular yogurt.

- **Dairy-free option:** Instead of yogurt and skim milk, combine ¼ cup (60 mL) lemon juice plus 3¾ cups (940 mL) soy milk.

DR. ED SAYS:

- **Yogurt,** in its low-fat form, is a great source of vitamin B12 (lacking in vegetarian-based diets) and also has good quantities of high-quality protein, zinc, and choline. Many yogurts are also fortified with vitamin D, so if you choose the fortified version, you will also get this important brain nutrient that is often missing from vegetarian diets. Yogurt's main claim to fame is its inclusion of active culture, which promotes a healthy gut and immune system.

- **Cucumbers** are mostly water and therefore do not provide much in the way of nutrition, although they do provide some fiber and antioxidants through the peel. On the other hand, they have a very refreshing taste, and cucumbers are often used in professional tasting panels to cleanse the mouth.

RECIPE CONTINUED . . .

COOL AS A CUCUMBER SOUP (continued)

- **Overall,** a serving of this recipe provides excellent quantities of vitamin B12, good amounts of vitamin C, magnesium, and zinc, and reasonable amounts of vitamin D and folate. Antioxidants are also provided by the parsley, dill, onions, and garlic. The only downside is the sugar content at 11 g per serving, primarily due to the yogurt. Substituting Greek yogurt is a good option.

> **DID YOU KNOW?** A lot of research is currently being done on the gut/brain axis, and it is thought that the impact of healthy bioactive cultures, such as are found in yogurt, help control inflammation, which is a factor in cognitive decline.

QUICK PEA & SPINACH SOUP

DAIRY OPTION | PAREVE | GLUTEN-FREE | REHEATS AND/OR
FREEZES WELL | MAKES ABOUT 11 CUPS (2.75 L)

This fabulous, fiber-filled soup uses frozen peas and is sure to "ap-peas" your hunger. The original recipe came from Sandra Gitlin. I substituted spinach for iceberg lettuce, added garlic and fresh basil, and reduced the cooking time from 1½ hours to just 30 minutes to retain more nutrients.

1. Heat oil in a large soup pot over medium heat. Add onion and sauté for about 5–7 minutes, until golden.

2. Add all remaining ingredients, except basil, to the soup pot and bring to a boil. Reduce heat to low and simmer, partially covered, for 30 minutes, until vegetables are tender. Remove from heat and cool slightly.

3. Using an immersion blender, purée soup right in the pot, or purée in batches in a blender or food processor. Stir in basil and adjust seasonings to taste.

103 calories per 1-cup (250 mL) serving, 21 g carbohydrates, 5 g fiber, 7 g sugar, 6 g protein, 1 g fat (0 g saturated fat), 445 mg sodium, 271 mg potassium

NORENE'S NOTES:

- **Frozen assets:** Most people keep green peas in their freezer. Frozen peas have additional benefits besides acting as an ice pack!

- **Sodi-yum!** Consider making your own Vegetable Broth (p. 207) without salt.

- **Dairy option:** For a calcium boost, add a swirl of plain Greek yogurt (skim or 1%) or a dollop of low-fat sour cream at serving time.

DR. ED SAYS:

- **Spinach** is a great substitute for iceberg lettuce as it is packed with brain-maintaining nutrients. It is an excellent source of vitamin C, folate, magnesium, and manganese, and is a good source of vitamins E and B6. Best of all, its antioxidant content shines—it contains a

RECIPE CONTINUED . . .

---

1 Tbsp (15 mL) olive oil

1 large onion, thinly sliced

4 cups (1 L) lightly packed baby spinach leaves

2 medium carrots, cut into chunks

1 medium potato, peeled and cut into chunks

1 pkg (2 lb/1 kg) frozen green sweet peas or baby peas (no need to defrost)

8 cups (2 L) vegetable broth (preferably low-sodium or no-salt-added)

3–4 cloves garlic (about 1 Tbsp/ 15 mL minced)

2 tsp (10 mL) curry powder (or 1 tsp/5 mL ground cumin)

1 tsp (5 mL) salt (or to taste)

½ tsp (2 mL) freshly ground black pepper

3–4 Tbsp (45–60 mL) minced fresh basil

whopping 12.2 mg per 100 g of the important carotenoid antioxidants lutein and zeaxanthin, which makes it an excellent source for these important brain molecules. It is also an excellent source of the flavonoid antioxidant kaempferol, which is believed to be an important antioxidant for the brain.

· **Curry powder** is a common ingredient in India that contains turmeric as one of its main components. Curcumin is the major chemical in turmeric, and because of its anti-inflammatory properties, it has been shown to be helpful for maintaining brain and general health. Curcumin is one of the recommended supplements in this book.

· **Overall,** this recipe provides excellent levels of vitamin C and fiber, good amounts of folate, and reasonable amounts of vitamin B6 and magnesium. It is somewhat high in sugar at 7 g per serving, primarily due to the peas, but is acceptable. (I usually consider any level above 7 g per serving as the cut-off point.)

DID YOU KNOW? Lutein and zeaxanthin were first found to be useful for slowing down macular degeneration in the eyes of aged individuals. Because the eyes are connected directly to the brain, research was conducted on the benefit of these compounds for brain health and the results were positive.

SPLIT PEA & PORTOBELLO MUSHROOM SOUP

PAREVE | GLUTEN-FREE | REHEATS AND/OR FREEZES WELL |
MAKES ABOUT 7 CUPS (1.75 L)

This decadent, velvety soup is full of fiber and flavor. Children's cook-book author Frieda Wishinsky uses shallots rather than garlic in her cooking because they add another dimension of flavor. Frieda refers to herself as "The Lady of Shallots." I'm sure Lord Tennyson would have poetic praise for her heavenly soup.

1. Combine split peas, water, and broth in a large pot. Bring to a boil. Reduce heat to low, cover partially, and simmer for 35 minutes.

2. While peas are cooking, heat oil in a large nonstick skillet over medium-high heat. Add onion, shallots, and mushrooms; sauté until golden brown, about 5 minutes. Reduce heat and cook slowly until onion has caramelized, about 5–10 minutes.

3. Add onion mixture to the cooked peas. Add carrot and simmer 15 minutes longer, until tender. Stir in paprika and remove from heat. Let cool slightly.

4. Using an immersion blender, purée soup right in the pot, or purée in batches in a blender or food processor. If too thick, add a little water or broth. Season with salt and pepper to taste, and serve.

152 calories per 1-cup (250 mL) serving, 26 g carbohydrates, 9 g fiber, 7 g sugar, 8 g protein, 3 g fat (0 g saturated fat), 194 mg sodium, 445 mg potassium

1 cup (250 mL) dried green split peas, rinsed and drained

5 cups (1.25 L) water

1 cup (250 mL) vegetable or chicken broth (preferably low-sodium or no-salt-added)

1 Tbsp (15 mL) canola or olive oil

1 large sweet onion, chopped (red or Vidalia)

2 medium shallots (about ½ cup/125 mL chopped)

2 cups (500 mL) sliced portobello mushrooms (about 5 mushrooms)

1 medium carrot, chopped

¼ tsp (1 mL) sweet paprika

½ tsp (2 mL) salt

Freshly ground black pepper

NORENE'S NOTES:

• **Variations:** Use a combination of split peas and lentils, using either green or yellow split peas. Cook ¼ cup (60 mL) pearl barley, rinsed and drained, along with peas and/or lentils. Or, substitute barley for half the peas. This makes a thicker soup, so thin as needed with additional broth. Instead of portobello mushrooms, try shiitake, oyster, or button mushrooms, or a combination.

RECIPE CONTINUED . . .

- **No shallots?** Use 2 or 3 garlic cloves. Shallots look like small elongated onions, with a garlic flavor. When peeled, they divide into cloves like garlic.

DR. ED SAYS:

- **Onions and shallots** are both from the same onion family. Both have reasonable amounts of brain nutrients and fiber, but nothing extraordinary. They also have relatively high levels of sugar, at about 8 g per 100 g. Their main claim to fame is that they are high in the flavonoid antioxidant quercetin, which in preliminary (but unconfirmed) research has been shown to be beneficial for brain and heart health, as well as for prevention of cancer and arthritic pain. This is thought to be due to its anti-inflammatory properties.

- **Portobello mushrooms** are a good source of potassium, protein, and fiber. They are low in sugar, digestible carbs, fat, and sodium, and have reasonable levels of magnesium, folate, vitamin B6, and, depending on light exposure, can also provide vitamin D. Even better, they provide unique antioxidants not usually found in vegetables.

- **Overall,** each serving provides good quantities of vitamin B6, zinc, and potassium, reasonable quantities of magnesium, and excellent levels of fiber and protein.

> DID YOU KNOW? Fiber, especially soluble fiber, is good for beneficial gut bacteria, which in turn can enable the gut immune system to control inflammation and brain decline.

CREAMY SQUASH SOUP

PAREVE | GLUTEN-FREE | PASSOVER | REHEATS AND/OR FREEZES
WELL | MAKES ABOUT 12 CUPS (3 L)

When the weather turns cooler, this satisfying squash soup is a perfect starter for chilly days. Toasted pumpkin seeds add a brain-healthy boost.

1. Heat oil in a large soup pot over medium heat. Add onion and ginger and sauté for 5 minutes, until translucent.

2. Stir in squash cubes, apple, and potato; sauté 3–4 minutes longer. Add broth plus enough water to cover the vegetables. Season with salt and pepper.

3. Bring to a boil. Reduce heat and simmer, covered, for 30 minutes, until squash and potato are tender.

4. Remove from heat and cool slightly. Using an immersion blender, purée soup right in the pot, until silky smooth. Add more broth or water if you prefer a thinner soup.

5. Reheat before serving. Adjust seasonings to taste. Sprinkle with pumpkin seeds.

127 calories per 1-cup (250 mL) serving, 25 g carbohydrates, 4 g fiber, 7 g sugar, 3 g protein, 3 g fat (trace saturated fat), 368 mg sodium, 512 mg potassium

NORENE'S NOTES:

- **Frozen assets:** Store fresh ginger in the freezer—it keeps for about 6 months. When needed, grate as much as you need (no need to thaw first). A microplane is excellent for grating fresh ginger.

- **Shopping tip:** Butternut squash cubes can be found in the produce department of most supermarkets. A 14-oz (398 g) package contains about 2 cups (500 mL).

RECIPE CONTINUED . . .

1 Tbsp (15 mL) olive oil

1 large onion, diced

2 tsp (10 mL) minced ginger

2 pkg (14 oz/398 g each) butternut squash cubes (see Norene's Notes)

1 large apple, peeled, cored, and cut into chunks

1 medium potato, peeled and cut into chunks

4 cups (1 L) vegetable broth (preferably low-sodium or no-salt-added)

1 cup (250 mL) water

1 tsp (5 mL) salt

¼ tsp (1 mL) freshly ground black pepper

½ cup (125 mL) toasted pumpkin seeds (omit for Passover)

- **Butternut squash cubes:** Slash a butternut squash in several places with a sharp knife. Either microwave on high for 5 minutes, or bake on a parchment-lined baking sheet at 350°F (175°C) for 15–20 minutes. Cool slightly. Cut squash into 2 pieces at the neck. Cut the round bottom part in half and use a large spoon or ice cream scoop to remove pulp and stringy fibers. Peel squash with a vegetable peeler and cut it into cubes. One medium squash yields about 5 cups (1.25 L) cubes.

DR. ED SAYS:

- **Butternut squash** is a great source of antioxidants, vitamin C, magnesium, and plant Omega-3 fats (although of a lower quality than fish Omega-3 fats), which are all important for cognition. It also contains good levels of vitamin E, and vitamins B6 and folate. Butternut squash is very low in saturated fat, salt, and available sugar, all of which can be harmful to cognition.

- **Ginger** has been shown to reduce cognitive decline. Its anti-inflammatory and positive blood circulation properties also contribute to the prevention of heart disease.

- **Pumpkin seeds,** or pepitas, are a very nutritionally dense food for the brain. Because they only contain about 5% moisture, they are very rich in protein and fiber, and very low in sugar and digestible carbs. They are also excellent sources of fiber, potassium, magnesium, manganese, zinc, and vitamin E (especially the brain relevant gamma tocopherol), and good sources of vitamin B6, folate, and choline.

- **Overall,** this recipe provides good sources of vitamin C, Omega-3 fats, folate, magnesium, and zinc. This tasty soup is also low in total fat and saturated fat.

> DID YOU KNOW? The oil in pumpkin seeds has been shown to reduce the symptoms of benign prostate hyperplasia (BPH). BPH causes men to urinate frequently.

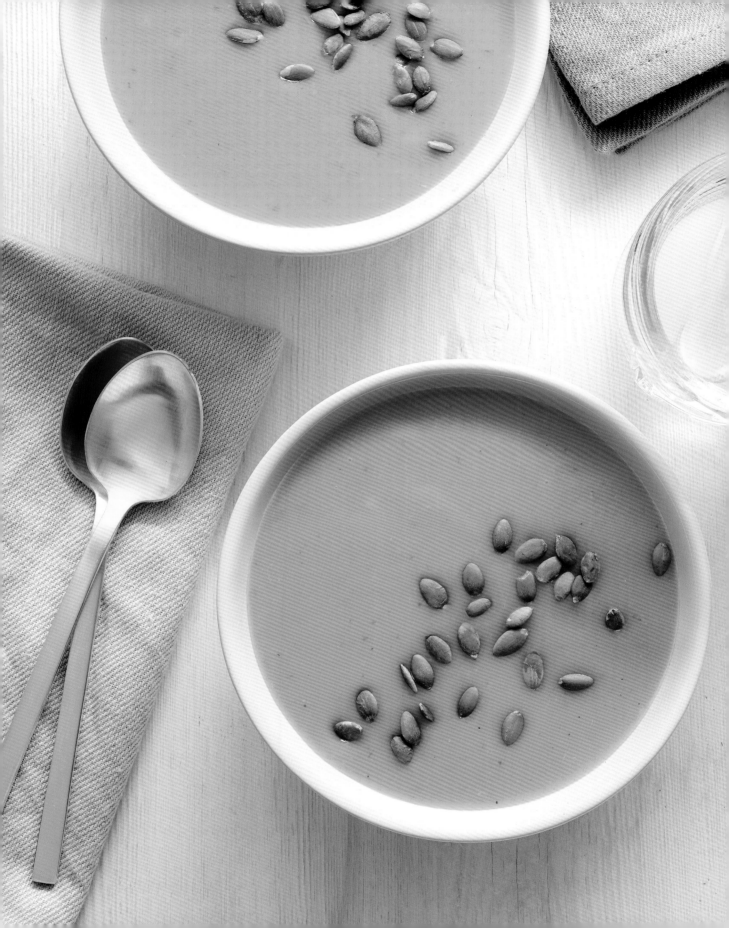

ROASTED TOMATO SOUP

DAIRY OPTION | PAREVE | GLUTEN-FREE | PASSOVER | REHEATS
AND/OR FREEZES WELL | MAKES ABOUT 10 CUPS (2.5 L)

3 lb (1.5 kg) Italian (Roma) plum tomatoes, halved lengthwise (12–14 tomatoes)

3 red bell peppers, cut into chunks

2 medium onions, cut into chunks

2 Tbsp (30 mL) olive oil

2 Tbsp (30 mL) balsamic vinegar

¾ tsp (4 mL) salt

Freshly ground black pepper

2 Tbsp (30 mL) fresh minced basil (or 2 tsp/10 mL dried)

1 Tbsp (15 mL) fresh minced thyme (or 1 tsp/5 mL dried)

2 heads garlic (about 30 cloves of garlic)

4 cups (1 L) vegetable broth or water (preferably low-sodium or no-salt-added)

Sweetener equivalent to 2 tsp (10 mL) sugar (or to taste)

Roasting brings out the full flavor of tomatoes and also increases the lycopene—and we like that! It's a perfect way to use up the last of your summer tomatoes. This low-cal soup tastes delicious hot or cold and is tastier and healthier than canned tomato soup!

1. Preheat oven to 400°F (200°C). Line a large, rimmed baking sheet with parchment paper.

2. Combine tomatoes, red peppers, and onions in a large bowl. Drizzle with olive oil and balsamic vinegar. Sprinkle with salt, pepper, basil, and thyme; mix well. Spread vegetables in a single layer on the prepared sheet, placing tomatoes cut side up.

3. Cut a ¼-inch (0.5 cm) slice from the top of each head of garlic, wrap each head in foil, and place on a baking sheet. Roast vegetables, uncovered, for 35–45 minutes, until nicely browned, stirring occasionally.

4. Transfer roasted vegetables to a large pot. Squeeze roasted garlic cloves into the pot. Add broth and bring to a boil.

5. Reduce heat to low and simmer, uncovered, for 10 minutes, stirring occasionally. Stir in sweetener. Remove from heat and cool slightly.

6. Using an immersion blender, purée soup right in the pot, or purée in batches in a blender or food processor. If too thick, add a little water or broth. Serve hot or cold.

93 calories per 1-cup (250 mL) serving, 15 g carbohydrates, 3 g fiber, 7 g sugar, 3 g protein, 3 g fat (0 g saturated fat), 196 mg sodium, 473 mg potassium

NORENE'S NOTES:

- **Roasted tomato gazpacho:** Prepare soup as directed above. Once cooled, cover and refrigerate. To serve, stir in 1 chopped, unpeeled English cucumber, ½ cup (125 mL) chopped green pepper, 6 minced green onions, ½ tsp (2 mL) chili powder, 2 Tbsp (30 mL) minced fresh basil, and the juice of half a lemon. Serve chilled.

- **Can do!** If you don't have enough fresh tomatoes, canned ones will do. In Step 2, prepare and roast tomatoes as directed, using 6–8 fresh tomatoes. In Step 4, add 1 can (28 oz/796 g) drained tomatoes to the roasted tomato mixture, along with the broth. Simmer for 10–15 minutes.

- **Flavor boost!** Add a spoonful of pesto to each bowl of soup at serving time.

- **Dairy option:** Add ½ cup (125 mL) milk (skim or 1%) or a dollop of Greek yogurt (skim or 1%) to each bowl of soup. Serve hot or cold.

DR. ED SAYS:

- **Tomatoes,** which are in the fruit-vegetable category because of their sugar content, are a wonderful source of both carotenoid (mainly lycopene) and phenolic antioxidants, though the carotenoids, which are fat-soluble, tend to provide most of the antioxidant activity. Soup is an excellent vehicle for tomatoes because the temperature and maceration used in their preparation maximizes the availability of the lycopene for the body. Because tomatoes are very high in moisture at 95%, they tend to be modest in most nutrients, but are still excellent sources of vitamin C.

- **Bell Peppers** are excellent sources of vitamin C and beta carotene antioxidants, and are good sources of vitamins B6, E, and folate. They also supply good quantities of fiber, though as fruit-vegetables their sugar content is higher than most vegetables, at about 4 g per 100 g.

- **Overall,** a serving of this soup provides excellent levels of vitamin C, and good amounts of vitamin E and folate, as well as some magnesium and zinc.

> **DID YOU KNOW?** Tomatoes belong to the deadly nightshade family and immature fruit and leaves still contain a toxin called tomatin. Because of this, and because the acidity in tomatoes causes pewter plates to corrode, Europeans at first thought them to be poisonous.

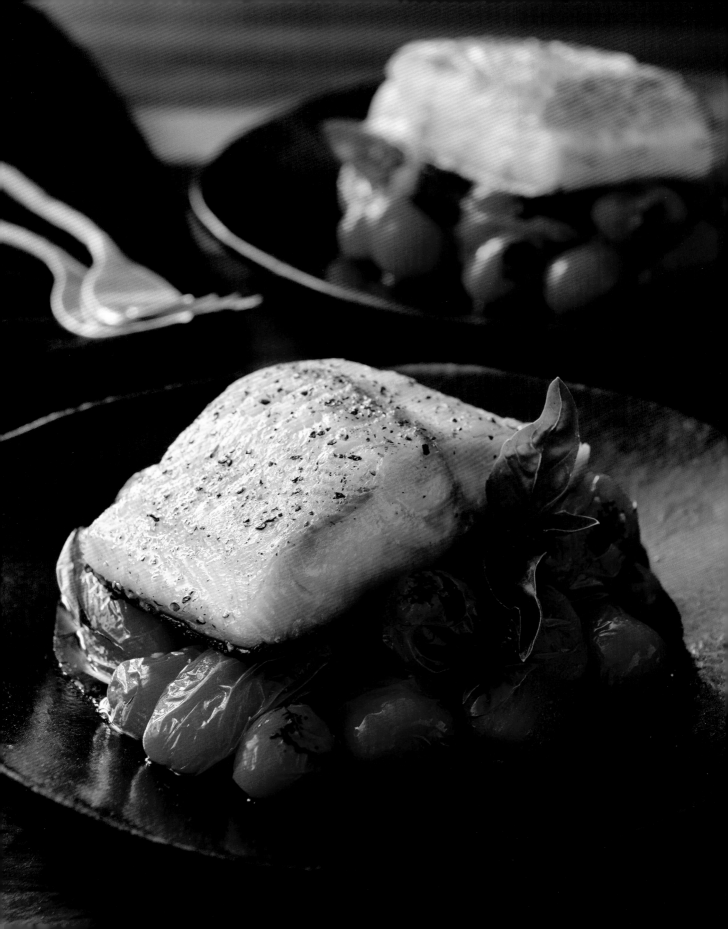

FISHFUL THINKING

THE DAILY CATCH: Fresh is best, but frozen is also an excellent option.

HOOK, LINE, AND STINKER! Fresh fish should smell sweet and vaguely like the ocean. If it has a strong, fishy, or ammonia-like smell, either it's not fresh or it may have been mishandled. The smell of ammonia usually occurs when frozen fish has been thawed and then refrozen.

EAT SMART: The following recommended brain-healthy varieties of fish are grouped according to their Omega-3 content:

- **High Omega-3:** Salmon, sardines, herring, mackerel, anchovies, tuna (bluefin), whitefish (especially black cod/sablefish)
- **Moderate Omega-3:** Rainbow trout, arctic char, pollock, tuna (canned)
- **Low Omega-3:** Snapper, sole, halibut

Did you know? Fish eggs, commonly known as caviar, roe, or ikura, have the highest concentration of Omega-3 fats, which can constitute up to 30% of the total fatty acids in these eggs.

GO WILD! Wild salmon is a better choice than farmed. Fresh wild salmon is available fresh or frozen. Canned sockeye salmon, which is usually wild, is affordable and convenient, so enjoy it often. Wild salmon gets its Omega-3 fatty acids and color from eating natural prey, while farmed salmon gets its color from supplements in its feed. Without that added pigment, farmed salmon would be a pale grey. Pacific salmon is mostly wild, while Atlantic salmon is usually farmed.

Did you know? Black cod has the highest Omega-3 content of any white fish—even higher than many species of salmon.

STORE IT RIGHT: Store lean fish such as halibut or sole in the coldest part of the refrigerator (40°F) for 2–3 days, or freeze up to 6 months at 0°F. Fatty fish such as salmon can be stored in the refrigerator for 2–3 days, or frozen for 2–3 months at 0°F.

NO COOKING REQUIRED: Canned salmon, tuna, sardines, anchovies, and jarred marinated herring are great choices for a no-cook meal. As an added bonus, the bones from sardines and salmon provide calcium. Add anchovy fillets to salads or puréed anchovies to Caesar salad dressing.

FROSTY FACTS: To thaw fish quickly, unwrap it and place on a microwaveable plate. Allow 4–5 minutes per pound on the "defrost" setting (30% power), turning the fish over at half-time. A few ice crystals should still remain—these will disappear after the fish stands at room temperature for a few minutes. If you plan to cook fish in the microwave, thaw it completely before cooking so it will cook evenly.

CHILL OUT! You can thaw still-wrapped fish under cold running water, or overnight in the refrigerator. Don't refreeze fish after defrosting. However, once it has been cooked, it can then be frozen.

MARINE-AIDES! Marinating fish gives it great flavor. However, don't marinate fish longer than 1 hour or it will start to "cook." If you are planning to cook fish on the barbecue, marinating it first will help protect it from forming cancer-causing substances while it is being grilled.

THE SKINNY TRUTH: Fish fillets such as halibut and salmon are usually sold with their skin on, but are also available skinless. It's fine to buy fish with the skin on, just remove the skin and visible fat from cooked fish before eating it to reduce any trace amounts of PCBs (polychlorinated biphenyls). Bake, broil, poach, or grill fish instead of frying.

TIMELY TIPS: Measure a fillet at its thickest point. Allow 10 minutes per inch (2.5 cm) of thickness and cook at 425–450°F (220–230°C). If one end is thinner than the other, fold that end underneath so it is uniform in thickness. If the fish is being cooked in a sauce or wrapped in foil, cook it 5 minutes longer. This rule applies to baking, broiling, grilling, poaching, and steaming. Cooking times for frying and microwaving are generally quicker. If the fish is frozen, double the cooking time, allowing 20 minutes per inch (2.5 cm) of thickness.

MICROWAVE MAGIC: Calculate 4 minutes per pound on high power. One serving of fish will cook in 2–3 minutes, depending on the wattage of your microwave. To "stop the pop" and save on cleanup, cook fish between lettuce or spinach leaves, or wrap it in parchment paper.

FINNY GRILL! To cook salmon on an indoor electric grill, preheat your grill according to the manufacturer's instructions. Season salmon fillets as desired. To save on cleanup, either spray the grill with nonstick cooking spray or line it with parchment paper—it's heatproof up to 400°F (200°C). Place salmon in a single layer on parchment paper, if using. Cover with another sheet of parchment. In a closed grill, cook 5–6 minutes per inch (2.5 cm) of thickness. In an open grill, cook 10–12 minutes per inch (2.5 cm).

SKILL AT THE GRILL: To cook salmon directly on the grill, season salmon fillets as desired, oiling them lightly to prevent sticking. Place fillets, flesh side down, on the well-oiled grill. At the beginning, fish will cling to the grate until it has cooked about 7–8 minutes. Turn fish over carefully using a wide spatula and cook the second side 2–3 minutes longer, until it flakes. This is known as the 70/30 timing rule, which results in a beautiful presentation with great grill marks.

IS IT DONE YET? Fish is done if it's opaque yet still moist in the center. It should just flake when pressed gently with a fork. On an instant-read thermometer, the interior temperature should reach 145°F (63°C). If overcooked, the fish will become dry.

PAN-TASTIC! To transfer a large salmon fillet to a serving platter, use a rimless baking sheet as a giant spatula.

LETTUCE COOK FISH FOR DINNER!

PAREVE | PASSOVER | GLUTEN-FREE | MAKES 4 SERVINGS

Simply dill-icious! Dinner's done in minutes!

½ head Romaine lettuce

4 salmon fillets (about 6 oz/
180 g each)

Salt and freshly ground
black pepper

2 Tbsp (30 mL) chopped fresh dill
+ extra dill for garnish

4 tsp (20 mL) lemon juice

Lemon slices (for garnish)

1. Wash lettuce well; shake off excess water. Arrange a layer of lettuce leaves in the bottom of a 7- × 11-inch (18 × 28 cm) glass baking dish. Arrange salmon in a single layer on top of the lettuce, folding any thin ends under so the fish cooks evenly. Sprinkle with salt, pepper, dill, and lemon juice. Cover with another layer of lettuce.

2. Microwave on high for about 4 minutes, or until fish is no longer opaque. Let stand, covered, for 2 minutes. Fish should flake when lightly pressed. Discard lettuce leaves.

3. Garnish with lemon slices and additional dill. Delicious hot or cold.

231 calories per serving, 3 g carbohydrates, 2 g fiber, 1 g sugar, 36 g protein, 8 g fat (1 g saturated), 134 mg sodium, 823 mg potassium

NORENE'S NOTES:

- **Dinner for one:** For a single serving, microwave in a small casserole on high for 2½ minutes.

- **Paper-poached fish:** Omit lettuce leaves. Arrange salmon in a single layer in a glass baking dish; sprinkle with seasonings and lemon juice. Moisten parchment paper under running water for about 20 seconds and squeeze gently to remove excess moisture. It will now be flexible so you can mold it around the baking dish!

- **Change it up:** Instead of dill, use basil, thyme, or rosemary—fresh or dried herbs work equally well.

DR. ED SAYS:

- **Salmon** is one of the best choices for getting your Omega-3 fats. A single serving provides an excellent 1.3 g Omega-3s. In addition, salmon is also an excellent source of vitamin D and vitamin B12, two important nutrients that are difficult to get through plant foods.

RECIPE CONTINUED . . .

- **Romaine lettuce and dill** are leafy vegetables that provide excellent amounts of vitamins B6 and folate, as well as the important brain minerals magnesium and zinc, which work together with the Omega-3 fats.

> **DID YOU KNOW?** Combining Omega-3 fats with B vitamins from leafy vegetables enhances the brain-saving effects of the Omega-3 fats—one study showed that brain atrophy in older-age subjects could be reduced by 40% by combining these foods in their diets.

CHIMICHURRI SALMON

PAREVE | GLUTEN-FREE | PASSOVER | SAUCE FREEZES WELL | MAKES 6 SERVINGS

Chimichurri, an herb sauce from Argentina, pairs perfectly with salmon, but is also delicious with beef, chicken, tofu, or vegetables (see Chimichurri Cauliflower Steaks, p. 457). It takes moments to prepare the gorgeous green sauce in your food processor—or just use a chef's knife and a cutting board. Either bake the salmon in your oven or cook it on the grill (see Norene's Notes), depending on the weather.

---

1. **CHIMICHURRI SAUCE:** In a food processor fitted with the steel blade or a mini prep, process garlic, green onions, and parsley until minced, about 8–10 seconds. Add olive oil, vinegar, oregano, red pepper flakes, and salt. Process until combined, 5–10 seconds. Transfer sauce to a large glass measure. Cover and refrigerate up to 48 hours. Bring to room temperature before serving.

2. Spray a 9- × 13-inch (23 × 33 cm) baking dish with nonstick cooking spray.

3. **SALMON:** Arrange salmon, skin side down, in a single layer on the prepared baking dish. Sprinkle lightly with salt and pepper. Spread half the sauce evenly over the top of the salmon; reserve the remaining sauce.

4. Preheat oven to 375°F (190°C). Let salmon stand 10–15 minutes while oven is preheating.

5. Bake uncovered for 12–15 minutes. Salmon is done if it flakes when gently pressed with a fork.

6. Serve salmon with reserved sauce. Delicious hot or cold.

331 calories per serving, 2 g carbohydrates, 1 g fiber, trace sugar, 35 g protein, 20 g fat (3 g saturated), 328 mg sodium, 701 mg potassium

NORENE'S NOTES:

- **Buffet beauty:** For a pretty presentation, buy a side of salmon that is filleted (about 2½-3 lb/1.1-1.4 kg). Cooking time will be 15-18 minutes at 400°F (200°C).

RECIPE CONTINUED . . .

CHIMICHURRI SAUCE:

3 cloves garlic

4 green onions, trimmed

¾ cup (185 mL) tightly packed fresh flat-leaf parsley (washed and well dried, stems trimmed)

⅓ cup (80 mL) extra virgin olive oil

3 Tbsp (45 mL) white wine vinegar

½ tsp (2 mL) dried oregano

¼–½ tsp (1–2 mL) red pepper flakes (or to taste)

½ tsp (2 mL) salt

SALMON:

6 salmon fillets (6–8 oz/ 180–235 g each)

Salt and freshly ground black pepper

- **Sheet pan dinner:** Arrange fillets in a single layer at one end of a prepared baking sheet. Spread out 1 sliced zucchini, 1 sliced red or yellow bell pepper, and 4 Campari tomatoes that have been cut into wedges at the other end. Spoon some Chimichurri sauce on top. Bake as directed above. Garnish with toasted sliced almonds.

- **Skill at the grill:** To grill salmon, preheat the barbecue or grill, setting it to medium-high. Coat salmon with half the sauce and let it marinate while the grill is preheating. Remove salmon from the marinade and discard the remaining marinade. Place salmon, skin side down, on the grill for 7–8 minutes. Turn the salmon over carefully and cook on the second side for 2–3 minutes. Serve with the reserved sauce.

DR. ED SAYS:

- **Salmon:** Similar to Lettuce Cook Fish for Dinner (p. 247), we have the same positive nutritional benefits of the salmon. Also, as with most fish sources, we have low carbs, sugar, and saturated fats. So, we benefit from both what the fish contains as well as what it doesn't contain. How good can it get?

- **Chimichurri sauce** is another way to provide the unique nutritional benefits of plant foods that are missing from the fish, including some of the B vitamins, the antioxidants in the oregano, parsley, onions, and garlic, and the brain-conserving properties of the olive oil.

> DID YOU KNOW? Despite fish being the main source of the major Omega-3 fats DHA and EPA, a study in 2015 found that 95% of Americans have sub-optimal levels of Omega-3 fats.

CHUTNEY-GLAZED SALMON

PAREVE | GLUTEN-FREE | REHEATS AND/OR FREEZES WELL | MAKES 4 SERVINGS

This combination of flavors is amazing, and it makes for an "en-chutneyed" evening!

---

1. Preheat oven to 425°F (220°C). Line a rimmed baking sheet with foil and spray with nonstick cooking spray.

2. Arrange fillets in a single layer on the prepared baking sheet. Sprinkle lightly with salt and pepper. Spread about 2 Tbsp (30 mL) chutney evenly overtop of each fillet, then sprinkle with curry powder, cumin, and paprika. Let stand for 15–20 minutes.

3. Bake, uncovered, for 10–12 minutes, until salmon is glazed and golden. Salmon is done when it flakes when gently pressed with a fork. Serve hot or cold.

233 calories per serving, 4 g carbohydrates, 1 g fiber, 3 g sugar, 35 g protein, 8 g fat (1 g saturated), 129 mg sodium, 676 mg potassium

NORENE'S NOTES:

- **Sheet pan dinner:** Arrange fillets in a single layer at one end of the prepared baking sheet; place 1 lb (500 g) trimmed asparagus and 1 thinly sliced red bell pepper at the other end. Bake as directed above. Garnish with toasted slivered almonds.

- **Buffet beauty:** For a large crowd, buy a large salmon fillet (about 3 lb/1.4 kg). Use double the amount of the other ingredients and bake on a parchment-lined, rimless baking sheet at 425°F (220°C) for 15–18 minutes. Serve hot or at room temperature. Garnish with parsley, sliced lemon, and tomatoes.

DR. ED SAYS:

- **Salmon,** the major ingredient in this recipe, is the main contributor of Omega-3 fats as well as the other nutrients mentioned in the previous two recipes.

RECIPE CONTINUED . . .

4 salmon fillets (6–8 oz/ 180–235 g each)

Salt and freshly ground black pepper

½ cup (125 mL) mango or apricot chutney (preferably low-sugar or all-fruit)

1 tsp (5 mL) curry powder

1 tsp (5 mL) ground cumin

1 tsp (5 mL) sweet paprika

- **Spices:** Curry, cumin, and paprika provide a good source of antioxidants that complement the nutrients from the salmon.

- **Mango and/or apricot chutney:** Although these fruits are high in sugar, the contribution per serving is only 3 g, which is quite manageable.

> DID YOU KNOW? Omega-3 fats from fish are not just good for the brain and heart—studies have shown that they can reduce depression and boost muscle function in older-age women.

MAPLE-GLAZED SALMON

PAREVE | GLUTEN-FREE | PASSOVER OPTION | REHEATS AND/OR
FREEZES WELL | MAKES 10 SERVINGS

Whenever I prepare this show-stopping dish at my cooking demon-
strations, it gets rave reviews. Don't tell anyone that it includes simple,
easily available ingredients that are good for your brain: salmon, dark
leafy greens, and rosemary. Always a winner!

1. Line a large rimless baking dish with aluminum foil and spray with
nonstick cooking spray.

2. Place salmon, skin side down, on the prepared baking sheet.

3. In a small bowl, combine mustard, jam, maple syrup, oil, and rosemary; mix well. Reserve and refrigerate ¼ cup (60 mL) glaze. Spread
the remaining glaze evenly on the top of the salmon, then sprinkle with
pepper and paprika. Marinate for 20–30 minutes.

4. Preheat oven to 425°F (220°C). Bake salmon, uncovered, for 15–18
minutes, or until glazed and golden, basting occasionally with pan
juices. Cool slightly.

5. Carefully transfer salmon to a large serving platter lined with baby
spinach leaves. Garnish with lemon slices and rosemary. Drizzle salmon
with the reserved glaze mixture. Serve hot or cold.

217 calories per serving, 6 g carbohydrates, 0 g fiber, 4 g sugar, 29 g
protein, 8 g fat (1 g saturated), 250 mg sodium, 524 mg potassium

1 large salmon fillet, with skin
(about 3 lb/1.4 kg)

¼ cup (60 mL) Dijon mustard
(for a Passover option, see
Norene's Notes)

¼ cup (60 mL) apricot jam
(low-sugar or all-fruit)

2 Tbsp (30 mL) maple syrup

1 Tbsp (15 mL) olive oil

2 Tbsp (30 mL) minced fresh
rosemary (or 2 tsp/10 mL dried) +
extra for garnish

Freshly ground black pepper

Sweet paprika

Baby spinach and lemon slices
(for garnish)

NORENE'S NOTES:

- **Passover option:** Replace Dijon mustard with 2 Tbsp (30 mL) white
horseradish.

- **Fishing for compliments?** For a large party, calculate that each pound
of salmon will feed 3-4 people. Allow 4-5 oz (115-150 g) per person for
a buffet.

- **Big or small:** Instead of a large salmon fillet, use individual salmon fillets or steaks (6-8 oz/180-235 g each).

RECIPE CONTINUED . . .

MAPLE-GLAZED SALMON (continued)

- **No bones about it:** To check for pin bones, drape a salmon fillet over a drinking glass or the palm of your hand so that the ends extend and hang downwards. The layers of fish will spread, making it easy to see and remove the bones. Tweezers are a terrific tool for removing fish bones.

- **Maple-glazed chicken breasts:** Substitute 6 boneless, skinless chicken breasts for salmon. Bake, uncovered, at 400°F (200°C), for 25–30 minutes, until glazed and golden. Baking time will depend on thickness of the chicken breasts.

DR. ED SAYS:

- **Salmon,** the main ingredient in this recipe, offers the same major Omega-3 benefits as the other recipes in this book that feature it. Most of these recipes contain antioxidants and B vitamins, providing the maximum benefit from the Omega-3s, along with the other valuable nutrients previously mentioned.

- **Rosemary,** in addition to being a flavorful herb, is an extremely potent natural antioxidant. Its properties are so powerful that it is used as a protective agent against the effects of oxygen in processed foods.

- **Spinach:** Although spinach is only used as a garnish in this recipe, this leafy green has been shown to help boost cognitive health.

- **Overall,** this delicious dish is an excellent choice for brain health because of its high Omega-3 content, which is combined with high levels of vitamin D, B12, and B6, and magnesium. Rosemary also provides high levels of antioxidants.

> DID YOU KNOW? An analysis of five studies from Western countries showed the lowest mortality rates for ischemic heart disease in those vegetarians who also ate fish (pescatarians). This was significantly even lower for vegans who introduced fish into their diet.

MARMALADE-GLAZED SALMON SHEET PAN DINNER

PAREVE | GLUTEN-FREE OPTION | REHEATS AND/OR FREEZES WELL |
MAKES 4 SERVINGS

This one-pan dinner is simple enough for your family but festive enough for company. For variety, substitute apricot or peach jam for the marmalade. It's jam-good!

4 salmon fillets or steaks (6–8 oz/180–235 g each)

3 cups (750 mL) sliced assorted mushrooms

1 red bell pepper, sliced

1 yellow bell pepper, sliced

⅓ cup (80 mL) orange marmalade (preferably low-sugar or all-fruit)

2 Tbsp (30 mL) soy sauce or tamari (preferably low-sodium)

1 Tbsp (15 mL) Asian (toasted) sesame oil

Freshly ground black pepper

¼ cup (60 mL) sesame seeds (optional)

1. Preheat oven to 425°F (220°C). Line a rimmed baking sheet with foil and spray with nonstick cooking spray.

2. Arrange fillets in a single layer at one end of the prepared baking sheet and mushrooms and peppers at the other.

3. Combine marmalade, soy sauce, and sesame oil in a bowl and mix well. Using a pastry or barbecue brush, spread glaze evenly overtop of the fillets and vegetables. Season with pepper and sprinkle with sesame seeds, if using. Let stand for 20–30 minutes.

4. Bake, uncovered, for 10–12 minutes, until salmon is glazed and just flakes when gently pressed with a fork. Serve hot or cold.

319 calories per serving, 16 g carbohydrates, 1 g fiber, 9 g sugar, 38 g protein, 11 g fat (2 g saturated), 636 mg sodium, 1044 mg potassium

NORENE'S NOTES:

- **Leftovers?** Break salmon into chunks and place on a bed of chilled salad greens, or add it to cooked whole grain or vegetable pasta along with thinly sliced onions and bell peppers. Drizzle with your favorite homemade or bottled Asian salad dressing.

- **Wrap-ture!** Leftover flaked cooked salmon makes an excellent filling for wraps.

- **Eggs-actly!** Leftover flaked cooked salmon is also delicious in frittatas or omelets.

RECIPE CONTINUED . . .

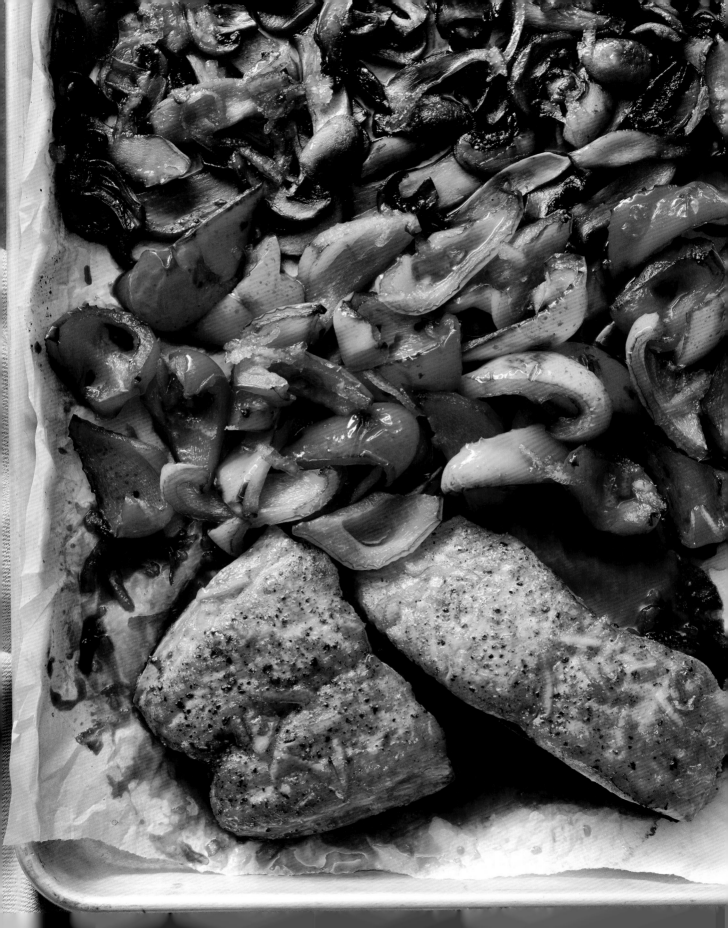

MARMALADE-GLAZED SALMON SHEET PAN DINNER (continued)

DR. ED SAYS:

- **Salmon,** the main ingredient, offers all the benefits described in the previous salmon recipes.

- **Mushrooms** are a great source of protein and have unique antioxidants not found in other plants. They are also low in digestible carbs and a good source of fiber, B vitamins, and magnesium.

- **Bell peppers** are always a great source of vitamin C and other antioxidants, and a good source of vitamins B6 and folate.

- **Overall,** this recipe is an excellent source of vitamin C, phytoantioxidants, vitamins D, B6, and B12, and is well balanced in providing many of the brain-friendly nutrients required to stave off cognitive decline. It is somewhat high in sugar, but this can be reduced by controlling the amount of orange marmalade used.

> DID YOU KNOW? Mushrooms have some of the highest concentrations of naturally occurring phytosterols. These act similarly to the statins, which are a class of drugs prescribed to reduce harmful cholesterol.

PANKO-CRUSTED SESAME SALMON

PAREVE | GLUTEN-FREE OPTION | REHEATS AND/OR FREEZES WELL | MAKES 4 SERVINGS

4 salmon fillets (6–8 oz/
180–235 g each)

Salt and freshly ground black
pepper

¼ cup (60 mL) panko crumbs
(for a gluten-free option,
see Norene's Notes)

2 Tbsp (30 mL) sesame seeds

1 tsp (5 mL) dried basil

4 tsp (20 mL) light mayonnaise
or honey mustard

Nonstick cooking spray

Lemon slices (for garnish)

Easy and elegant, this simple salmon dish is perfect for quick weeknight suppers, yet is also ideal for special occasions. See Norene's Notes.

1. Preheat oven to 400°F (200°C). Line a rimmed baking sheet or casserole with parchment paper.

2. Arrange salmon in a single layer on the prepared baking sheet. Sprinkle lightly with salt and pepper.

3. In a small bowl, mix together panko crumbs, sesame seeds, and basil.

4. Spread 1 tsp (5 mL) mayonnaise or honey mustard on top of each fillet. Sprinkle a generous tablespoon of the panko mixture overtop, then press lightly so crumbs will stick. Lightly spray crumb topping with nonstick cooking spray.

5. Bake, uncovered, for 10–12 minutes, until golden.

6. Transfer salmon to serving plates and garnish with lemon slices. Delicious hot or cold.

199 calories per serving, 5 g carbohydrates, <1 g fiber, trace sugar, 26 g protein, 8 g fat (1 g saturated fat), 145 mg sodium, 441 mg potassium

NORENE'S NOTES:

- **Gluten-free option:** Use gluten-free panko crumbs or quinoa flakes.

- **Dinner for one?** Use 1 salmon fillet (6–8 oz/180–235 g), 1 tsp (5 mL) mayonnaise, 1 Tbsp (15 mL) panko, 1½ tsp (7 mL) sesame seeds, and a pinch of salt, pepper, and basil.

- **Company's coming?** Use a large boneless fillet of salmon (about 3 lb/1.4 kg) instead of individual portions. Double all ingredients. Baking time will be 16–18 minutes. Makes 8–10 servings.

- **Frozen assets:** Use frozen salmon fillets (no need to thaw first) and double the cooking time.

- **Panko-crusted tofu:** Instead of salmon fillets, substitute 1 lb (500 g) firm tofu cut into ½-inch (5 cm) thick slices. Prepare as directed above.

DR. ED SAYS:

- **Salmon** is an excellent source of fish Omega-3 fats, which have been shown to reduce the risk of AD/dementia more than any other food component. It is difficult to obtain Omega-3 fats other than by eating fatty fish. Salmon also provides almost a full day's supply of the important vitamin B12, which is noted for reducing cognitive decline. The combination of vitamin B12 with Omega-3 fats makes it even more effective. Salmon is also rich in vitamin B6 and has good amounts of magnesium.

- **Tahini** provides high levels of fiber, magnesium, and vitamins B6 and folate.

- **Overall,** this simple salmon dish is an outstanding choice for brain health due to the combination of high levels of fish Omega-3 fats and B vitamins. It contains good amounts of magnesium, and is low in sugar and sodium.

> **DID YOU KNOW?** You get a much higher concentration of Omega-3 fats in fatty fish such as salmon or herring as compared with low-fat fish such as pollock or haddock. Higher-fat fish tend to be darker in color as compared to low-fat fish which are whiter in color.

SESAME SALMON SHEET PAN DINNER

PAREVE | GLUTEN-FREE | REHEATS AND/OR FREEZES WELL |
MAKES 10 SERVINGS

4 cups (1 L) sliced mushrooms

2 red bell peppers, cut into thin strips

1 yellow bell pepper, cut into thin strips

1 medium red onion, halved and thinly sliced

3 Tbsp (45 mL) extra virgin olive oil

1 large salmon fillet, with skin (about 3 lb/1.4 kg)

Salt and freshly ground black pepper

Asian Dressing/Marinade (p. 422)

⅓–½ cup (80–125 mL) black or white sesame seeds (or a combination)

Easy prep, easy clean-up! Sheet pan dinners are an excellent solution for time-starved cooks. So versatile, so delicious, and so many options— see Norene's Notes.

---

1. Line a large baking sheet with foil and spray with nonstick cooking spray.

2. Spread mushrooms, peppers, and onion in a single layer at one end of the prepared baking sheet and drizzle with oil. Place salmon, skin side down, at the other end of the baking sheet. Lightly sprinkle salmon and vegetables with salt and pepper. Drizzle with marinade and sprinkle with sesame seeds. Let stand for 30–60 minutes.

3. Preheat oven to 425°F (220°C). Bake, uncovered, for 15–18 minutes. Salmon will be glazed and golden and vegetables will be tender-crisp when done.

4. Cool slightly. Transfer salmon carefully to a large serving platter using a wide spatula. Surround salmon with vegetables. Serve hot or cold.

349 calories per serving, 12 g carbohydrates, 2 g fiber, 7 g sugar, 31 g protein, 20 g fat (3 g saturated), 507 mg sodium, 757 mg potassium

NORENE'S NOTES:

- **The daily catch:** This is also delicious with rainbow trout, orange roughy, red snapper fillets, pickerel, or halibut. Reduce temperature to 400°F (200°C) and bake for 10–12 minutes, until fish flakes when gently pressed with a fork and vegetables are tender. Vegetables may require an extra few minutes of cooking.

- **Veggie heaven:** Roast other quick-cooking vegetables, such as asparagus or broccoli spears, French green beans (*haricots verts*), sliced zucchini, or halved baby bok choy along with the fish. Portobello or other types of mushrooms are a tasty addition.

- **Go nuts!** Instead of sesame seeds, use slivered almonds, chopped cashews, walnuts, or pistachios.

DR. ED SAYS:

- **Salmon** has been the fish of choice for many of the recipes in this section, and for good reason. It is one of the best sources of fish Omega-3s among the different species of fish. It is freely available, very popular, and easy to prepare. In addition, it is a great source of vitamin D and vitamin B12, which are deficient in older-age adults and important for the brain. Nevertheless, Norene has offered fish alternatives for those who may get bored with salmon all the time.

- **Mushrooms** are always good to see in a recipe. Aside from providing unique antioxidants not usually found in plants, they are also a significant source of naturally occurring statins for cholesterol control called phytosterols. They are also a good source of fiber and protein.

- **Sesame seeds** are a nutrient-dense ingredient with high fiber, protein, and low digestible carb content. They have high concentrations of B vitamins as well as magnesium, potassium, and zinc, which are important for brain health.

- **Overall,** this recipe is an excellent source of Omega-3 fats, vitamin C, vitamin D, vitamin B6, and vitamin B12. It is also a good source of folate, magnesium, and zinc. The sugar content is somewhat high primarily because of the Asian dressing, which tends to contain larger quantities of sugar, but one can experiment with dressings containing less sugar.

> **DID YOU KNOW?** There at least 25,000–35,000 (depending on the source) species of fish on earth, but only a small fraction are commonly eaten by humans.

SPICY SESAME SALMON

PAREVE | GLUTEN-FREE | REHEATS AND/OR FREEZES WELL | MAKES 10 SERVINGS

1 large salmon fillet (about 3 lb/1.4 kg)

2–3 Tbsp (45 mL) maple syrup or honey

SPICE RUB:

2 cloves garlic (about 2 tsp/10 mL minced)

2 tsp (10 mL) fresh minced ginger (or ½ tsp/2 mL powdered ginger)

1 tsp (5 mL) Kosher or sea salt (to taste)

1 tsp (5 mL) coarsely ground black pepper

2 tsp (10 mL) sweet or smoked paprika

2 tsp (10 mL) crumbled dried cilantro leaves or thyme

2 tsp (10 mL) ground cumin

2 tsp (10 mL) ground cinnamon

2 Tbsp (30 mL) olive oil

2 Tbsp (30 mL) lemon juice (preferably fresh)

¼ cup (60 mL) sesame seeds (for sprinkling on top)

Parsley sprigs, lemon wedges, and cucumber slices (for garnish)

This will definitely rub you the right way! Season a side of salmon with this exotic, aromatic rub, then top with sesame seeds and marinate briefly before roasting. Try this with individual fillets, or even chicken (see Norene's Notes).

1. Line a large baking sheet with foil and spray with nonstick cooking spray.

2. Place salmon on the prepared baking sheet and brush lightly on both sides with maple syrup.

3. **SPICE RUB:** In a small bowl, combine all ingredients except the sesame seeds. Mix well and spread spice evenly over the salmon.

4. Sprinkle sesame seeds on top of the salmon. Marinate for 30 minutes at room temperature, or refrigerate, covered, for 1–2 hours.

5. Preheat oven to 425°F (220°C). Bake, uncovered, for 15–18 minutes. Salmon is done when it just flakes when gently pressed with a fork. Cool slightly.

6. Transfer to a serving platter using a wide spatula. Serve hot or cold. Garnish with parsley, lemon, and cucumber slices.

236 calories per serving, 5 g carbohydrates, 1 g fiber, 3 g sugar, 29 g protein, 11 g fat (2 g saturated), 297 mg sodium, 563 mg potassium

NORENE'S NOTES:

- **Fishful thinking:** Make half the recipe for a small family or multiply it for a large crowd, allowing 6 oz (180 g) fish per person. Individual fillets will take 8–12 minutes to cook, depending on thickness.

- **The daily catch:** This aromatic rub is also excellent for trout, red snapper, orange roughy, or any thick fish fillets. Rub-a-dub-dub!

- **Spicy sesame chicken:** Brush 10 boneless, skinless single chicken breasts with maple syrup, coat with spice rub, and sprinkle with sesame seeds. Cover and refrigerate up to 24 hours. Bake, uncovered, for 20–25 minutes, until firm but springy to the touch.

DR. ED SAYS:

- **Salmon:** Once again, salmon is our fish of choice because it is a poster child for brain nutrition. Other fatty fish, as described in Appendix 1, are also quite suitable. Even non-fatty fish will offer significant benefits.

- **Spices:** This recipe offers a large variety of different spices for brain health. The advantages of this are twofold: (1) Spices are known to have high concentrations of plant antioxidants that help in reducing oxidative stress of the brain, and (2) the variety of spices in this recipe provides a diverse range of antioxidants, which is important because we cannot be sure which antioxidants are the most effective.

- **Overall,** this recipe is a powerful source of Omega-3 fats from the fish and strong antioxidants from the spices. It is also an excellent source of vitamin D, vitamins B6 and B12, and a good source of vitamin E, magnesium, and zinc.

DID YOU KNOW? Although it is relatively well known that Omega-3 fats from fish are important for brain maintenance and for keeping triglyceride levels low for heart health, it has also been discovered that they can improve the symptoms of depression.

STEAK-SPICED PLANKED SALMON

PAREVE | GLUTEN-FREE | REHEATS AND/OR FREEZES WELL |
MAKES 6 SERVINGS

One 8- × 12-inch (20 × 30 cm) or larger untreated cedar plank (about 1 inch/2.5 cm thick)

6 salmon fillets, with skin (6–8 oz/180–235 g each)

2 Tbsp (30 mL) lemon juice (preferably fresh)

1 Tbsp (15 mL) extra virgin olive oil

1–2 Tbsp (15–30 mL) Montreal steak spices (to taste)

2 tsp (10 mL) dried basil

Lemon slices (for garnish)

Feeling "board" with the same old salmon? Try this technique and everyone will be saying "planks" for the memories!

1. Soak cedar plank in cold water for about 1 hour before grilling. (To keep the plank submerged, place a couple of unopened cans or other heavy objects on top of it.)

2. Season salmon fillets with lemon juice, olive oil, steak spices, and basil.

3. Remove soaked plank from water and shake well to remove any excess water. Heat plank on grill over indirect heat until hot, about 6–8 minutes.

4. Place salmon fillets, skin side down, on the preheated plank (careful, it will be very hot!). Grill for about 7–8 minutes. Turn salmon over and grill on the other side for 2–3 minutes longer. Keep lid closed for even cooking.

5. When done, carefully remove hot plank from grill and place on a heatproof surface. Slide a flexible wide spatula between the skin and flesh of the fillets, then transfer to a serving platter.

6. Garnish with lemon slices and serve hot or cold.

238 calories per serving, <1 g carbohydrates, trace fiber, trace sugar, 35 g protein, 10 g fat (2 g saturated), 128 mg sodium, 634 mg potassium

NORENE'S NOTES:

- **No plank?** Oil grates of the grill and preheat. Season salmon fillets as directed in Step 2, oiling them lightly on both sides to prevent sticking. Place fillets, flesh side down, on grill. Fillets will stick to the grate until they've cooked for about 7–8 minutes. Turn salmon over carefully, using a wide spatula. Grill the second side 2–3 minutes longer, or until fish flakes. (This is known as the 70/30 timing rule, which results in a beautiful presentation with great grill marks.)

- **Spice it up!** Instead of Montreal steak spices, use the coating mix from "Everything but the Bagel" Chicken Breasts (p. 297) or store-bought "Everything but the Bagel" seasoning blend.

- **Is it done yet?** Fish is done if it's opaque yet still moist in the center. It should just flake when gently pressed with a fork. On an instant-read thermometer, the interior temperature should reach 145°F (63°C). If overcooked, fish will become dry.

- **Grate tip:** If you've cooked the fish with its skin on, just slide a flexible metal spatula between the flesh and skin, leaving the skin behind on the cooking grate or pan.

DR. ED SAYS:

- **Salmon** is the major ingredient here without too much extra. Because of this, the recipe is very high in protein and low in carbs and sugar, while providing all the benefits of fatty fish, including high Omega-3s and high vitamin D, B6, and B12.

THYME FOR LIME SALMON

PAREVE | GLUTEN-FREE | PASSOVER | REHEATS AND/OR FREEZES
WELL | MAKES 4 SERVINGS

4 salmon fillets or steaks
(6–8 oz/180–235 g each)

Salt and freshly ground
black pepper

1–2 tsp (5–10 mL) minced fresh
thyme (or 1 tsp/5 mL dried)

Juice of 1 lime (about
2 Tbsp/30 mL)

1 Tbsp (15 mL) extra virgin
olive oil

2 tsp (10 mL) honey

This takes very little time to prepare and tastes terrific. I love to use fresh lime juice because of its light, vibrant flavor, but you can easily substitute bottled juice. Did you know that limes don't contain any seeds? The pit stops here!

1. Preheat oven to 425°F (220°C). Line a baking sheet with foil and spray with nonstick cooking spray.

2. Place salmon, skin side down, on the prepared baking sheet. Sprinkle with salt, pepper, and thyme. In a small bowl, whisk together lime juice, oil, and honey. Drizzle over salmon and use back of a spoon to evenly spread the mixture.

3. Bake, uncovered, for 10–12 minutes, until fish just flakes when gently pressed with a fork. Serve hot or cold.

259 calories per serving, 4 g carbohydrates, 0 g fiber, 3 g sugar, 35 g protein, 11 g fat (2 g saturated), 128 mg sodium, 635 mg potassium

NORENE'S NOTES:

- **The daily catch:** This is also delicious with rainbow trout, Arctic char, halibut, or black cod (sablefish).

- **Variations:** Instead of lime and thyme, use lemon and dill. Instead of honey, use maple syrup. For a spicy kick, sprinkle lightly with red pepper flakes before baking.

- **Cindy's sheet pan dinner:** Cut 1 bunch asparagus into 2-inch (5 cm) pieces. Cut 12–16 parboiled baby new potatoes in quarters. Place vegetables and salmon on a large baking sheet. Use double the amount of seasonings, lime juice, oil, and honey to coat both the salmon and the vegetables. Bake as directed in Step 3. Thanks to Cindy Beer for this terrific time-saving tip!

- **Salmon:** Similar to Steak-Spiced Planked Salmon (p. 264), the brain-healthy nutrients all come primarily from the salmon because the other ingredients are used in relatively small quantities. However, we do get some antioxidants from the thyme, pepper, and olive oil.

DID YOU KNOW? Before modern refrigeration and shipping techniques, fish tended to have off-flavors because the fat oxidized during the long transit times from catch to table. To overcome this, people would squeeze lemon or lime juice on fish, a tradition that has endured despite the fact that most fish are now fresh and mild-tasting.

APRICOT-GLAZED RAINBOW TROUT

PAREVE | GLUTEN-FREE | PASSOVER OPTION | REHEATS AND/OR
FREEZES WELL | MAKES 4 SERVINGS

4 rainbow trout fillets (about
5 oz/150 g each)

1 Tbsp (15 mL) Dijon mustard

2 Tbsp (30 mL) apricot jam
(low-sugar or all-fruit)

1 tsp (5 mL) dried basil or thyme
or 1 Tbsp (15 mL) chopped fresh

Salt and freshly ground
black pepper

Paprika

It doesn't get much easier or better than this! If you're in a jam and out
of apricot jam, substitute with marmalade, peach, or mango jam, or
preserves.

1. Preheat oven to 425°F (220°C). Line a rimmed baking sheet with foil
and spray with nonstick cooking spray.

2. Arrange fillets in a single layer on the prepared baking sheet. In a
small bowl, combine mustard, jam, and basil; mix well. Spread evenly
overtop of the fish. Sprinkle with salt, pepper, and paprika. Let stand
for 20 minutes.

3. Bake, uncovered, for 10–12 minutes, until fillets are glazed and
cooked through. Fish is done when it just flakes when gently pressed
with a fork. Serve hot or cold.

217 calories per serving, 3 g carbohydrates, 0 g fiber, 3 g sugar, 28 g
protein, 9 g fat (2 g saturated), 162 mg sodium, 539 mg potassium

NORENE'S NOTES:

- **Meal deal:** Oven-Roasted Asparagus (p. 441) makes an excellent
  accompaniment and can be roasted in the oven with the rainbow
  trout at the same time.

- **Passover option:** Instead of mustard and apricot jam, substitute
  3 Tbsp (45 mL) jarred Passover sweet & sour duck sauce.

- **Rainbow trout** does not have quite as high an Omega-3 content as salmon, which exceeds 1000 mg per 3-oz serving, but is still excellent at slightly less than 1000 mg per 3-oz serving. It also has a similar nutritional profile to salmon for the important brain nutrients vitamins D, E, B6, and B12. Magnesium and zinc are also quite acceptable. All in all, rainbow trout is a suitable substitute, nutritionally, for salmon.

DID YOU KNOW? Compared to similarly sized vertebrates such as birds or mammals, fish have about 1/15th the brain mass.

SNAPPER BALSAMICO WITH GRAPE TOMATOES & MUSHROOMS

PAREVE | GLUTEN-FREE | PASSOVER | DO NOT FREEZE | MAKES
6 SERVINGS

6 red snapper fillets (about
8 oz/235 g each)

1 container (1 pint/550 mL) grape
or cherry tomatoes (about
2 cups/500 mL)

½ lb (250 g) mushrooms, coarsely
chopped (about 2½ cups/625 mL)

6–8 cloves garlic, peeled
and sliced

1 tsp (5 mL) dried thyme
(or 1 Tbsp/15 mL fresh)

Salt and freshly ground
black pepper

2 Tbsp (30 mL) chopped fresh
basil (for garnish)

MARINADE:

¼ cup (60 mL) balsamic vinegar

2 Tbsp (30 mL) olive oil

1–2 Tbsp (15–30 mL) honey or
maple syrup

1 Tbsp (15 mL) lemon juice
(preferably fresh)

These snapper fillets are so scrumptious they'll get snapped up in a minute! Cooking the fish and vegetables together in one pan saves time and cleanup. This potassium-packed dish is also delicious made with whitefish, sole, pickerel, or any mild-flavored fish fillet.

1. Line a large baking sheet with foil and spray with nonstick cooking spray.

2. Arrange fillets in a single layer on the prepared baking sheet. Scatter tomatoes, mushrooms, and garlic around the fish. Season with thyme, salt, and pepper to taste.

3. MARINADE: In a glass measure, combine vinegar, oil, honey, and lemon juice; mix well. Drizzle mixture over the fish and vegetables until all are well coated. Marinate for 30–60 minutes.

4. Preheat oven to 425°F (220°C). Bake fish and vegetables, uncovered, for 12–15 minutes. Fish is done when it just flakes when gently pressed with a fork. Garnish with basil and serve immediately.

310 calories per serving, 10 g carbohydrates, 1 g fiber, 6 g sugar, 48 g protein, 8 g fat (1 g saturated), 153 mg sodium, 1282 mg potassium

NORENE'S NOTES:

- **What's in store:** Red snapper gets its name because of its reddish-pink skin and flesh, as well as its red eyes. It has a mild, sweet flavor, and its flesh is tender, firm, moist, and lean.

- **Cook it right:** Red snapper is delicious broiled, baked, grilled, poached, steamed, or pan-fried. Try it seasoned with pungent Cajun spices or with a delicate lemon, olive oil, and herb marinade. Red snapper's mild flavor matches well with mango, pineapple, or tomato and herb salsa.

- **Red snapper** is in the group of fish that is lowest in Omega-3 content. At less than 500 mg per 3-oz serving, one would have to consume about 4–5 times the weight of this fish as compared to salmon or rainbow trout to get the same content of Omega-3s. However, the larger portion sizes in this recipe tend to compensate for the lower Omega-3s. The high content of brain-healthy nutrients, vitamins E, D, B6, and B12, and magnesium and zinc, is in the same quantity as salmon and rainbow trout.

- **Mushrooms** are advantageous in brain-healthy recipes because of their unique antioxidant profile and contribution of phytosterols to control cholesterol. As an added bonus, they contain fiber and protein.

- **Garlic** is an excellent source of vitamin B6, vitamin C, and antioxidants.

- **Overall,** this recipe is very similar in brain-healthy nutrients to the other fish recipes.

> DID YOU KNOW? People who consume fish regularly, even fish with low Omega-3 content, have shown improved cognitive benefits as compared with those who consume low quantities of fish. This indicates that there may be components in the fish aside from the Omega-3 fats that help reduce the risk of AD/dementia and help preserve memory.

FISH FILLETS FLORENTINE

PAREVE | GLUTEN-FREE OPTION | PASSOVER OPTION | DO NOT FREEZE | MAKES 8 SERVINGS

SPINACH STUFFING:

1 Tbsp (15 mL) olive oil

½ Spanish onion, diced

1 red or yellow bell pepper, diced

2 cloves garlic (about 2 tsp/10 mL minced)

1 pkg (10 oz/300 g) frozen chopped spinach, thawed and squeezed dry

Salt and freshly ground black pepper

¼ cup (60 mL) chopped fresh parsley

1 tsp (5 mL) dried basil or thyme

TOPPING:

½ cup (125 mL) seasoned panko crumbs (see Norene's Notes)

1 Tbsp (15 mL) olive oil

FISH:

8 sole or pickerel fillets (about 6 oz/180 g each)

Salt and freshly ground black pepper

1 tsp (5 mL) dried basil or thyme

Heart and 'sole' I fell in love with you! Whether you make fish "sandwiches" or roll-ups, this brain-boosting dish is sure to please. This dish multiplies easily, so it's great if you're expecting company.

---

1. **SPINACH STUFFING:** In a large nonstick skillet, heat oil on medium. Add onion, bell pepper, and garlic and sauté for 5 minutes, until softened. Stir in spinach and cook 2–3 minutes longer, until most of the moisture disappears. Sprinkle lightly with salt and pepper; stir in parsley and basil.

2. **TOPPING:** Combine panko crumbs and oil in a small bowl; mixture should resemble wet sand.

3. Preheat oven to 375°F (190°C). Spray an oven-to-table baking dish with nonstick cooking spray.

4. **FISH:** Lightly season fish with salt and pepper; sprinkle with basil. Arrange half the fillets in a single layer in the prepared baking dish. Top each fillet with 3–4 Tbsp (45–60 mL) spinach filling. Place the remaining fillets on top, making 4 "sandwiches." Cut in half crosswise, making 8 "sandwiches." Sprinkle with topping. (Can be assembled in advance and refrigerated for a few hours. Remove from refrigerator while oven is preheating.)

5. Bake, uncovered, for 25–30 minutes, until golden. Serve immediately.

214 calories per serving, 7 g carbohydrates, 2 g fiber, 1 g sugar, 28 g protein, 8 g fat (1 g saturated), 654 mg sodium, 517 mg potassium

NORENE'S NOTES:

- **Gluten-free/passover option:** Both matzo meal and panko crumbs are available in gluten-free form, as well as for Passover.

- **Fish roll-ups:** In Step 4, lightly sprinkle fish with salt, pepper, and basil. Spread each fillet with about 2 Tbsp (30 mL) spinach stuffing. Roll up and place seam side down in the prepared baking dish. Sprinkle with topping and bake as directed above.

- **Sole,** as well as pickerel, is low in fat, and therefore has a low Omega-3 content, below 500 mg per 3-oz serving. However, like Snapper Balsamico (p. 270), the larger serving compensates somewhat for this, resulting in an acceptable Omega-3 content. The low fat, combined with the addition of other ingredients, results in about a quarter to a third of the nutrient intake per serving for vitamin D as compared with fish containing higher fat and Omega-3 content. Vitamins B6 and B12 are also significantly lower per serving.

- **Spinach stuffing:** Spinach is one of the best foods for brain health because of its high content of antioxidants (especially lutein and zeaxanthin), folate, magnesium, and vitamin E. And because it is a leafy vegetable, it acts synergistically to enhance the beneficial effects of the Omega-3s on the brain.

- **Overall,** this recipe is lower in Omega-3, vitamin D, and vitamins B12 and B6 than the other fish recipes, but is still quite acceptable. Also, due to the folate content of the spinach, it is higher in this component than most of the other fish recipes.

DID YOU KNOW? Fish do not produce their own Omega-3 fatty acids but need to get it from their diet. The Omega-3s actually originate in algae and phytoplankton, and work their way up the fish food chain.

FISH FILLETS IN PARCHMENT

PAREVE | GLUTEN-FREE | PASSOVER | REHEATS AND/OR FREEZES
WELL | MAKES 2 SERVINGS

2 sole, whitefish, or pickerel fillets
(about 6 oz/180 g each)

2 tsp (10 mL) extra virgin olive oil

2 tsp (10 mL) lemon or lime juice
(preferably fresh)

1 clove garlic (about 1 tsp/
5 mL minced)

Salt and freshly ground
black pepper

Paprika to taste

2 tsp (10 mL) minced fresh
basil, dill, or thyme (or ½ tsp/
2 mL dried)

Whether you're cooking for two or a crowd, this dish is true "wrap-ture!" Cooking in parchment paper saves on cleanup. If you don't have parchment paper, wrap fish in foil—foiled again!

1. Preheat oven to 400°F (200°C). Cut 2 large squares of parchment paper. Place a fish fillet in the center of each piece of parchment.

2. In a small bowl, whisk together oil and lemon juice. Drizzle each fillet with the oil/lemon mixture. Sprinkle with garlic and seasonings, coating fish on both sides.

3. Seal parchment paper packets by folding up the top, bottom, and sides; crimp edges closed with your fingers. Place packets on a baking sheet and let marinate for 15 minutes.

4. Bake for 10 minutes. Place each packet on a dinner plate and cut open at the table. Be careful not to scald yourself when the hot steam escapes once the packets are opened. Serve immediately.

272 calories per serving, 1 g carbohydrates, 0 g fiber, trace sugar, 33 g protein, 15 g fat (2 g saturated), 87 mg sodium, 553 mg potassium

NORENE'S NOTES:

- **Microwave magic:** Instead of baking, microwave parchment paper packets on high power for 3½-4 minutes.

- **Fish and vegetables in parchment:** Season fillets as directed in Step 2. Top each fillet with broccoli or cauliflower florets, cherry tomatoes, chopped red bell pepper, sliced mushrooms, green onions, or zucchini. Sprinkle with a little white wine or salsa, then seal packets. Either bake at 400°F (200°C) for 12-15 minutes or microwave on high for 5 minutes.

DR. ED SAYS:

- **Fish:** If you want the maximum content of Omega-3s choose white-fish, as pickerel and sole are in the grouping of fish with the lowest content of Omega-3s. Nevertheless, the amount of Omega-3 per serving is still reasonable in the lower-fat sole and pickerel, at 500 mg per serving (about half the level of the whitefish). This is because the serving sizes are higher than the typical 3 oz (90 g).

- **Antioxidants:** Basil, thyme, dill, pepper, and paprika provide an assortment of antioxidants, but keep in mind that basil provides the highest concentration of antioxidants per unit weight. Olive oil, which is a mainstay of the Mediterranean diet, also provides essential anti-oxidants and oils.

- **Overall,** this recipe is reasonable but provides significantly less Ome-ga-3s and essential B vitamins than fattier fish such as salmon and rainbow trout.

SOLE, MEDITERRANEAN STYLE

PAREVE | GLUTEN-FREE | PASSOVER | DO NOT FREEZE | MAKES
6–8 SERVINGS

This company-worthy dish comes together very quickly to make a heart-healthy meal. The fish is topped with a garden-fresh tomato salsa that tastes like a trip to the Mediterranean!

SALSA:

2 cloves garlic

3 medium Roma (plum) tomatoes, quartered

3 green onions, cut into chunks

1 yellow or orange bell pepper, cut into chunks

¼ cup (60 mL) fresh basil (or 1 tsp/5 mL dried)

1 Tbsp (15 mL) lemon juice (preferably fresh)

1 Tbsp (15 mL) extra virgin olive oil

Salt and freshly ground black pepper

FISH:

6–8 sole, pickerel, or whitefish fillets (about 6 oz/180 g each; see Norene's Notes)

2 cloves garlic, minced

Salt and freshly ground black pepper

2 Tbsp (30 mL) lemon juice (preferably fresh)

2 Tbsp (30 mL) olive oil

⅓ cup (80 mL) pitted, sliced black olives

2 Tbsp (30 mL) capers, rinsed and drained (optional)

---

1. **SALSA:** In a food processor fitted with the steel blade, drop garlic through the feed tube while the machine is running; process until minced. Add tomatoes, green onions, bell pepper, and basil; process with quick on/off pulses until coarsely chopped. Add lemon juice, oil, salt, and pepper. Transfer to a serving bowl.

2. **FISH:** Preheat oven to 425°F (220°C). Coat a large, rimmed baking sheet with nonstick cooking spray.

3. Arrange fillets in a single layer on the prepared baking sheet. Season with garlic, salt, and pepper. Drizzle with lemon juice and olive oil, coating the fish on both sides. Let marinate for 10 minutes.

4. Bake, uncovered, for 8–10 minutes, until fish flakes when lightly pressed with a fork.

5. Spoon salsa over fillets and sprinkle with olives and capers, if using.

209 calories per serving, 5 g carbohydrates, 1 g fiber, 1 g sugar, 22 g protein, 11 g fat (2 g saturated), 544 mg sodium, 453 mg potassium

NORENE'S NOTES:

- **Be prepared:** Salsa can be prepared in advance and refrigerated, covered, up to 1 day. Just bring it to room temperature before serving.

- **Sheet pan dinner:** In Step 3, scatter 2 cups (500 mL) sliced mushrooms, zucchini, and/or asparagus spears around the fish. Sprinkle vegetables with salt and pepper, then drizzle lightly with olive oil and lemon juice. Bake as directed.

- **Salmon, mediterranean style:** Instead of sole, use 6–8 individual salmon fillets or 1 large salmon fillet (about 3 lb/1.4 kg). Prepare Salsa as directed and spread evenly over the seasoned salmon; marinate for 30–60 minutes. Individual fillets take about 10–12 minutes to bake and a large fillet takes about 15 minutes.

- **Fish:** Similar to Fish Fillets in Parchment (p. 274), you may want to choose the whitefish for maximum Omega-3 and vitamin D content. Choosing other varieties of fish will still give you good amounts of Omega-3s and B vitamins, but less than fattier fish.

- **Salsa:** The main contributors to the salsa are tomatoes, basil, and bell peppers, which supply a good quantity and variety of antioxidants, including lycopene, as well as excellent amounts of vitamin C and fiber. The salsa also provides good amounts of magnesium, zinc, and folate.

> **DID YOU KNOW?** There are Antarctic fish that can live in water below the freezing point because there is an antifreeze chemical in their blood to prevent them from freezing.

BLACK COD WITH TINY ROASTED TOMATOES

PAREVE | GLUTEN-FREE | PASSOVER | DO NOT FREEZE | MAKES
4 SERVINGS

TINY ROASTED TOMATOES:

4 cups (1 L) (about 2 pints)
cherry or grape tomatoes (remove
any stem ends)

2 cloves garlic (about 1 tsp/
5 mL minced)

Salt and freshly ground
black pepper

2 Tbsp (30 mL) olive oil

FISH:

4 black cod fillets
(5 oz/150 g each)

Salt and freshly ground
black pepper

2 cloves garlic (about 1 tsp/
5 mL minced)

2 Tbsp (30 mL) chopped fresh
basil + extra for garnish

One oven, two pans—this easy and elegant meal is excellent for entertaining. You won't have to fish for compliments!

1. Preheat oven to 400°F (200°C). Place an oven rack in the lower third
of the oven and a second rack in the middle of the oven.

2. **TINY ROASTED TOMATOES:** Line a rimmed baking sheet with parchment paper. Add tomatoes and sprinkle with garlic, salt, and pepper.
Drizzle with olive oil and, using your hands, mix well, coating tomatoes
on all sides. Spread out evenly and roast, uncovered, in the lower third
of the oven for 6–8 minutes.

3. **FISH:** Meanwhile, coat a 9- × 13-inch (23 × 33 cm) glass baking dish
with nonstick cooking spray. Place fish in the prepared dish and sprinkle lightly with salt and pepper. Top with garlic and basil.

4. Place fish on the middle rack of the oven and bake, along with the
tomatoes, for an additional 10–12 minutes. When done, fish will flake
when gently pressed with a fork and tomatoes will be tender.

5. Spoon roasted tomatoes over fish and garnish with additional basil.
Serve hot or at room temperature.

368 calories per serving, 7 g carbohydrates, 2 g fiber, 4 g sugar, 21 g
protein, 29 g fat (6 g saturated), 88 mg sodium, 877 mg potassium

NORENE'S NOTES:

· **Black cod,** also known as sablefish, has a delicate, silky texture and a
rich, buttery flavor, which is why it is sometimes called butterfish. It's
delicious poached, baked, or grilled, and goes well with Asian flavors.

· **Halibut with tiny roasted tomatoes:** For a different twist, use halibut
fillets instead of black cod. Chilean sea bass also makes a scrumptious substitution.

· **Meal deal:** For a delicious, nutritious dinner, serve with steamed cauliflower or broccoli florets.

RECIPE CONTINUED . . .

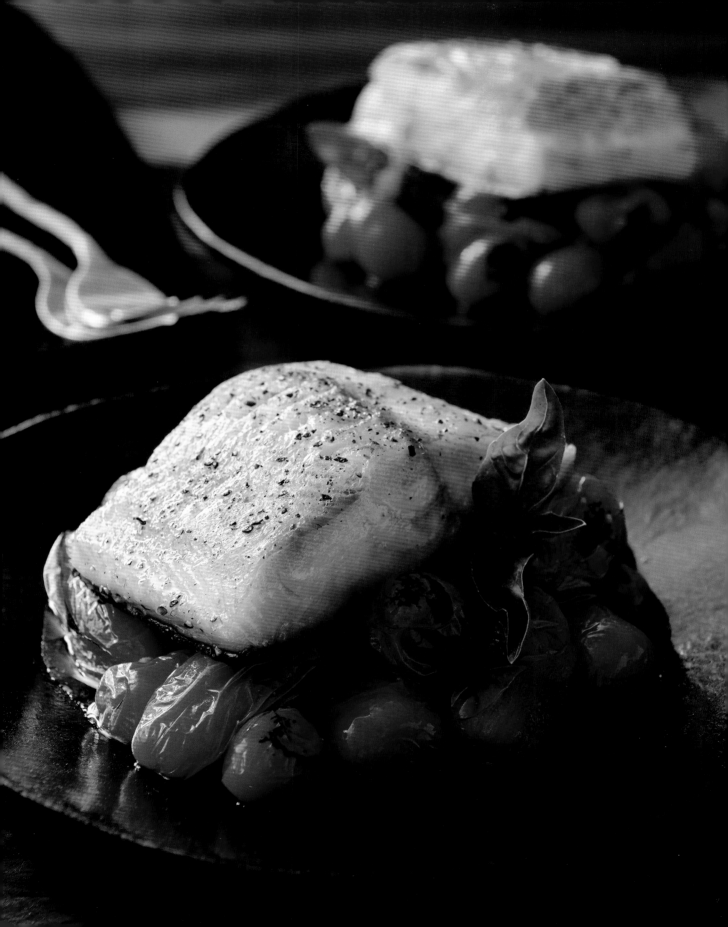

BLACK COD WITH TINY ROASTED TOMATOES (continued)

DR. ED SAYS:

- **Black cod** is a fish with one of the highest Omega-3 concentrations available, at an average of 1.4 g per serving. Compared with halibut, at less than 500 mg per serving, it's a no-brainer to choose black cod.

- **Tomatoes,** the other major component of this recipe, are primarily known for their high content of carotenoid antioxidants, especially lycopene. They also provide excellent amounts of vitamin C and good amounts of fiber, potassium, and zinc.

- **Overall,** black cod makes this recipe an excellent source of Omega-3 fat, as well as vitamin D and vitamin B12.

> DID YOU KNOW? Because of their long lives in deep cold waters, black cod store much of their fat in the form of Omega-3s. They have the highest Omega-3 content of any white fish—even higher than many species of salmon.

PESTO HALIBUT WITH PISTACHIOS

PAREVE | PASSOVER | DO NOT FREEZE | MAKES 4 SERVINGS

Everyone will "go nuts" over this easy, elegant dish. If you're expecting guests, you can double or triple the recipe easily. To switch it up, make either black cod with pesto or pesto salmon (see Norene's Notes).

4 halibut fillets (6–8 oz/ 180–235 g each)

¼ cup (60 mL) Power Pesto (p. 492)

Salt and freshly ground black pepper

½ cup (125 mL) shelled pistachios, coarsely chopped

1. Preheat oven to 425°F (220°C). Line a baking sheet with parchment paper.

2. Arrange fish fillets in a single layer on the prepared baking sheet. Spread about 1 Tbsp (15 mL) pesto evenly on top of each fillet. Sprinkle with salt, pepper, and pistachios.

3. Bake, uncovered, for 10–12 minutes, or until fish flakes when gently pressed with a fork. Serve hot or cold.

315 calories per serving, 5 g carbohydrates, 1 g sugar, 2 g fiber, 35 g protein, 17 g fat (2 g saturated), 155 mg sodium, 923 mg potassium

NORENE'S NOTES:

- **Black cod with pesto:** Black cod (also known as sablefish), with its silky, buttery texture, is an excellent substitute for halibut. You can also use Chilean sea bass. Instead of pistachios, sprinkle with sesame seeds.

- **Pesto salmon:** Substitute salmon fillets for halibut. Instead of pistachios, sprinkle fillets with grated Parmesan cheese or slivered almonds, using 1 Tbsp (15 mL) per fillet.

- **Leftovers?** Use leftover cooked fish to make the Fast Fish Salad (p. 282). It's a fabulous filling for tortilla wraps—just add baby spinach leaves and roasted red bell pepper strips. Pure wrap-ture!

DR. ED SAYS:

- **Pesto** is a rich source of vitamin E and carotenoid antioxidants, especially lutein and zeaxanthin.

- **Pistachios:** It's always good to see a nutritionally dense nut ingredient in a recipe. Pistachios are an excellent source of fiber, good fats, potassium, magnesium, zinc, vitamin B6, and a variety of antioxidants including lutein and zeaxanthin.

- **Overall,** this is a great recipe, supplying reasonable levels of Omega-3, along with excellent levels of vitamins E, D, B6, and B12, as well as good levels of folate, magnesium, and zinc.

FAST FISH SALAD

PAREVE | GLUTEN-FREE | PASSOVER | DO NOT FREEZE | MAKES
4 SERVINGS

2 green onions, trimmed

1 stalk celery

1 small carrot, peeled and
trimmed

2–3 radishes, trimmed

2 Tbsp (30 mL) fresh dill

2 cups (500 mL) leftover cooked
fish (skin and bones removed)

¼ cup (60 mL) light mayonnaise
(approx.)

Salt and freshly ground
black pepper

This is a terrific way to use up any leftover cooked fish like halibut, salmon, sole, or whitefish. It's delicious on top of salad greens, in wraps, or as a stuffing for hollowed-out tomatoes or peppers. If you don't have enough fish, add one or two hard-boiled eggs to the mixture.

1. In a food processor fitted with the steel blade, process green onions, celery, carrot, radishes, and dill for 8–10 seconds, until minced.

2. Add fish and mayonnaise. Process with quick on/off pulses, until combined. Season with salt and pepper to taste.

3. Transfer mixture to a bowl, cover, and refrigerate. Serve chilled.

184 calories per serving, 10 g carbohydrates, 3 g fiber, 6 g sugar, 21 g protein, 7 g fat (1 g saturated), 218 mg sodium, 929 mg potassium

NORENE'S NOTES:

· **Quick crab salad:** Substitute 1 lb (500 g) flaked surimi (imitation crab) for fish. Add ½ cup (125 mL) chopped red bell pepper, 2 Tbsp (30 mL) lemon juice, and 4–6 drops of hot pepper sauce or Sriracha.

· **Quickie chicken salad:** Substitute 2 cups (500 mL) cooked chicken for fish. Replace radishes with ½ cup (125 mL) each chopped celery and red bell pepper.

DR. ED SAYS:

· **Fish:** Because this recipe can be made with either fish or chicken, it is difficult to calculate the Omega-3 contribution. On average, it should still work out to at least 300 mg per serving, which is low but not unreasonable.

· **Vegetables:** A variety of vegetables are added, which help boost the folate, magnesium, and zinc content.

- **Overall,** although not providing as high a concentration of brain-healthy nutrients as the previous recipes in this section, there are still reasonable amounts of essential brain nutrients.

DID YOU KNOW? Although we have been highlighting the benefit of Omega-3s for brain health, these nutrients are also important in preventing and alleviating other chronic diseases. The body needs a dietary source of two essential groups of unsaturated fats—Omega-3s and Omega-6s—for proper functioning, and these need to be in balance. Unfortunately, while we take in plenty of Omega-6s in the form of linoleic acid (found in most vegetable oils), we don't get enough Omega-3s (found in fish in their most efficient form), which help in controlling inflammation.

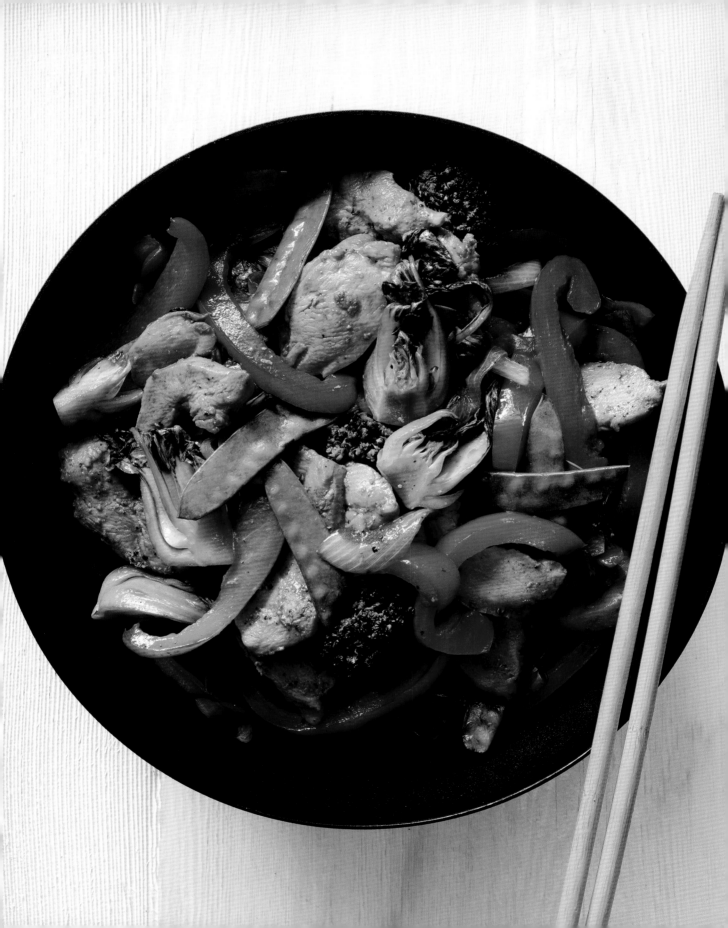

MARVELOUS MAINS: POULTRY & MEAT

CHICK-INFORMATION!

THE SKINNY ON SKIN: Cooking chicken with the skin on keeps it moist and prevents it from drying out. Remove the skin at serving time to reduce calorie and fat content.

SKINNY SECRETS: When cooking chicken in a sauce, remove the skin before cooking if you plan to serve it immediately—otherwise, the fat from the skin will melt and drain into the sauce. However, if you plan to serve it the next day, cook it with the skin on, then refrigerate it overnight. Discard congealed fat before reheating and remove skin before eating.

TO COVER OR NOT TO COVER? Skinless chicken on the bone should be cooked covered to prevent it from drying out. Uncover during the last 20–30 minutes, to thicken any pan juices, and baste occasionally. If the skin is on you can either cook it covered or uncovered—your choice.

NO BONES ABOUT IT: Boneless, skinless single chicken breasts that have been marinated should be cooked uncovered at 400°F (200°C) for 20–25 minutes, until juices run clear. If grilling, allow 4–6 minutes per side on medium-high, until grill marks appear and juices run clear.

FROZEN ASSETS: Marinate several batches of raw chicken in resealable freezer bags and freeze uncooked. When needed, thaw in the refrigerator overnight; cook as directed.

LEFTOVERS? Chilled leftover breasts can be thinly sliced against the grain and added to salads or used in wraps, whole grain pita pockets, or tacos. Add veggies and leafy greens to increase your intake of brain-boosting antioxidants.

HOW LONG WILL IT KEEP? Uncooked poultry is safe in the refrigerator for 1–2 days and safe in the freezer for 9 months in pieces (or up to 12 months for a whole chicken or turkey). Cooked poultry is safe in the refrigerator for 3–4 days or for 3–4 months in the freezer. Refrigerate or freeze cooked poultry as soon as possible after cooking or serving. Reheat to 165°F (74°C), until piping hot.

SALT ALERT: If sodium intake is a concern, soak kosher raw poultry in cold water up to 2 hours, changing the water every half hour. Most of the salt is in the skin, so removing it helps to reduce sodium levels.

GROUNDS FOR CONCERN: Kosher ground chicken contains more salt than kosher ground turkey. A pound of ground chicken contains about ¼ tsp (1 mL per 500 mg) sodium, whereas a pound of ground turkey contains about ⅛ tsp (0.5 mL per 250 mg).

TURKEY TALK!

TURKEY TIME: Calculate 20–25 minutes per pound at 350°F (175°C) for turkey breast, bone-in, with or without skin.

NO BONES ABOUT IT: Calculate 25–30 minutes per pound at 350°F (175°C) for either rolled turkey breast or boneless, skinless turkey breast.

TEST FOR DONENESS: When done, juices will run clear when turkey is pierced with a fork. A meat thermometer inserted into the thickest part of a turkey should register an internal temperature of 165°F (74°C) after turkey has rested for 15 minutes.

LEFTOVERS? Combine leftover turkey with chopped vegetables and whole grain pasta or grains for a quick meal. Or use it in soups, wraps, or stir-fries. They'll gobble it up!

WHAT'S YOUR BEEF?

REDUCE THE RED: Limit your intake of red meat, especially processed meats. Save beef recipes for special occasions. Our dietician, Sharon Abramovitch, suggests limiting red meat to twice a month, or maximum once a week. When possible, replace beef with lean cuts of poultry.

LEANER CUISINE: Be a savvy buyer and check the nutrition label when shopping. Choose leaner cuts of beef (e.g., flank steak/London broil, extra lean ground beef). Remember, meats with a higher percentage of fat will shrink more when cooked. When making fattier dishes such as briskets, stews, or spaghetti sauce, make them a day in advance. Refrigerate overnight, then lift off and discard congealed fat before reheating.

SIZE COUNTS: Reduce portion sizes of meats by cutting them into thin slices or pieces and cooking them with hearty helpings of vegetables in stir-fries, stews, and chili. Add grated vegetables such as zucchini, onions, carrots, squash, or mashed beans to replace a portion of the ground meat in recipes.

THE DAILY GRIND: When buying ground beef, choose the lowest percentage of fat—10% or lower.

SWITCH A-GROUND: You can use lean ground turkey, chicken, or veal in any recipe calling for ground beef. Ground turkey breast is a leaner choice than ground turkey, which often includes dark meat and has an average fat content of 8%. If you don't want to switch meat types entirely, mix lean ground turkey/chicken with veal or extra-lean beef.

CLEAN CUISINE: Always wash your hands when handling raw meat or poultry. Use separate dishes and utensils for raw and cooked meat or poultry.

SAFE STORAGE: Use or freeze raw ground meat within 1–2 days of purchase.

THAW IT RIGHT: Ground meat or poultry will take approximately 6 hours per pound to thaw in the refrigerator. It's not recommended to thaw it on the counter. You can also defrost it in the microwave—check your manual for times. Once thawed, cook as soon as possible.

SALT ALERT: Kosher meat has already been salted, so take this into account when adding seasonings.

POMEGRANATE CHICKEN

MEAT | GLUTEN-FREE | PASSOVER | REHEATS AND/OR FREEZES
WELL | MAKES 12 SERVINGS

This fragrant dish contains honey, carrots, and pomegranate—traditional foods served with hope for a sweet and fruitful New Year. This popular recipe comes from *Norene's Healthy Kitchen*, now out of print. According to ancient lore, the number of seeds in the pomegranate is exactly the same number (613) as the mitzvot (good deeds) found in the Torah (Jewish Bible). If you're curious, count away!

---

1. Spray a large roasting pan with nonstick cooking spray. Scatter onions and carrots in the bottom of pan. Place chicken on top of the vegetables and sprinkle under skin and on top with salt, pepper, thyme, and turmeric, if using. Tuck apricots and prunes between chicken pieces.

2. Whisk marinade ingredients together in a bowl. (If using juice of a whole pomegranate, reserve some seeds for garnish.) Pour over the chicken and sprinkle with paprika. Marinate, covered in the refrigerator, for at least 1 hour or up to 24 hours.

3. Preheat oven to 350°F (175°C). Cook chicken, covered, for 1½ hours or until tender. Uncover and cook for 30 minutes longer, basting occasionally, until golden.

4. Transfer to a large serving platter and sprinkle pomegranate seeds overtop. Remove chicken skin before eating.

433 calories per serving, 24 g carbohydrates, 17 g sugar, 3 g fiber, 58 g protein, 11 g fat (3 g saturated), 227 mg sodium, 947 mg potassium

NORENE'S NOTES:

- **Do-ahead:** Follow Steps 1–3. Let chicken cool, then refrigerate. About 30 minutes before serving, remove and discard any congealed fat from the chicken. Reheat, covered, for 25–30 minutes at 350°F (175°C). Garnish with pomegranate seeds.

- **Good to know:** One pomegranate contains about ¾ cup (185 mL) seeds and yields ½ cup (125 mL) juice.

RECIPE CONTINUED . . .

2 medium onions, sliced

2 cups (500 mL) baby carrots (or 2 cups/500 mL sliced medium carrots)

2 whole chickens (3.5 lb/1.6 kg each), cut into pieces

Kosher salt and freshly ground black pepper

1 tsp (5 mL) dried thyme

½ tsp (2 mL) turmeric (optional)

1 cup (250 mL) dried whole apricots, loosely packed

1 cup (250 mL) pitted dried prunes, loosely packed

2 tsp (10 mL) sweet paprika

MARINADE:

½ cup (125 mL) pomegranate juice (or juice of 1 pomegranate)

2 cloves garlic (about 2 tsp/ 10 mL minced)

Juice and rind of 1 lemon

⅓ cup (80 mL) balsamic vinegar

2 Tbsp (30 mL) extra virgin olive oil

2 Tbsp (30 mL) honey

POMEGRANATE CHICKEN (continued)

- **No pomegranates?** Substitute with bottled pomegranate or cranberry juice, or even red wine (e.g., Cabernet Sauvignon). If desired, garnish chicken with toasted pumpkin or sesame seeds (but not during Passover).

DR. ED SAYS:

- **Chicken,** as a meat protein, is in the upper tier of quality proteins. The main dishes featured in this chapter provide needed protein for the body and this recipe doesn't disappoint, with 58 g protein per serving. (The recommended daily intake for a 2000 calories per day diet is 60 g).

- **Overall,** aside from the protein, the tasty accoutrements of this low-sodium recipe provide a good serving of needed antioxidants (especially carotenoids), fiber, magnesium, folate, and potassium. The dried prunes and apricots are a double-edged sword, with high antioxidants and fiber, but also very high sugar levels (so for those who are trying to cut back on sugar, you may want to cut back on the dried fruit).

DID YOU KNOW? Not all proteins are the same, with some being better than others based on composition and digestibility.

GRILLED MOROCCAN CHICKEN

MEAT | GLUTEN-FREE | REHEATS AND/OR FREEZES WELL | MAKES
6 SERVINGS

Grill-y delicious! Use your outdoor grill in the summertime or an electric indoor grill the rest of the year. Quinoa Tabbouleh (p. 414) and
grilled vegetables make great accompaniments.

1. Lightly sprinkle chicken with salt and pepper and place in a resealable plastic bag.

2. In a small bowl, combine garlic, mint, thyme, cumin, paprika, turmeric, olive oil, and lemon juice; mix well. Pour marinade over the
chicken in the plastic bag, seal tightly, and shake to coat all sides. (Can
be prepared in advance up to this point and marinated up to 2 days in
the refrigerator.)

3. Preheat barbecue or grill. Remove chicken from the marinade and
drain well; discard marinade.

4. Grill chicken over indirect heat about 4–6 minutes per side, until grill
marks appear and juices run clear. (A two-sided indoor grill will cook in
half the time of a gas or charcoal grill. Chicken breasts will be done in
4–6 minutes total time, depending on thickness. They will register at
165°F/74°F (on an instant-read thermometer.)

189 calories per serving, 2 g carbohydrates, trace sugar, <1 g fiber, 27 g
protein, 8 g fat (1 g saturated), 55 mg sodium, 425 mg potassium

NORENE'S NOTES:

- **Herb-alicious:** Instead of mint, use coriander, basil, or parsley. If you
  don't have fresh herbs, substitute 1 tsp (5 mL) dried for 1 Tbsp (15 mL)
  fresh.

- **Variation:** Instead of lemon juice, use orange, lime, or pomegranate
  juice.

RECIPE CONTINUED . . .

---

6 boneless, skinless single chicken
breasts (or 12 boneless, skinless
chicken thighs)

Salt and freshly ground
black pepper

3 cloves garlic (about 1 Tbsp/
15 mL minced)

3 Tbsp (45 mL) minced fresh mint
(see Norene's Notes)

1 Tbsp (15 mL) minced
fresh thyme

1 tsp (5 mL) ground cumin

1 tsp (5 mL) sweet paprika

½ tsp (2 mL) turmeric

2 Tbsp (30 mL) olive oil

2 Tbsp (30 mL) lemon juice
(preferably fresh)

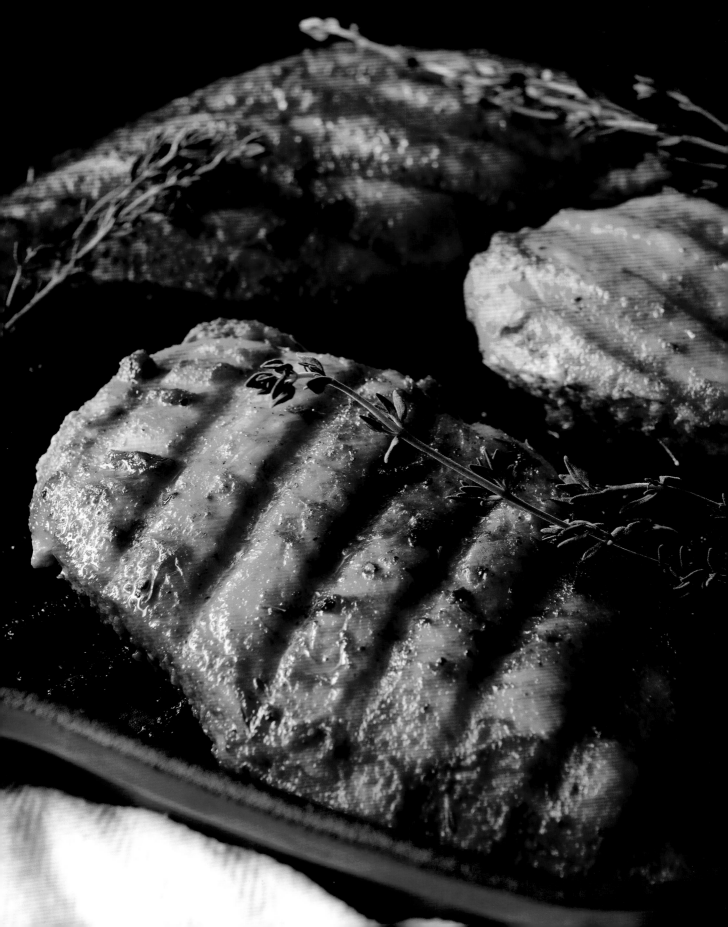

DR. ED SAYS:

- **Protein power:** The chicken in this recipe provides a high percentage of your daily protein requirement, with minimal calories. The saturated fat per serving is well below the government guideline of 10% of calories and well within the American Heart Association recommendation of a maximum of 7% of calories. Chicken also has excellent levels of vitamin B6 and potassium, as well as reasonable levels of magnesium and zinc, while being low in sodium and sugar.

- **Overall,** this recipe contains an abundance of spices, which boost the flavor in addition to being rich in antioxidants.

MARINATED GRILLED CHICKEN BREASTS

MEAT | GLUTEN-FREE | REHEATS AND/OR FREEZES WELL | MAKES
4 SERVINGS

Shake-It-Up Vinaigrette
(p. 432) or your favorite vinaigrette dressing

4 boneless, skinless single
chicken breasts

Cook once—serve twice! Grill an extra batch or two of chicken breasts
the first night to serve hot or cold along with your favorite side dishes.
Then, refrigerate or freeze any leftovers, slice leftover chicken across
the grain, and add it to your favorite salad!

1. Prepare Shake-It-Up Vinaigrette as directed.

2. Place chicken breasts in a resealable plastic bag and add ¼ cup
(60 mL) dressing. Refrigerate the remaining dressing. Marinate chicken
for at least 30 minutes at room temperature, or up to 24 hours in the
refrigerator.

3. Preheat barbecue or grill. Remove chicken from the marinade. Discard leftover marinade.

4. Grill chicken over indirect medium-high heat for 4–6 minutes per
side, until grill marks appear and juices run clear. When done, chicken
will spring back when lightly touched and will register at 165°F (74°C)
on an instant-read thermometer.

187 calories per serving, 2 g carbohydrates, 1 g sugar, 0 g fiber, 27 g protein, 8 g fat (1 g saturated), 121 mg sodium, 408 mg potassium

NORENE'S NOTES:

- **Two-sided electric grills:** These cook in half the time of a gas or charcoal grill. Chicken breasts will be done in 4-6 minutes total time,
depending on thickness.

- **No grill?** Bake, uncovered, in a preheated 400°F (200°C) oven for
20-25 minutes, until chicken is cooked through and juices run clear.

DR. ED SAYS:

- **Overall,** this is another good chicken recipe that is high in protein,
relatively low in calories, low in carbs, sugar, saturated fat, and salt—a
great way to get needed protein without excessive calories or harmful nutrient intake.

CHICKEN SATAY

MEAT | GLUTEN-FREE OPTION | CHICKEN REHEATS AND FREEZES
WELL (DO NOT FREEZE SAUCE) | MAKES ABOUT 30 SKEWERS

This Indonesian favorite is excellent as a main dish or appetizer. If you're expecting a crowd, just double the recipe! The peanut sauce does double-duty as both a marinade and a dipping sauce.

1. **PEANUT SAUCE:** In a food processor fitted with the steel blade, combine garlic, ginger, soy, peanut butter, honey, vinegar, sesame oil, and cayenne. Process until blended, about 15 seconds. If sauce is too thick, thin with a little water. (Can be prepared in advance and refrigerated for 1–2 months in a covered container.)

2. **CHICKEN:** Cut chicken into long strips. Place in a resealable plastic bag along with ½ cup (125 mL) peanut sauce and seal bag tightly. Refrigerate the remaining sauce. Marinate chicken for 30 minutes at room temperature, or up to 24 hours in the refrigerator.

3. Remove chicken from marinade; discard marinade.

4. Thread chicken onto soaked skewers and sprinkle with sesame seeds.

5. Preheat grill to medium-high. Grill skewers 3–4 minutes per side over indirect heat. Don't overcook.

6. Transfer skewers to a serving platter and serve with reserved sauce for dipping. Delicious hot or cold.

69 calories per skewer, 2 g carbohydrates, <1 g sugar, trace fiber, 7 g protein, 4 g fat (<1 g saturated), 49 mg sodium, 87 mg potassium

NORENE'S NOTES:

• **Peanut butter:** The healthiest kind of peanut butter lists only peanuts on the label. Stir well before using. Store in the refrigerator to avoid rancidity.

• **Peanut sauce:** Use in stir-fries or as a dipping sauce for steamed veggies such as broccoli or cauliflower. Try it with fish, tofu, or beef.

• **Skewing around:** Soak the whole package of wooden skewers in cold water for 20 minutes. Transfer to a resealable freezer bag and freeze for future use.

RECIPE CONTINUED . . .

PEANUT SAUCE:

1 Tbsp (15 mL) minced fresh garlic

1 Tbsp (15 mL) minced fresh ginger

2 Tbsp (30 mL) soy sauce or tamari (preferably low-sodium)

½ cup (125 mL) natural peanut butter (see Norene's Notes)

1–2 Tbsp (15–30 mL) honey

2 Tbsp (30 mL) rice vinegar

2 tsp (10 mL) toasted sesame oil

¼ tsp (1 mL) cayenne pepper

CHICKEN:

6 boneless, skinless single chicken breasts (or 12 boneless, skinless chicken thighs)

Thirty 8-inch (20 cm) wooden skewers (presoak in cold water for 20 minutes)

¼ cup (60 mL) sesame seeds

CHICKEN SATAY (continued)

- **No skewing around:** Instead of cutting chicken breasts or thighs into strips, marinate them whole. Sprinkle with sesame seeds. Either grill 4-6 minutes per side, or bake, uncovered, at 400°F (220°C), for 20-25 minutes. Slice across the grain and serve with reserved sauce.

DR. ED SAYS:

- **Peanut butter** is a great source of protein, fiber, and nutrients, and combining it with ginger and garlic gives it an extra antioxidant punch.

- **Sesame seeds** are a very dense nutrient source, with high B vitamin levels as well as fiber, magnesium, and zinc. They are also very low in carbs—so sprinkle them freely on the skewers.

- **Overall,** each skewer is very low in calories and harmful ingredients while providing 10% of your daily protein needs. Of course, the main protein source is the chicken.

"EVERYTHING BUT THE BAGEL" CHICKEN BREASTS

MEAT | GLUTEN-FREE | REHEATS AND/OR FREEZES WELL | MAKES
4 SERVINGS

This crunchy coating is popular on bagels. Try it on chicken for a
scrumptious main course—it's a winner!

---

1. **COATING MIX:** Combine poppy seeds, sesame seeds, onion flakes,
garlic flakes, salt, and pepper on a flat plate; mix well.

2. **CHICKEN:** In a shallow bowl, blend honey with mustard. Coat each
breast with honey-mustard, then dip in the seed mixture to coat on
both sides. Arrange in a single layer on a parchment-lined rimmed
baking sheet. (Can be prepared up to a few hours in advance and refrigerated up to 24 hours.)

3. Preheat oven to 400°F (200°C). Bake, uncovered, for 25–30 minutes,
turning chicken over halfway through cooking, until golden on both
sides. Baking time will depend on thickness of chicken breasts. Serve
hot or cold.

351 calories per serving, 29 g carbohydrates, 4 g fiber, 19 g sugar, 32 g
protein, 12 g fat (2 g saturated fat), 243 mg sodium, 601 mg potassium

NORENE'S NOTES:

- **Dinner for one?** For one serving, combine 1 Tbsp (15 mL) each of
poppy seeds, sesame seeds, onion flakes, and garlic flakes, plus a
pinch each of salt and pepper. In a small bowl, blend 1 Tbsp (15 mL)
honey with 1½ tsp (7 mL) Dijon mustard. Prepare as directed above.

- **Company coming?** This recipe doubles or triples easily.

- **Chicken fingers:** Cut breasts into strips about 1 inch (2.5 cm) wide.
Prepare and bake as directed above. Total baking time is about
15 minutes.

- **Test for doneness:** Chicken will be springy when lightly touched with
your fingertips. If overcooked, chicken will be tough.

- **"Everything but the Bagel" salmon:** Substitute salmon fillets for
chicken. Prepare as directed above. Bake, uncovered, for 10–12 minutes.

RECIPE CONTINUED . . .

"EVERYTHING BUT THE BAGEL" COATING MIX:

¼ cup (60 mL) poppy seeds

¼ cup (60 mL) sesame seeds (try a
combination of black and white)

¼ cup (60 mL) dehydrated
onion flakes

¼ cup (60 mL) dehydrated
garlic flakes

Pinch of kosher salt and freshly
ground black pepper

CHICKEN:

4 boneless, skinless single
chicken breasts

¼ cup (60 mL) honey

2 Tbsp (30 mL) Dijon mustard

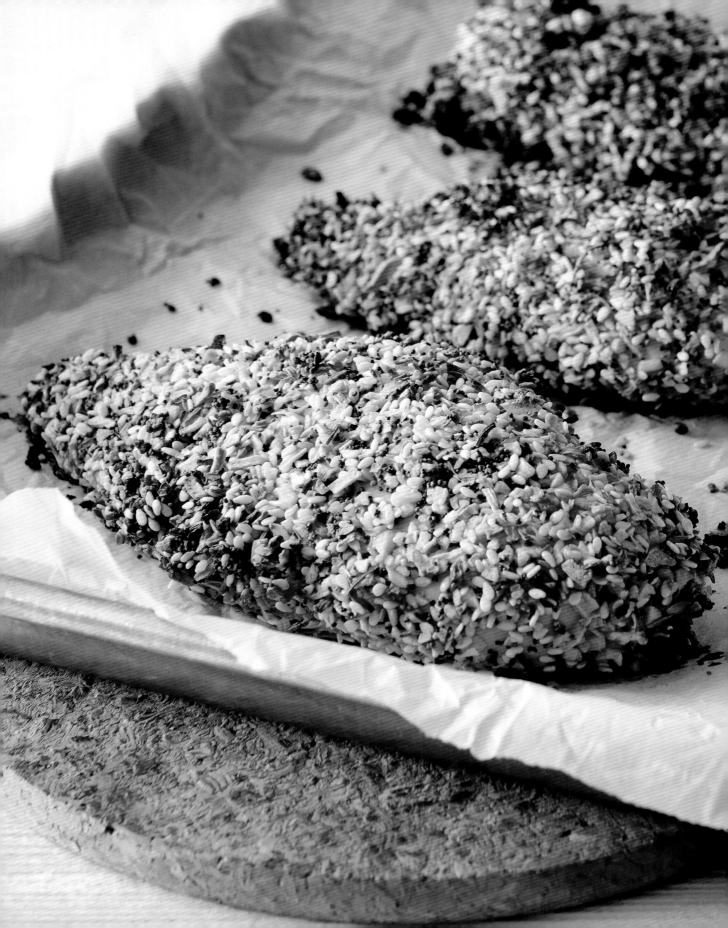

"EVERYTHING BUT THE BAGEL" CHICKEN BREASTS (continued)

- **"Everything but the Bagel" coating mix:** Combine 1 cup (250 mL) each of poppy seeds, sesame seeds, onion flakes, and garlic flakes in a resealable container. Add ½ tsp (2 mL) each of salt and pepper and mix well. Store in the pantry for 2–3 months. Refrigerate or freeze for longer storage. You can also use "Everything but the Bagel" seasoning blend.

DR. ED SAYS:

- **Chicken:** This crispy chicken is comparable in brain-boosting nutrients to Rosemary Chicken (p. 310)—and equally delicious! Although it has more carbs and sugar than some of the other chicken recipes, the crispy coating offers variety, texture, and taste.

- **Sesame seeds and poppy seeds** are very nutrient-dense and are very high in the important brain nutrients magnesium, manganese, fiber, and vitamin E. They are also high in vitamins B6 and folate. As an added bonus, they contain good levels of natural phytosterols, which can lower cholesterol by 5–15%.

NO-FRY CHICKEN SCHNITZEL

MEAT | GLUTEN-FREE | PASSOVER OPTION | REHEATS AND/OR FREEZES WELL | MAKES 4 SERVINGS

1 cup (250 mL) almond flour

½ tsp (2 mL) salt

½ tsp (2 mL) freshly ground black pepper

½ tsp (2 mL) garlic powder

½ tsp (2 mL) cumin

½ tsp (2 mL) dried mint

⅓ cup (80 mL) sesame seeds

2 large eggs

4 boneless, skinless single chicken breasts (or 8 boneless, skinless chicken thighs)

Lemon wedges (for garnish)

You'll go nuts for these crispy, crunchy chicken breasts! The coating is healthy because of the good fat in the almonds and sesame seeds. Expecting guests? Just multiply the recipe accordingly. Feel free to change up the seasonings.

1. Preheat oven to 400°F (200°C). Spray a rimmed baking sheet with nonstick cooking spray.

2. Place almond flour in a wide, shallow bowl. Add salt, pepper, garlic powder, cumin, mint, and sesame seeds; mix well. Lightly whisk eggs in a second bowl.

3. Cut each chicken breast in half crosswise to make 8 thin cutlets.

4. Dip each cutlet first in egg, then in the almond mixture, coating both sides. Arrange in a single layer on the prepared baking sheet. (Can be prepared up to this point, covered, and refrigerated overnight.)

5. Bake, uncovered, for 20–25 minutes, flipping cutlets over halfway through cooking, until crisp and golden.

6. Transfer to a serving platter and garnish with lemon wedges.

412 calories per serving, 10 g carbohydrates, 1 g sugar, 5 g fiber, 38 g protein, 26 g fat (3 g saturated), 387 mg sodium, 496 mg potassium

NORENE'S NOTES:

- **Almond-crusted chicken fingers:** Cut each chicken breast into 5 or 6 strips (or use chicken tenders). Coat as instructed above. Bake for 15–18 minutes, until crisp and golden.

- **Pan-fried schnitzel:** Instead of baking schnitzel as directed in Step 5, brown in a large nonstick skillet in a little hot oil over medium-high heat for 3-4 minutes per side.

- **Turkey schnitzel:** Substitute 8 turkey scaloppini for chicken and omit Step 3.

- **Passover option:** Omit sesame seeds and increase almond flour to 1⅓ cups (310 mL).

- **Nut allergies?** Omit almonds and use matzo meal, panko crumbs, or quinoa flakes—all are available in gluten-free form, and for Passover, too.

DR. ED SAYS:

- **Nuts and seeds** are some of my favorite ingredients because they are brain-nutrient-dense. They provide a great balance of protein, fiber, good unsaturated fat and natural vitamin E (almond flour is one of the richest sources of natural vitamin E), as well as magnesium and B vitamins.

- **Almond flour and sesame seeds** provide a healthy, crispy coating without excessive digestible carbs or sugar.

- **Overall,** this recipe provides an excellent source of protein, especially due to the egg.

CHICKEN FABULOSA

MEAT | GLUTEN-FREE | PASSOVER | REHEATS AND/OR FREEZES
WELL | MAKES 4 SERVINGS

4 boneless, skinless single chicken breasts (or 8 boneless, skinless chicken thighs)

Salt and freshly ground black pepper

1 tsp (5 mL) dried basil

1 tsp (5 mL) garlic powder

½ tsp (2 mL) dried oregano or thyme

8 cloves garlic, peeled

½ cup (125 mL) dried mangoes, cut into strips (use scissors)

¼ cup (60 mL) dry-packed, sun-dried tomatoes, cut into strips (use scissors)

¼ cup (60 mL) dry white wine or chicken or vegetable broth (preferably low-sodium or no-salt-added)

2 Tbsp (30 mL) balsamic vinegar

2 Tbsp (30 mL) honey

2 tsp (10 mL) olive oil

Chopped fresh parsley (for garnish)

This fabulous chicken dish is perfect for any occasion, especially the Jewish High Holidays as it contains honey, wine, and dried fruit. Expecting a crowd? It can be doubled or tripled easily, and can be prepared in advance. Rave reviews guaranteed!

1. Spray a 7- × 11-inch (18 × 28 cm) baking dish with nonstick cooking spray. Arrange breasts in a single layer. Season with salt, pepper, basil, garlic powder, and oregano on all sides. Tuck garlic cloves, mangoes, and sun-dried tomatoes in between breasts.

2. Combine wine, vinegar, honey, and oil in a glass measure and mix well. Drizzle over the chicken mixture. If you have time, cover and refrigerate for several hours or overnight.

3. Remove marinated chicken from the refrigerator. Preheat oven to 375°F (190°C).

4. Bake, uncovered, for 35–40 minutes, basting occasionally. Juices will run clear when chicken is pierced with a fork.

5. Transfer to a serving platter and sprinkle with parsley.

279 calories per serving, 26 g carbohydrates, 18 g sugar, 2 g fiber, 29 g protein, 6 g fat (1 g saturated), 61 mg sodium, 574 mg potassium

NORENE'S NOTES:

- **Switch it up:** Prepare as directed in Steps 1–2. Bake, covered, at 350°F (175°C), for 1 hour. Uncover and bake 20–30 minutes longer, basting occasionally. When done, juices will run clear.

- **Variations:** Instead of honey, use maple syrup. Instead of dried mango, use dried apricots or prunes.

- **Garlic** provides great levels of vitamin B6 and reasonable levels of vitamin C.

- **Tomatoes** also add significant quantities of vitamin C, magnesium, and carotenoid and lycopene antioxidants. These antioxidants are also boosted by the variety of herbs and spices used, which themselves provide different types of antioxidants.

- **Overall,** although this high-protein recipe contains more sugar than I would like to see in a recipe at 18 g per serving (mostly due to the mangoes), it does satisfy a person's sweet tooth and contributes to a flavorful recipe.

> **DID YOU KNOW?** Lycopene, as found naturally in foods, is not only beneficial for the brain, but has been found to help prevent or slow the development of prostate, renal, and breast cancers. As well, it reduces the risk of cardiovascular disease.

STUFFED CHICKEN BREASTS

MEAT | GLUTEN-FREE | PASSOVER | REHEATS AND/OR FREEZES
WELL | MAKES 8 SERVINGS

This elegant, luscious, low-carb dish can be doubled for a crowd or halved for a small family. The super stuffing is packed with phytonutrients, vitamins, and flavor.

STUFFING:

1 Tbsp (15 mL) olive oil

2 medium onions, coarsely chopped

½ cup (125 mL) coarsely chopped red bell pepper

2½ cups (625 mL) coarsely chopped mushrooms

2–3 cloves garlic (or 2 tsp/ 10 mL minced)

2 cups (500 mL) packed fresh baby spinach

1 Tbsp (15 mL) orange juice

2 Tbsp (30 mL) minced fresh basil (or 2 tsp/10 mL dried)

Salt and freshly ground black pepper

CHICKEN:

8 boneless, skinless single chicken breasts

Salt and freshly ground black pepper

¼ cup (60 mL) orange juice

2 Tbsp (30 mL) olive oil

2 tsp (10 mL) honey

1 Tbsp (15 mL) minced fresh basil (or 1 tsp/5 mL dried)

1. **STUFFING:** Heat oil in a large nonstick skillet over medium heat. Add onions and sauté for 5 minutes, until tender. Stir in red pepper, mushrooms, and garlic. Sauté for 5 minutes longer. If the mixture starts to stick, add a little water.

2. Stir in spinach and cook for 2–3 minutes, until most of the moisture has disappeared. Stir in orange juice, basil, salt, and pepper. Let cool before using.

3. **CHICKEN:** Butterfly chicken by cutting horizontally through the middle of each breast, leaving it hinged on one side so that it opens flat like a book. Sprinkle with salt and pepper. Spread 3–4 Tbsp (45–60 mL) stuffing on one side, then fold the other side over to cover the stuffing. Repeat with the remaining breasts and stuffing.

4. Place in a single layer in a sprayed 9- × 13-inch (23 × 33 cm) baking dish.

5. Combine orange juice, olive oil, honey, and basil in a measuring cup; mix well. Drizzle over chicken. Cover and refrigerate for 1 hour or up to 24 hours.

6. Preheat oven to 375°F (190°C). Bake, uncovered, for 35–45 minutes, basting occasionally. Juices should run clear when chicken is pierced with a fork.

220 calories per serving, 7 g carbohydrates, 4 g sugar, 1 g fiber, 28 g protein, 8 g fat (1 g saturated), 67 mg sodium, 581 mg potassium

NORENE'S NOTES:

• **The right stuff!** Use this versatile stuffing for turkey, salmon, or omelets.

- **Variation:** Instead of fresh spinach, use a 10-oz (300 g) package of frozen, chopped spinach, thawed and squeezed dry (or use chopped broccoli instead of spinach).

DR. ED SAYS:

- **Super stuffing:** Aside from the protein that the chicken contributes, most of the other good nutrients come from the ingredients in the stuffing. Onions provide the antioxidant quercetin, which helps in the absorption of other plant antioxidants. Mushrooms provide additional protein and fiber.

- **Spinach** is extremely rich in the brain-important antioxidants lutein and zeaxanthin, as well as other carotenoid antioxidants and vitamin C. It is also an excellent source of folate and vitamins B6 and B12, as well as the minerals magnesium and zinc. Spinach is one ingredient where you may want to consider an organic source, since it is known to be among the top foods for pesticide contamination.

- **Overall,** this recipe is low-calorie, low-sugar, low-carb, and low-sodium, as well as a low–saturated fat source of protein.

HOISIN SESAME CHICKEN

MEAT | REHEATS AND/OR FREEZES WELL | MAKES 6 SERVINGS

6 boneless, skinless single chicken breasts (or 12 boneless, skinless chicken thighs)

Freshly ground black pepper

¼ cup (60 mL) hoisin sauce

1 Tbsp (15 mL) apricot preserves (reduced-sugar or all-fruit)

1 Tbsp (15 mL) minced garlic

1 Tbsp (15 mL) orange juice

¼ cup (60 mL) sesame seeds

Sinfully good! Enjoy this chicken baked or grilled, hot or cold, or transform it into a sheet pan dinner (see Norene's Notes). Since it doubles easily, why not make extra for another day?

1. Place chicken on a parchment-lined, rimmed baking sheet. Sprinkle lightly with pepper on both sides.

2. In a medium bowl, combine hoisin sauce, apricot preserves, garlic, and orange juice; mix well.

3. Brush sauce evenly over chicken on both sides, then sprinkle sesame seeds on top. Let marinate for 30 minutes or refrigerate, covered, for 24 hours.

4. Preheat oven to 400°F (200°C). Bake, uncovered, for 20–25 minutes, or until juices run clear when chicken is pierced with a fork. Serve hot or cold.

212 calories per serving, 7 g carbohydrates, 4 g sugar, 1 g fiber, 28 g protein, 7 g fat (1 g saturated), 226 mg sodium, 440 mg potassium

NORENE'S NOTES:

- **Grilled hoisin sesame chicken:** Prepare and marinate chicken as directed in Steps 1–3. Preheat barbecue to medium-high. Grill chicken over indirect heat for 4–6 minutes per side, or until juices run clear and grill marks appear. (If using a two-sided indoor grill, spray with nonstick cooking spray. Place chicken on the grill and close the lid. Total grilling time will be 4–6 minutes.)

- **Sheet pan dinner:** Make a double batch of the sauce mixture in a large bowl. Add assorted sliced vegetables (e.g., 2 onions, 2 red or yellow bell peppers, 1 zucchini, or 2 cups/500 mL mushrooms) and mix well. Spread out in a single layer on the same baking sheet as the chicken. Bake, uncovered, for 20–25 minutes, stirring vegetables once or twice.

- **Hoisin sauce** typically includes substantial quantities of soy, sugar, and wheat, so when you use it, try to source a version that is gluten-free and low in sugar. For those that are at risk of breast cancer, you may also want to minimize the soy content because of its phytoestrogen content and the controversy associated with phytoestrogens.

- **Sesame seeds** are a great accompaniment to many recipes because of their very high fiber, high protein, high unsaturated fat, high B vitamin, high magnesium, zinc, manganese, and other minerals, as well as low sugar and digestible carbohydrates. The more you use, the better it is.

- **Garlic, orange juice, and apricot preserves** round out the antioxidant profile.

LEMON CHICKEN & VEGETABLE PACKETS

MEAT | GLUTEN-FREE | PASSOVER | REHEATS AND/OR FREEZES
WELL (BUT VEGETABLES WON'T BE AS CRISP WHEN THAWED) |
MAKES 6 SERVINGS

6 boneless, skinless single
chicken breasts

Salt and freshly ground
black pepper

Sweet paprika to taste

2 Tbsp (30 mL) minced fresh
basil or dill

6 Tbsp (90 mL) fresh lemon juice

2 Tbsp (30 mL) olive oil

3 cups (750 mL) chopped
vegetables (e.g., bell peppers,
broccoli and/or cauliflower
florets, cherry tomatoes,
mushrooms, red onions)

2 Tbsp (30 mL) chopped
fresh parsley

Versatile and easy! Perfect for a crowd, or just for one or two. Bonus?
Clean-up is a snap!

1. Place chicken in a bowl and sprinkle lightly with salt, pepper, and
paprika. Rub chicken with basil, lemon juice, and olive oil. Marinate for
20–30 minutes at room temperature or up to 24 hours, covered, in the
refrigerator.

2. Preheat oven to 400°F (220°F). Cut 6 large squares of parchment
paper or foil. Place a chicken breast on each piece of paper and reserve
marinade. Top with vegetables and parsley and drizzle marinade overtop. Seal each packet by crimping edges closed and place on a rimmed
baking sheet. Bake for 20–25 minutes.

3. To serve, place each packet on a dinner plate. Carefully cut open at
the table.

202 calories per serving, 5 g carbohydrates, 2 g sugar, 1 g fiber, 28 g
protein, 8 g fat (1 g saturated), 60 mg sodium, 567 mg potassium

NORENE'S NOTES:

- **Dinner for one?** Season chicken with salt, pepper, and paprika. Use
  1 tsp (5 mL) basil or dill, 1 Tbsp (15 mL) lemon juice, 1 tsp (5 mL) oil, and
  ½ cup (125 mL) chopped vegetables. Prepare and bake as directed
  above.

- **Variations:** Instead of basil, use rosemary and thyme (fresh or dried).
  Use white wine instead of lemon juice. For a spicy version, season
  chicken with a pinch of chili powder, sweet paprika, and cayenne.

- **The complete package:** The unique feature of this recipe is the blend of vegetables placed on each chicken portion. All the vegetables chosen are brain-healthy and rich in vitamin C, B vitamins, magnesium, and zinc, as well as the brain-friendly antioxidants lutein and zeaxanthin. As a bonus, broccoli and cauliflower are also known for their anti-cancer properties.

- **Overall,** this recipe is an excellent source of vitamin C, as well as the lutein and zeaxanthin antioxidants. It also provides good quantities of B vitamins, especially folate and B6, as well as magnesium and zinc. Low sodium, low carbs, and low calories round out its benefits.

ROSEMARY CHICKEN & VEGETABLES

MEAT | GLUTEN-FREE | REHEATS AND/OR FREEZES WELL | MAKES
6 SERVINGS

6 boneless, skinless single chicken breasts (or 12 boneless, skinless chicken thighs)

Kosher salt and freshly ground black pepper

Sweet paprika to taste

3 cloves garlic (about 1½ tsp/ 7 mL minced)

6 Tbsp (90 mL) apricot jam (low-sugar or all-fruit)

2 Tbsp (30 mL) Dijon mustard

1 Tbsp (15 mL) olive oil

1 tsp (5 mL) fresh rosemary, minced (or ½ tsp/10 mL dried)

2 red bell peppers, thinly sliced

1 medium onion, quartered and thinly sliced

Fresh rosemary (for garnish)

This scrumptious chicken and vegetable combo comes together quickly. Simple and elegant, it multiplies easily, so it's great when you're having guests. Since rosemary is a memory booster, everyone will remember this dish!

1. Line a 9- × 13-inch (23 × 33 cm) baking dish with parchment paper. Arrange breasts in a single layer in the prepared baking dish and sprinkle lightly with salt, pepper, and paprika.

2. Combine garlic, jam, mustard, oil, and rosemary in a small bowl and mix well. Spread evenly over the chicken on both sides. If you have time, marinate chicken for 20 minutes at room temperature or up to 24 hours, covered, in the refrigerator.

3. Preheat oven to 400°F (200°C). Tuck pepper and onion slices in between chicken breasts.

4. Bake, uncovered, for 25–30 minutes, turning chicken over at half time and stirring the vegetables. When done, chicken will spring back when lightly touched and vegetables will be tender-crisp. If overcooked, chicken will be tough.

5. Arrange chicken and vegetables on a serving platter and garnish with fresh rosemary.

209 calories per serving, 11 g carbohydrates, 1 g fiber, 7 g sugar, 27 g protein, 6 g fat (1 g saturated fat), 111 mg sodium, 511 mg potassium

NORENE'S NOTES:

- **Variation:** In Step 3, add 1 unpeeled sliced zucchini and 1 cup (250 mL) cherry tomatoes. Cook as directed above.

- **Frozen assets:** Combine seasoned chicken with marinade in a resealable freezer bag and freeze. When needed, thaw overnight in the refrigerator. Transfer contents to a parchment-lined baking dish, add vegetables, and cook as directed above.

- **Kitchen hack:** To strip rosemary leaves off their stems, hold the stem in one hand, needles pointing upright. With the fingers of your other hand, pull downwards, stripping the leaves off their tough, woody stems. Discard stems. Mince or chop leaves with a chef's knife.

DR. ED SAYS:

- **Rosemary,** the feature ingredient of this dish, is a powerful natural antioxidant that has been linked to better brain function (see Maple-Glazed Salmon, p. 253).

- **Bell peppers** also provide significant fiber, antioxidants, and vitamins C, E, and B6. They also have a low sodium and saturated fat content. (See Grilled Corn, Red Pepper, and Snap Pea Salad, p. 416).

- **Chicken** is an excellent source of protein and vitamin B6. It has reasonable amounts of magnesium, zinc, vitamin B12, and Omega-3 fat. Chicken is low in fat and sodium.

- **Garlic, onion, and olive oil** all add important components of the Mediterranean diet.

- **Overall,** this easy chicken dish is a good source of vitamins C, B6, and folate, as well as magnesium and antioxidants.

> DID YOU KNOW? Rosemary is so powerful that it has been used as a food additive to prevent spoilage of foods.

SHAWARMA-STYLE CHICKEN

MEAT | REHEATS AND/OR FREEZES WELL | MAKES 6 SERVINGS

2 lb (1 kg) boneless, skinless chicken thighs

½ tsp (2 mL) kosher salt (or to taste)

½ tsp (2 mL) freshly ground black pepper

2 tsp (10 mL) ground cumin

2 tsp (10 mL) sweet paprika

½ tsp (2 mL) turmeric

Pinch allspice

5–6 cloves garlic, crushed (about 2 Tbsp/30 mL minced)

Juice of 2 lemons (6–8 Tbsp/ 90–120 mL)

¼ cup (60 mL) olive oil + 2 Tbsp (30 mL), for frying

¼ cup (60 mL) chopped fresh parsley

Thanks to my niece, Merav Barr, for her "spit-free" recipe for this marvelous Mediterranean delight. Shawarma is typically roasted on a rotating spit and the cooked chicken is then shaved off in coarse shreds. In warm weather, Merav barbecues the chicken thighs, but in wintery weather she fries them in a cast iron skillet. If you prefer crunchy crispy bits, try shaved-style (see Norene's Notes).

1. Place chicken thighs in a large bowl. Season chicken on all sides with salt, pepper, cumin, paprika, turmeric, and allspice. Add garlic, lemon juice, and ¼ cup (60 mL) olive oil and mix well. Cover and marinate in the refrigerator for at least 1 hour or overnight.

2. When ready to cook, heat 2 Tbsp (30 mL) oil in a large skillet on medium-high. Brown chicken thighs on both sides until golden, about 5 minutes per side, working in batches if necessary.

3. Transfer to a baking dish and cover loosely with foil. Bake at 350°F (175°C) for 20 minutes, until cooked through.

4. Place on a platter, sprinkle with parsley, and serve.

308 calories per serving, 3 g carbohydrates, <1 g sugar, <1 g fiber, 31 g protein, 19 g fat (3 g saturated), 329 mg sodium, 64 mg potassium

NORENE'S NOTES:

- **Shaved-style shawarma:** Cook chicken as directed in Step 2. Slice thighs into small bits. Fry them again in a large skillet with hot oil over medium-high heat until brown and crispy, 4–5 minutes. Transfer to a platter and top with chopped parsley.

- **No-fry method:** Preheat oven to 425°F (220°C). Line a rimmed baking sheet with parchment. Prepare chicken as directed in Step 1. Arrange in a single layer on the prepared baking sheet. Bake, uncovered, for 30-35 minutes, or until the edges of the chicken thighs are crisp and golden and juices run clear.

- **Aside from the protein** contributed by the chicken, the main brain-friendly nutrients here are the antioxidants provided by the spices and herbs.

- **Garlic** provides excellent quantities of vitamin C.

- **Olive oil** supplies a substantial quantity of beneficial monounsaturated fatty acids as well as vitamin E. I would recommend you use extra virgin first press olive oil to get the most brain-healthy antioxidants and nutrients of this major component of the Mediterranean diet.

- **Overall,** this recipe is a good source of vitamin C, vitamin E, antioxidants, and protein, while being low in carbs and sugar. If you have sodium concerns, you could use a salt substitute.

QUICK CHICKEN CACCIATORE

MEAT | GLUTEN-FREE | PASSOVER | REHEATS AND/OR FREEZES
WELL (BUT VEGETABLES WON'T BE AS CRISP WHEN THAWED) |
MAKES 6 SERVINGS

6 boneless, skinless single
chicken breasts

Salt and freshly ground
black pepper

2 Tbsp (30 mL) olive oil, divided

2–3 cloves garlic (1 Tbsp/
15 mL minced)

2 medium onions, sliced

1 red bell pepper, seeded
and sliced

1 yellow bell pepper, seeded
and sliced

2½–3 cups (625–750 mL) sliced
mushrooms

3 cups (750 mL) tomato basil
sauce (preferably low-sodium)

½ cup (125 mL) red wine
(e.g., Cabernet Sauvignon)

1 tsp (5 mL) dried basil

½ tsp (2 mL) dried oregano

Pinch of red pepper flakes

¼ cup (60 mL) minced fresh basil
and/or parsley

Dinner's done in 30 minutes! When you're short on time and need something simple for dinner, this dish is great for guests, or makes perfect family fare. Serve it over quinoa or golden strands of Spaghetti Squash Noodles (p. 478) or any vegetable spirals, such as zucchini noodles, to keep the carbs at bay.

1. Cut chicken into thin strips. Sprinkle lightly with salt and pepper.

2. Heat 1 Tbsp (15 mL) oil in a large nonstick wok or deep skillet over medium-high heat. Add chicken strips and garlic and stir-fry until chicken is no longer pink. Transfer to a bowl.

3. Heat the remaining oil in the wok. Add onions, peppers, and mushrooms. Stir-fry for 4–5 minutes, or until golden.

4. Return chicken to wok. Add tomato sauce, wine, basil, oregano, and red pepper flakes; stir well. Heat to simmering, then reduce heat and cover partially. Simmer for 15 minutes, or until tender, stirring occasionally. Season with additional salt and pepper, if needed.

5. Transfer to a serving platter and sprinkle with basil and/or parsley.

326 calories per serving, 20 g carbohydrates, 9 g sugar, 4 g fiber, 31 g protein, 12 g fat (2 g saturated), 348 mg sodium, 664 mg potassium

NORENE'S NOTES:

- **Variation:** Substitute 12 boneless, skinless chicken thighs for breasts. In Step 2, add 1 medium unpeeled zucchini, trimmed and chopped.

DR. ED SAYS:

- **Benefits:** This dish has many of the same benefits as Stuffed Chicken Breasts (p. 304) as it calls for similar ingredients. It is extremely high in vitamin C antioxidant at 98 mg per serving, but also very high in other antioxidants from the spices and herbs, especially lycopene from the tomato basil sauce.

- **Onions** provide the antioxidant quercetin, which enhances the activity of the other antioxidants.

- **Wine** provides the important brain antioxidant resveratrol, as well as other nutrients known to reduce the risk of AD/dementia.

- **Overall,** aside from the antioxidants, protein, and vitamin C, this recipe is rich in vitamin E, B vitamins, magnesium, zinc, and fiber. It is somewhat high in sugar, due to the peppers and wine, so I suggest choosing a dry wine instead of a sweeter wine.

> DID YOU KNOW? Scientists have attributed an anti-aging effect to resveratrol.

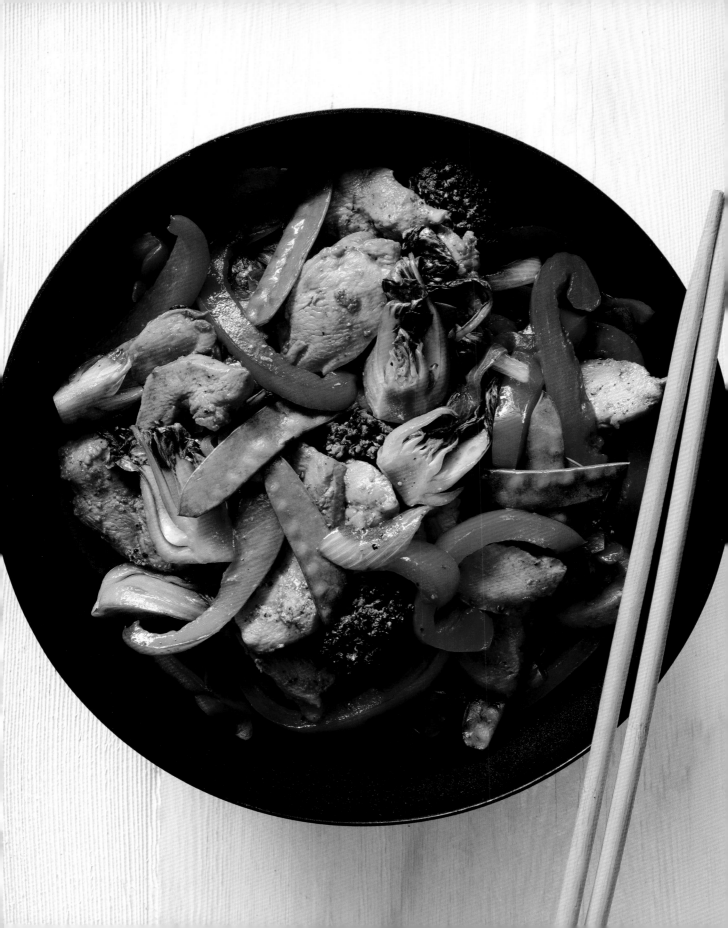

STIR-FRY CHICKEN & VEGETABLES

MEAT | REHEATS WELL | VEGETABLES WILL BECOME SOGGY IF FROZEN | MAKES 6 SERVINGS

Don't go stir-crazy when you read the list of ingredients for this simple stir-fry. It comes together quickly, so prepare everything in advance. Experiment using different vegetables, use lean beef instead of chicken, or try it with tofu. Faux-Fried Rice (p. 463) is a perfect accompaniment.

1. **MARINADE:** In a medium bowl, combine hoisin sauce, preserves, soy sauce, rice vinegar, garlic, ginger, and sesame oil (if using); mix well.

2. **CHICKEN AND VEGETABLES:** Place chicken strips in a large bowl. Add half the marinade and stir to coat, reserving the remaining marinade. Let chicken marinate while you prepare the vegetables. (Chicken and vegetables can be prepared up to 24 hours in advance and refrigerated.)

3. Heat oil in a nonstick wok or large skillet over medium-high heat.

4. Stir-fry chicken for 2 minutes, or until no longer pink. Add vegetables and stir-fry 2 minutes longer.

5. Stir in reserved marinade and cook 2–3 minutes longer, until heated through. Serve immediately.

246 calories per serving, 24 g carbohydrates, 11 g sugar, 4 g fiber, 25 g protein, 7 g fat (1 g saturated), 239 mg sodium, 232 mg potassium

NORENE'S NOTES:

- **Go nuts!** Stir-fry 1 can (8 oz/250 g) sliced water chestnuts, rinsed and drained, along with the vegetables in Step 4. Garnish with ½ cup (125 mL) toasted sliced almonds to serve.

- **Beef variation:** Replace chicken with 1½ lb (750 g) lean boneless beef, cut into strips. (Freeze beef or chicken for a few minutes for easier slicing.)

- **Vegetarian version:** Replace chicken with 1 lb (500 g) extra-firm tofu. Place tofu between layers of paper toweling on a plate, and top with another plate. Weigh down with cans and let absorb for 20 minutes. Cut tofu into strips.

RECIPE CONTINUED . . .

MARINADE:

¼ cup (60 mL) hoisin sauce

2 Tbsp (30 mL) apricot or peach preserves (preferably low-sugar or all-fruit)

2 Tbsp (30 mL) soy sauce (preferably low-sodium)

1 Tbsp (15 mL) rice vinegar or lemon juice

2 tsp (10 mL) minced garlic

2 tsp (10 mL) minced fresh ginger (or 1 tsp/5 mL powdered ginger)

2 tsp (10 mL) toasted sesame oil (optional)

CHICKEN AND VEGETABLES:

4 boneless, skinless single chicken breasts, cut into thin strips (about 1½ lb/750 g)

2 Tbsp (30 mL) canola or grapeseed oil

1 medium onion, halved and thinly sliced

1 red bell pepper, halved and thinly sliced

1 yellow bell pepper, halved and thinly sliced

2 cups (500 mL) broccoli florets

2 baby bok choy (about 2 cups/500 mL thinly sliced)

1 cup (250 mL) snow peas, ends trimmed

- **As you like it stir-fry:** Instead of baby bok choy, substitute thinly sliced cabbage. Instead of bell peppers, use 2 cups (500 mL) sliced mushrooms. Instead of snow peas, use pea pods or green peas. If desired, add pineapple tidbits, mandarin orange segments, or sliced mango.

DR. ED SAYS:

- **Veggie power:** Most of the key brain nutrients in this recipe, other than protein, are found in the added vegetables—the main contributors here are the bok choy and broccoli florets. These are part of the cruciferous vegetable family, which is known for its high fiber and low calories. Nutritionally, these veggies are rich in carotenoid antioxidants and vitamin C, and contain ample quantities of B vitamins and minerals important for the brain and heart. An added bonus is their well-known cancer prevention properties due to the glucosinolate that they contain.

> DID YOU KNOW? Raw cruciferous vegetables should be eaten in moderation as they contain an enzyme that can interfere with thyroid function and is inactivated by cooking.

TURKEY MUSHROOM SCALOPPINI

MEAT | GLUTEN-FREE | PASSOVER OPTION | REHEATS AND/OR FREEZES WELL | MAKES 8 SERVINGS

Cheryl Goldberg of Toronto inspired the recipe for this tender, juicy turkey dish. I've modified it to reduce the carbs. Simply delicious!

1. Arrange turkey scaloppini in a single layer in a large, oblong baking dish. Sprinkle with salt, pepper, paprika, rosemary, and thyme. Drizzle with lemon juice and 2 Tbsp (30 mL) oil. Turn scaloppini over to coat on all sides. Marinate, covered, for 30 minutes at room temperature, or up to 24 hours in the refrigerator. Transfer scaloppini to a large plate and discard the marinade.

2. Heat 2 Tbsp (30 mL) oil in a large, nonstick skillet over medium-high heat. Add onions, mushrooms, and garlic. Sauté for 8–10 minutes, until golden. Transfer to a bowl.

3. Heat the remaining oil in the skillet. Working in batches, brown scaloppini for 2 minutes per side, until no longer pink. If needed, add a little more oil. Remove from pan.

4. Combine wine, broth, and cornstarch in a 2-cup (500 mL) measure and stir well. Add to the skillet and scrape up any brown bits from the bottom of the pan with a wooden spoon. Heat to simmering.

5. Return scaloppini, onions, and mushrooms to the skillet. Cook 2–3 minutes longer, until heated through, basting once or twice.

6. Transfer to a serving platter and top with parsley.

245 calories per serving, 7 g carbohydrates, 2 g sugar, 1 g fiber, 28 g protein, 10 g fat (2 g saturated), 139 mg sodium, 497 mg potassium

NORENE'S NOTES:

- **Variation:** Substitute boneless, skinless chicken fillets for scaloppini. In Step 3, brown chicken fillets for 2–3 minutes per side.

- **Company's coming?** In Step 5, instead of returning the scaloppini/mushroom mixture to the skillet, transfer to a sprayed ovenproof casserole. Cover tightly with foil and bake in a preheated 350°F (175°C) oven for 20–25 minutes, until heated through. Garnish with parsley.

RECIPE CONTINUED . . .

---

2 lb (1 kg) thinly sliced turkey scaloppini (8–12 slices)

Salt and freshly ground black pepper

½ tsp (2 mL) sweet paprika

½ tsp (2 mL) dried rosemary

½ tsp (2 mL) dried thyme

¼ cup (60 mL) lemon juice (preferably fresh)

5 Tbsp (75 mL) olive oil, divided

2 medium onions, thinly sliced

3 cups (750 mL) sliced mushrooms

3 cloves garlic, thinly sliced

½ cup (125 mL) dry white wine

½ cup (125 mL) chicken broth (preferably low-sodium or no-salt-added)

1 Tbsp (15 mL) cornstarch (use potato starch for Passover)

½ cup (125 mL) minced fresh parsley

TURKEY MUSHROOM SCALOPPINI (continued)

DR. ED SAYS:

- **Turkey and mushrooms** provide about half of our daily protein needs per serving in this recipe. Turkey also provides good quantities of the antioxidant selenium, B vitamins, and magnesium and zinc, while being low in carbs and fat.

- **Herbs and spices,** together with lemon juice and wine, give us a good variety of antioxidant sources, while the quercetin in the onions helps in their absorption.

- **Overall,** this recipe is a healthy, high-protein dish, with good levels of vitamin C, magnesium, and zinc, and a variety of antioxidants from different sources.

TURKEY PICCATA

MEAT | GLUTEN-FREE OPTION | PASSOVER OPTION | REHEATS AND/
OR FREEZES WELL | MAKES 6–8 SERVINGS

Elaine Kaplan of Toronto shared her recipe for this luscious lemony Turkey Piccata. Her husband, Marty, loves it—and so do their friends, who insist that she serve this dish when they're lucky enough to be invited for dinner. Winner, winner, turkey dinner!

½ cup (125 mL) flour (all-purpose or whole wheat)

½ tsp (2 mL) salt

½ tsp (2 mL) freshly ground black pepper

½ tsp (2 mL) garlic powder

½ tsp (2 mL) dried oregano

½ tsp (2 mL) dried rosemary

2 lb (1 kg) thinly sliced turkey scaloppini (8–12 slices)

2 Tbsp (30 mL) olive oil (approx.)

¾ cup (185 mL) chicken broth (preferably low-sodium or no-salt-added)

¼ cup (60 mL) lemon juice (preferably fresh)

¼ cup (60 mL) dry white wine

2 Tbsp (30 mL) fresh chopped dill + extra for garnish

Thinly sliced lemon (for garnish)

2 Tbsp (30 mL) capers (optional, for garnish)

1. Place flour in a large resealable bag. Add salt, pepper, garlic powder, oregano, and rosemary. Seal bag and shake well.

2. Add scaloppini to the bag, one slice at a time. Reseal bag and shake again, coating turkey well on both sides; shake off excess flour. Place on a parchment-lined tray.

3. Heat oil in a large nonstick skillet on medium-high. Working in batches, add scaloppini to the skillet and brown, about 2 minutes per side, just until no longer pink. If necessary, add a little more oil to prevent sticking.

4. Transfer scaloppini to a large plate, cover, and keep warm.

5. Add broth, lemon juice, and wine to the skillet. Scrape up any brown bits from the bottom of the skillet with a wooden spoon. Reduce heat and cook just until simmering, about 2 minutes, stirring occasionally.

6. Return scaloppini to the skillet along with dill. Simmer 2–3 minutes longer, until heated through, spooning sauce over scaloppini to keep moist.

7. Transfer scaloppini and sauce to a serving platter. Garnish with additional dill, lemon slices, and capers, if using.

267 calories per serving, 10 g carbohydrates, <1 g sugar, <1 g fiber, 38 g protein, 7 g fat (1 g saturated), 375 mg sodium, 429 mg potassium

NORENE'S NOTES:

- **Gluten-free/passover option:** Replace flour with potato starch.

- **Variation:** Substitute thinly sliced boneless, skinless chicken breasts for scaloppini. In Step 3, brown chicken for 3-4 minutes per side.

RECIPE CONTINUED . . .

TURKEY PICCATA (continued)

- **Company coming?** In Step 6, instead of returning scaloppini to the skillet along with the dill, transfer to a sprayed ovenproof casserole. Pour sauce over and cover tightly with foil. Refrigerate until shortly before serving. Reheat in a preheated 350°F (175°C) oven for 20–25 minutes, until heated through. Garnish as directed in Step 7.

DR. ED SAYS:

- **Turkey** packs a powerful wallop of good-quality protein per serving, supplying more than 50% of an average person's protein requirement. It is also a low source of digestible carbs, so that even adding flour to the recipe still keeps it in the lower range of carb intake.

- **Wine, lemon juice, and spices** provide a variety of antioxidants, especially rosemary, which is one of the more powerful plant antioxidants.

- **Dill,** aside from its antioxidant properties, is used as a digestive aid. It provides reasonably good levels of vitamin B6, folate, magnesium, and zinc.

DID YOU KNOW? Dill was used to defend against witchcraft and enchantment in the Middle Ages.

GLAZED TURKEY BREAST WITH VEGETABLES

MEAT | GLUTEN-FREE | PASSOVER | REHEATS AND/OR FREEZES
WELL | MAKES ABOUT 8 SERVINGS

This is an excellent option when you don't want to cook a whole turkey—cooking the vegetables alongside the turkey will save on time and cleanup. Cornbread Stuffing Mounds (p. 465) make a scrumptious side dish.

1. Spray a large roasting pan with nonstick cooking spray. Place turkey breast in the pan, skin side up. Loosen turkey skin, but don't remove it. Season turkey under the skin with salt, pepper, paprika, and basil.

2. In a measuring cup, combine vinegar, honey, olive oil, and garlic, and stir well. Drizzle mixture over the turkey breast and under the skin. Cover and marinate for 1 hour at room temperature, or up to 24 hours in the refrigerator.

3. Preheat oven to 350°F (175°C). Scatter mushrooms, peppers, and onions around the turkey. Drizzle wine and water over vegetables and cover loosely with foil.

4. Roast, covered, for 30 minutes. Remove foil and roast about 1 hour longer, basting turkey occasionally. Calculate 20–25 minutes per pound as your cooking time at 350°F (175°C).

5. Remove pan from oven and cover turkey loosely with foil to keep warm. Let stand for 15 minutes. Temperature of the turkey breast will rise to 165°F (74°C) as it rests.

6. Discard skin and slice turkey meat on an angle off the bone. Transfer to a serving platter and surround with vegetables. Spoon pan juices overtop.

320 calories per serving, 11 g carbohydrates, 8 g sugar, 1 g fiber, 49 g protein, 7 g fat (1 g saturated), 164 mg sodium, 628 mg potassium

NORENE'S NOTES:

- **Glazed roast chicken with vegetables:** Instead of turkey breast, substitute a whole chicken (about 4 lb/1.8 kg). Rub chicken with seasoning, both over and under the skin. Follow instructions as directed above. Cooking time will be about the same.

1 turkey breast, bone-in, skin-on (about 4½ lb/2 kg)

Salt and freshly ground black pepper

1 tsp (5 mL) sweet paprika

1 tsp (5 mL) dried basil

2 Tbsp (30 mL) balsamic vinegar

2 Tbsp (30 mL) honey

2 Tbsp (30 mL) olive oil

3 cloves garlic (about 1 Tbsp/ 15 mL minced)

2½ cups (625 mL) sliced mushrooms

2 red or yellow bell peppers, sliced

2 medium onions, sliced

⅓ cup (80 mL) dry white wine

⅓ cup (80 mL) water or chicken broth (preferably low-sodium or no-salt-added)

RECIPE CONTINUED . . .

DR. ED SAYS:

- **Protein power:** This dish is protein-packed, providing 49 g of protein, which is more than 80% of an average person's daily requirement. People with kidney disease should take this into consideration, as this amount could stress the kidneys.

- **Overall,** the combination of protein with vegetables offers an excellent source of vitamin C, vitamin B12, and zinc, as well as a very good source of folate and magnesium. Once again, the vegetables provide needed antioxidants from a variety of sources.

> **DID YOU KNOW?** We shouldn't rely on one source of antioxidants. In most cases, scientists still haven't identified which and how much of different plant antioxidants are most beneficial.

SALSA-TOPPED TURKEY BREAST

MEAT | GLUTEN-FREE | PASSOVER | REHEATS AND/OR FREEZES
WELL | MAKES 8 SERVINGS

Thanks to my amazing assistant, Renée Owieczka, who adapted my popular Sweet & Sour BBQ Brisket recipe. She lightened it up, cutting calories and fat, to create this delicious turkey dish. Renée serves it with fresh green beans or steamed broccoli, along with brown rice. If you don't want to cook a whole turkey, this is an excellent alternative.

3–4 medium onions, sliced

1 turkey breast, bone-in, skin-on
(about 4½ lb/2 kg)

Salt and freshly ground
black pepper

3–4 cloves garlic (about 1 Tbsp/
15 mL minced)

1 tsp (5 mL) sweet paprika

1 cup (250 mL) salsa (mild
or medium)

2 Tbsp (30 mL) honey

2 Tbsp (30 mL) lemon juice
(preferably fresh)

1 cup (250 mL) water (approx.)

1. Spray a large roasting pan with nonstick cooking spray. Scatter onions in the bottom of the pan. Place turkey breast on top of the onions and sprinkle with salt and pepper.

2. In a medium bowl, combine garlic, paprika, salsa, honey, and lemon juice; stir well. Pour over the turkey breast and spread evenly. Cover and marinate for 1 hour at room temperature, or up to 24 hours in the refrigerator.

3. Preheat oven to 350°F (175°C). Pour water into the bottom of the roasting pan and cover loosely with foil. Roast turkey for 1 hour. Remove foil and roast turkey about 25–30 minutes longer, basting occasionally, until golden (see "Turkey Time," p. 287).

4. Remove pan from oven and cover turkey loosely with foil to keep warm. Let rest for 15 minutes.

5. Discard skin and slice turkey meat on an angle off the bone. Transfer to a serving platter and spoon pan juices and onions overtop.

310 calories per serving, 11 g carbohydrates, 6 g sugar, 1 g fiber, 55 g protein, 4 g fat (1 g saturated), 310 mg sodium, 606 mg potassium

NORENE'S NOTES:

- **How much is enough?** Calculate 6 oz (180 g) raw turkey breast per person. An average whole turkey will serve 12 hungry people, plus leftovers if you are lucky!

- **Reheating hack:** To prevent turkey from drying out, place slices into an ovenproof casserole and cover with lettuce leaves. Reheat at 350°F (175°C) for 20-25 minutes, until heated through. Discard lettuce before serving.

RECIPE CONTINUED . . .

SALSA-TOPPED TURKEY BREAST (continued)

DR. ED SAYS:

- **Salsa** is rich in fiber and is an excellent source of the plant antioxidant lycopene. If sodium intake is a concern, either buy a low-sodium version or make your own (see Simple Salsa, p. 170).

- **Sweet news:** Since the sugar content is moderately high, replace honey with a low-sugar syrup if this is a concern.

- **Overall,** the B vitamins folate, B12, and B6, as well as the minerals magnesium and zinc, are provided in good quantities. Antioxidants are provided from the herbs, spices, onions, and lemon juice. In addition, the onions have a good wallop of quercetin, which helps in the absorption of the other antioxidants.

SPINACH-STUFFED TURKEY ROLL

MEAT | GLUTEN-FREE | PASSOVER | REHEATS AND/OR FREEZES
WELL | MAKES 8 SERVINGS

Looks complicated, cooks easy! This elegant dish is perfect for anyone who finds it challenging to carve a whole turkey but still wants tender white meat and flavorful stuffing, and it makes a beautiful addition to your holiday table. If you don't want to use the Spinach Stuffing, see Get Stuffed! (p. 477).

Spinach Stuffing (p. 477)

2 medium onions, sliced

1 boneless, skinless turkey breast (about 4 lb/1.8 kg; see Norene's Notes)

2 cloves garlic (about 2 tsp/ 10 mL minced)

Salt and freshly ground black pepper

Sweet paprika to taste

1 tsp (5 mL) dried basil

½ tsp (2 mL) dried thyme

¼ cup (60 mL) dry white wine

¼ cup (60 mL) chicken broth (preferably low-sodium or no-salt-added)

2 Tbsp (30 mL) olive oil

1. Prepare stuffing as directed. Spray a large roasting pan with nonstick cooking spray. Scatter onions in the bottom of the pan.

2. Butterfly turkey breast by slicing it almost in half horizontally and leaving it hinged on one side, so that it opens flat like a book. Cover with plastic wrap. Pound turkey with a heavy skillet to flatten it to about ½ inch (1 cm) thickness.

3. Spread stuffing mixture evenly onto the turkey to within 1 inch (2.5 cm) of the edges. Starting from the long edge, roll up tightly into a long cylinder. Tie roll with cooking twine about 2 inches (5 cm) apart. Place seam side down in the prepared pan. Season with salt, pepper, paprika, basil, and thyme.

4. In a measuring cup, combine wine, broth, and oil with a dash of salt and pepper; stir well. Drizzle mixture over the onions and around the turkey. Cover and marinate for at least 1 hour at room temperature, or up to 24 hours in the refrigerator. Remove from refrigerator about ½ hour before cooking.

5. Preheat oven to 350°F (175°C). Roast turkey, covered, for 1 hour. Uncover and roast about 30 minutes longer, basting occasionally. Calculate 25–30 minutes per pound as your cooking time. An instant read thermometer inserted into the thickest part of the roll should read 155°F (68°C).

6. Remove pan from oven, tent turkey loosely with foil, and let stand 15 minutes. Temperature of the turkey will rise to 165°F (74°C) after it has rested.

7. Transfer to a cutting board and cut into ¾-inch (2 cm) slices. Arrange on a serving platter and serve with pan juices.

RECIPE CONTINUED . . .

SPINACH-STUFFED TURKEY ROLL (continued)

369 calories per serving, 14 g carbohydrates, 8 g sugar, 3 g fiber, 57 g protein, 9 g fat (1 g saturated), 289 mg sodium, 917 mg potassium

NORENE'S NOTES:

- **No-roll stuffed turkey breast:** Use a bone-in, skin-on turkey breast (about 4½ lb/2 kg). Loosen turkey skin, but don't remove it. Spread stuffing evenly over the turkey breast and under the skin. Place turkey, bone side down, in the prepared pan on top of the onions. Season with salt, pepper, paprika, basil, and thyme. Continue as directed in Steps 4–7, cooking uncovered the whole time.

DR. ED SAYS:

- **Benefits:** In addition to the protein that the turkey contributes, most of the other benefits come from the stuffing ingredients.

- **Onions** provide the antioxidant quercetin, which helps in the absorption of other plant antioxidants.

- **Spinach** is rich in the brain-important antioxidants lutein and zeaxanthin, as well as other carotenoid antioxidants and vitamin C. It is also an excellent source of folate, B6 and B12 vitamins, as well as the minerals magnesium and zinc. Since spinach is known to be among the top foods for pesticide contamination, organic is your best choice. Spinach is the most documented for brain health, followed closely by parsley.

- **Parsley,** which is high in fiber, vitamin C, and folate, is a good source of magnesium, while being low in sugars and digestible carbs.

- **Overall,** this recipe is a low-carb, low-sodium, and low-saturated fat source of protein, while providing good amounts of brain-healthy nutrients.

TURKEY & BUTTERNUT SQUASH CHILI

MEAT | GLUTEN-FREE OPTION | REHEATS AND/OR FREEZES WELL |
MAKES 12 CUPS (3 L)

Thanks to Elana Abramovitch for sharing her homemade chili recipe with me. It's packed with a variety of vegetables and uses lean ground turkey, resulting in a hearty, healthy, tasty dish. Serve over brown rice, quinoa, couscous, or your favorite whole grain.

1. In a medium bowl, presoak beans in triple the amount of cold water for at least 1 hour or preferably overnight. Drain and rinse thoroughly.

2. Preheat oven to 400°F (200°C). Line a rimmed baking sheet with parchment paper.

3. Scatter squash cubes on the prepared pan and drizzle with a little olive oil. Roast, uncovered, for 15–20 minutes to give them some color.

4. Meanwhile, heat the remaining olive oil over medium heat in a large pot. Add onion and sauté for 5 minutes. Add celery and sauté 5 minutes more. Next, add carrot, peppers, and garlic and continue sautéing, about 20 minutes in total.

5. Increase heat to medium-high and add ground turkey. Brown slowly for 8–10 minutes, stirring often to break up the meat.

6. Add beans, squash, tomatoes, tomato sauce, broth, chili powder, cumin, cocoa powder, and chipotle peppers; mix well. Bring to a simmer. Cook, partially covered, for 1½–2 hours, stirring occasionally. Season with salt and pepper.

165 calories per 1-cup (250 mL) serving, 21 g carbohydrates, 5 g sugar, 6.5 g fiber, 14 g protein, 3.5 g fat (0.5 g saturated), 192 mg sodium, 709 mg potassium

NORENE'S NOTES:

- **Bean cuisine:** Instead of 1 cup (250 mL) dried beans, use 2 cans (15 oz/425 g each, preferably no-salt-added). Rinse and drain well before adding them in Step 6.

- **Variation:** Use minced chicken instead of turkey.

RECIPE CONTINUED . . .

---

1 cup (250 mL) dried red kidney or black beans (see Norene's Notes)

1 pkg (1 lb/454 g) butternut squash cubes

2–3 Tbsp (30–45 mL) olive oil, divided

1 large red onion, coarsely chopped

2 stalks celery, coarsely chopped

1 medium carrot, coarsely chopped

½ each red, yellow, and orange bell peppers, coarsely chopped

5 cloves garlic, chopped

1 lb (500 g) lean ground turkey

1 can (28 oz/796 g) + 1 can (14 oz/398 g) diced tomatoes, with their liquid

1 cup (250 mL) tomato sauce (preferably low-sodium or no-salt-added)

1 cup (250 mL) chicken or vegetable broth (preferably low-sodium or no-salt-added)

2–3 tsp (10–15 mL) chili powder (to taste)

2–3 tsp (10–15 mL) ground cumin (to taste)

1 Tbsp (15 mL) unsweetened cocoa powder

1½ Tbsp (22 mL) chopped chipotle peppers in adobo sauce (for a gluten-free option, see Norene's Notes)

Salt and freshly ground black pepper

- **Some like it hot:** If using chipotle peppers in adobe sauce, freeze leftovers in an ice cube tray. Add them to spaghetti sauce, soups, and stews for a little kick.

- **Gluten-free option:** Chipotle peppers in adobo sauce are not usually gluten-free. Just substitute with chipotle-flavored hot sauce, which has a lovely, smoky flavor. Start with 6–8 drops, then adjust as needed—it's really hot!

DR. ED SAYS:

- **This is a great way** to combine your main dish protein (turkey) with essential vegetable sources. I like that it provides a variety of vegetables known for their cognitive contributions, resulting in a variety of important components, each contributing their own unique nutrients.

- **The other important aspect** of this recipe is that it uses a combination of olive oil and water to extract important antioxidants from the vegetables, some of which are water soluble and some that are fat soluble. The net result is a good mix per serving of the important brain nutrients of antioxidant phytonutrients, natural vitamin E, vitamin C, B vitamins, magnesium, and zinc.

> DID YOU KNOW? Most dried or raw beans have a toxin called lectin which can cause a severe reaction. Red kidney beans have one of the highest levels of this toxin, so make sure to presoak the beans, drain thoroughly, then cook them completely. You can avoid the risk by using canned beans, which are harmless.

SWEET POTATO SHEPHERD'S PIE

MEAT | GLUTEN-FREE OPTION | PASSOVER | REHEATS AND/OR
FREEZES WELL | MAKES 8 SERVINGS

Shelley Sefton of Toronto served this award-winning meal for dinner
the night of the Academy Awards and everyone went back for second
helpings! This is perfect with a garden salad and roasted or steamed
vegetables. It's a winner!

1. **TOPPING:** Place sweet potatoes in a medium saucepan and cover
with water. Bring to a boil, reduce heat, and simmer, covered, for 18–20
minutes. Drain well. Add oil, salt, and pepper, and mash until very
smooth. Set aside.

2. Preheat oven to 350°F (175°C). Spray a 9- × 13-inch (23 × 33 cm) baking dish with nonstick cooking spray.

3. In a food processor fitted with the steel blade, process onions, carrots, and garlic with several quick on/off turns, until finely chopped.

4. **MEAT MIXTURE:** Heat oil in a large deep skillet or pot over medium
heat. Sauté onions, carrots, and garlic for 2–3 minutes, until soft. Add
ground chicken and brown for 6–8 minutes, stirring often. Remove
from heat. Add salt, pepper, basil, oregano, egg whites, tomato sauce,
and matzo meal; mix well.

5. **ASSEMBLY:** Spread meat mixture evenly in the prepared baking dish.
Top with the sweet potato mixture and sprinkle with paprika. (Can be
prepared in advance up to this point and refrigerated overnight.)

6. Bake, uncovered, for 50–60 minutes, or until golden. Cut into squares
and serve.

276 calories per serving, 23 g carbohydrates, 5 g sugar, 4 g fiber, 27 g
protein, 11 g fat (2 g saturated), 313 mg sodium, 351 mg potassium

NORENE'S NOTES:

- **Reduce the carbs:** Instead of sweet potatoes, use a combination of
sweet potato and butternut squash chunks.

RECIPE CONTINUED . . .

TOPPING:

4 medium sweet potatoes, peeled
and cut into chunks

2 tsp (10 mL) olive oil

Salt and freshly ground
black pepper

Sweet paprika (for garnish)

MEAT MIXTURE:

2 medium onions, cut into
chunks

1 cup (250 mL) baby carrots

2–3 cloves garlic (1–2 tsp/
5–10 mL minced)

1 Tbsp (15 mL) olive oil

2 lb (1 kg) lean ground chicken,
turkey, beef, or veal (or a
combination)

½ tsp (2 mL) salt (or to taste)

Freshly ground black pepper
to taste

½ tsp (2 mL) dried basil

½ tsp (2 mL) dried oregano

2 egg whites (or 1 egg)

¼ cup (60 mL) tomato sauce
(preferably low-sodium or
no-salt-added)

⅓ cup (80 mL) matzo meal

- **Veggie up!** To boost your fiber intake, add a layer of 2 cups (500 mL) lightly steamed mixed vegetables (e.g., broccoli or cauliflower florets, chopped bell peppers, sliced mushrooms, peas, etc.) between meat and sweet potato layers.

- **Gluten-free option:** Use gluten-free matzo meal.

- **Frozen dinners:** Prepare and assemble as directed above, using single-size foil pans. Bake, uncovered, for 40–45 minutes, until golden. Let cool. Cover and freeze up to 3 months.

DR. ED SAYS:

- **Veggie power:** Sweet potatoes, carrots, and tomato sauce are very high in carotenoid and vitamin A antioxidants, and the potatoes and carrots contribute a good amount of fiber to this recipe.

- **Sweet potatoes** boost the digestible carbs and sugar content, so replacing some of the potatoes with butternut squash is a good option (see Norene's Notes). Squash contains half the carbs and sugar of sweet potatoes, but is still very rich in carotenoid and vitamin A antioxidants, as well as fiber content.

- **Sauce options:** In addition to using low-sodium tomato sauce, also look for a low-sugar version, since many tomato sauces come with added sugar—or just make your own (see Oven-Roasted Tomato Sauce, p. 490).

DECONSTRUCTED CABBAGE ROLLS

MEAT | GLUTEN-FREE OPTION | PASSOVER OPTION | REHEATS AND/
OR FREEZES WELL | MAKES 10 SERVINGS

My friend Lela Kornberg used to make stuffed cabbage rolls, but her kids always unrolled the leaves and only ate the meat! This updated version solves that problem. If you use coleslaw mix, it almost disappears in the sauce when cooked. Perfect for fussy eaters.

---

1. Preheat oven to 350°F (175°C). Spray a large casserole with nonstick cooking spray.

2. **VEGETABLES:** Layer half the vegetables in the prepared casserole; reserve the remaining vegetables.

3. **SAUCE:** Combine tomato sauce, Splenda, and lemon juice in a medium bowl; mix well.

4. **MEATBALLS:** In a large bowl, combine all meatball ingredients and mix lightly. Wet your hands and shape mixture into 40 meatballs, about 1½ inch (4 cm) in diameter, then add to the casserole. Top with the remaining vegetables and bay leaves. Pour sauce over and cover the pan tightly with foil.

5. Bake for 1½ hours. Uncover and bake ½ hour longer to thicken the sauce. Discard bay leaves before serving.

299 calories per 4 meatballs, 26 g carbohydrates, 10 g sugar, 5 g fiber, 25 g protein, 12 g fat (2 g saturated), 523 mg sodium, 232 mg potassium

NORENE'S NOTES:

- **Passover option:** Instead of Splenda, use Passover sugar substitute.

- **Leftover quinoa?** Instead of uncooked quinoa, use 1 cup (250 mL) leftover cooked quinoa in the meatball mixture.

- **Variation:** Substitute rice for quinoa in the meatball mixture (but not during Passover).

- **Just the meatballs:** Omit vegetables. Prepare sauce and meatballs and cook as directed above. Kid-friendly!

- **Slow cooker method:** Layer ingredients in the sprayed insert of a 6-quart slow cooker. Cook on low for 8 hours.

RECIPE CONTINUED . . .

VEGETABLES:

2 medium onions, thinly sliced

2 cloves garlic (about 2 tsp/ 10 mL minced)

1 pkg (16 oz/454 g) coleslaw mix (or 6–8 cups/1.5–2 L thinly sliced cabbage)

SAUCE:

5 cups (1.25 L) tomato sauce (preferably low-sodium or no-salt-added)

¼ cup (60 mL) Splenda Brown Sugar Blend

2 Tbsp (30 mL) lemon juice or white vinegar

3 or 4 bay leaves

MEATBALLS:

2 lb (1 kg) lean ground turkey (or lean ground beef, chicken, or veal)

1 large egg + 2 egg whites (or 2 large eggs)

⅓ cup (80 mL) uncooked quinoa (see Norene's Notes)

¼ cup (60 mL) tomato sauce (preferably low-sodium or no-salt-added)

½ tsp (2 mL) salt (or to taste)

¼ tsp (1 mL) freshly ground black pepper

1 tsp (5 mL) dried basil

1 tsp (5 mL) garlic powder

½ cup (125 mL) rolled oats or matzo meal (gluten-free or whole wheat)

DECONSTRUCTED CABBAGE ROLLS (continued)

- **The cabbage/coleslaw mix** provides folate, fiber, magnesium, and zinc.

- **Tomato sauce** provides most of the antioxidants. It is especially rich in the carotenoid lycopene, which, in addition to preventing brain cell degeneration, also helps prevent heart disease and certain cancers including prostate.

- **Sweet news:** Many brands of tomato sauce contain added sugar, so pick one that is not only low in sodium but is also low in sugar. To make your own, see Oven-Roasted Tomato Sauce (p. 490).

- **Splenda brown sugar blend** was used to reduce the sugar content per serving from the original recipe, but maintains the flavor.

- **Overall,** this dish is an excellent source of protein, lycopene, vitamin C, and fiber, as well as being a reasonable source of folate, B6, magnesium, and zinc.

> **DID YOU KNOW?** Tomatoes have to be cooked for lycopene to be released. Tomato sauce is much better nutritionally than raw tomatoes.

MIGHTY GOOD MEATLOAF

MEAT | GLUTEN-FREE OPTION | PASSOVER OPTION | REHEATS AND/
OR FREEZES WELL | MAKES 8 SERVINGS

Meatloaf is comfort food no matter how you slice it. When you don't have time to roll meatballs, this is a quick alternative. You can also use the meat mixture for meatballs, individual meatloaf muffins, or even burgers. Have it your way!

1. Preheat oven to 375°F (190°C). Spray a 9- × 13-inch (23 × 33 cm) baking dish with nonstick cooking spray.

2. **MEAT:** In a large bowl, combine ground beef, egg, barbecue sauce, rolled oats, salt, pepper, garlic, and basil. Mix lightly (don't overmix or the meat will get tough).

3. Shape mixture into 2 oval-shaped loaves. Place in the prepared baking dish.

4. **SAUCE:** In another bowl, combine bell pepper, onion, mushrooms, barbecue sauce, and cola; stir well. Pour sauce over and around the meatloaves.

5. Bake, uncovered, for about 1 hour, or until cooked through. Let stand for 5 minutes to firm up, then slice and serve.

437 calories per serving, 13 g carbohydrates, 7 g sugar, 1 g fiber, 18 g protein, 35 g fat (14 g saturated), 578 mg sodium, 385 mg potassium

NORENE'S NOTES:

- **Lighter option:** If made with lean ground chicken or turkey breast instead of beef, the nutritional analysis is as follows: 223 calories per serving, 13 g carbohydrates, 7 g sugar, 1 g fiber, 21 g protein, 10 g fat (3 g saturated), 571 mg sodium, 730 mg potassium.

- **Mighty good meatballs:** Prepare meat mixture as directed in Step 2. Wet your hands and shape mixture into 1-inch (2.5 cm) meatballs, placing them in a single layer in a sprayed 15- × 10- × 2-inch (38 × 25 × 5 cm) baking dish. Prepare sauce and pour over meatballs. Bake, uncovered, at 350°F (175°F) for about 1 hour. Makes about 40 meatballs.

RECIPE CONTINUED . . .

MEAT:

2 lb (1 kg) extra-lean ground beef
(for a lighter option, see
Norene's Notes)

1 large egg

3–4 Tbsp (45–60 mL) barbecue
sauce (preferably sugar-free)

⅓ cup (80 mL) rolled oats
(preferably large flake)

½ tsp (2 mL) salt (or to taste)

Freshly ground black pepper

2 cloves garlic (about 2 tsp/
10 mL), minced

1 tsp (5 mL) dried basil

SAUCE:

1 yellow or red bell pepper,
quartered and sliced

1 large onion, sliced

1 cup (250 mL) sliced mushrooms

½ cup (125 mL) barbecue sauce
(preferably sugar-free)

⅓ cup (80 mL) diet cola or
ginger ale

- **Meatloaf muffins:** Prepare meat mixture as directed in Step 2. Divide evenly among sprayed compartments of a muffin pan. Top each one with some mashed potatoes or sweet potatoes and sprinkle lightly with paprika. Bake at 375°F (190°F) for 30–35 minutes, until golden. Makes 12. Perfect for kids!

- **Variation:** Instead of barbecue sauce, use chili sauce, spicy tomato sauce, or salsa.

- **Passover/gluten-free option:** Instead of rolled oats, use matzo meal (whole wheat or gluten-free) or quinoa flakes.

- **Mushroom meatloaf:** For a low-carb variation, substitute ground dried shiitake mushrooms for rolled oats or matzo meal. The mushrooms will add flavor and moisture, especially to ground turkey, which can be bland. One cup (250 mL) dried shiitake mushrooms will yield ½ cup (125 mL) when ground. Make extra and store in an airtight container in the refrigerator or freezer.

DR. ED SAYS:

- **What's your beef?** Enjoying an occasional beef dinner (one serving per week) should not be harmful, but keep in mind that many national health organizations have attributed a shorter life span and greater risk of cancer to those who eat red or processed meat on a regular basis. Nutritionally, the beef version is similar to the chicken version except for brain nutrition—the beef version contains four times the amount of vitamin B12 and about twice the amount of zinc as the chicken version.

- **Bell peppers** provide an excellent source of vitamin C in both versions.

LOW & SLOW BRISKET

MEAT | GLUTEN-FREE | PASSOVER | REHEATS AND/OR FREEZES
WELL | MAKES ABOUT 8 SERVINGS

Assemble all the ingredients in your slow cooker, plug it in, and walk away! There's usually no need to add water because the onions and meat juices create lots of gravy. Perfect for Shabbat, the major Jewish holidays, or any other special occasion.

1. Spray a slow cooker insert with nonstick cooking spray. Scatter onions in the bottom of the insert and place brisket on top.

2. Season brisket on both sides with salt, pepper, and garlic. Shmear tomato paste and apricot preserves on both sides and drizzle vinegar overtop. Tuck in carrots around the brisket. Cover and refrigerate up to 24 hours.

3. Cook brisket on low until tender, about 8–10 hours, depending on your slow cooker. (If you put the brisket into the slow cooker just before going to bed, your house will smell amazing in the morning!) Let cool in pan gravy for 1–2 hours.

4. Transfer brisket to a cutting board and slice across the grain into ¼-inch (0.5 cm) slices (an electric knife works well). Return sliced brisket to the slow cooker insert.

5. Cook, covered, for about 1 hour on low, until fork-tender. (If you plan to serve this the next day, refrigerate overnight, discard congealed fat, then reheat on low for 1–2 hours.)

375 calories per serving, 17 g carbohydrates, 10 g sugar, 2 g fiber, 50 g protein, 12 g fat (4 g saturated), 224 mg sodium, 1070 mg potassium

NORENE'S NOTES:

• **Flat or fat, double or single?** Beef brisket is divided into 2 sections. The flat cut has less fat and is usually more expensive than a point brisket, which is much fattier as well as more flavorful. A double brisket (second cut) has a thick layer of fat between the two sections. Ask your butcher to trim the meat, leaving a thin layer of fat.

RECIPE CONTINUED . . .

3–4 large onions, sliced

1 beef brisket (4 lb/1.8 kg)
(see Norene's Notes)

Salt and freshly ground black
pepper to taste

4 tsp (20 mL) minced garlic

¼ cup (60 mL) tomato paste
(freeze remaining paste in ice
cube tray compartments)

¼ cup (60 mL) apricot preserves
(reduced-sugar or all-fruit)

2 Tbsp (30 mL) balsamic vinegar,
wine, or water

24 baby carrots

LOW & SLOW BRISKET (continued)

- **Fat-saving tip:** Cook brisket a day in advance and refrigerate. Discard congealed fat before slicing and reheating.

- **Time-saving tip:** If your brisket is very large (8–10 lb/3.5–4.5 kg), cut it crosswise, creating 2 smaller briskets (4–5 lb/1.8–2.2 kg each). Cook, tightly covered in a large roasting pan, for 3–4 hours, until fork-tender.

- **Overnight oven method:** No slow cooker? Cook brisket, tightly covered, in a large roasting pan in a 250°F (120°C) preheated oven for 8 hours or overnight.

- **Variation:** Instead of apricot preserves, use duck sauce or cranberry sauce.

DR. ED SAYS:

- **Sweet news:** This recipe is relatively high in sugars at 10 g per serving, but anytime you use fruit or its concentrates you have to expect higher sugar levels. Onions also contribute some sugars. On the other hand, this dish is very low in sodium and high in potassium.

- **Baby carrots and onions** are major contributors of important antioxidants, specifically beta carotene and quercetin.

- **Beef brisket** provides a high protein content at 50 g per serving (about 80% of your daily requirement). Beef is also an excellent source of zinc, vitamin B6, vitamin B12, iron, and choline, which is used by the body to synthesize neurotransmitters.

TERIYAKI LONDON BROIL

MEAT | GLUTEN-FREE OPTION | FREEZES WELL | MAKES
6 SERVINGS

Great on the grill! This marinade is also terrific on salmon, chicken, tofu, or Miami ribs. Alternately, it can be transformed into teriyaki sauce (see Norene's Notes).

1. **TERIYAKI MARINADE:** Combine all marinade ingredients in a jar, cover tightly, and shake well. Refrigerate until ready to use. (Keeps about 2 weeks in the refrigerator.)

2. **MEAT:** Place London broil in a large resealable plastic bag. Add marinade, seal bag tightly, and massage meat with the marinade. Let meat marinate for 30 minutes at room temperature, or overnight in the refrigerator.

3. Preheat barbecue or grill.

4. Transfer meat to the hot grill. Pour marinade into a small saucepan.

5. Grill meat over indirect medium-high heat for 8–10 minutes per side, or until it reaches desired doneness. (For medium, cook to an internal temperature of 145°F/63°C.)

6. Meanwhile, bring marinade to a boil. Reduce heat and let simmer for 5 minutes. (To transform marinade into a sauce, see Norene's Notes.)

7. Transfer meat to a cutting board and let rest 5 minutes. Slice thinly across the grain. Transfer to a serving platter and pour hot marinade (or sauce) over meat.

380 calories per serving, 10 g carbohydrates, 7 g sugar, trace fiber, 56 g protein, 11 g fat (3 g saturated), 592 mg sodium, 564 mg potassium

NORENE'S NOTES:

- **No barbecue? No problem!** Preheat broiler. Spray the broiling rack with nonstick cooking spray and line the bottom tray with foil. Broil meat about 4 inches (10 cm) from the top, about 8–10 minutes per side.

RECIPE CONTINUED . . .

TERIYAKI MARINADE:

2 tsp (10 mL) minced garlic

2 tsp (10 mL) minced ginger

¼ cup (60 mL) soy sauce or tamari (preferably low-sodium)

¼ cup (60 mL) pineapple or orange juice

2 Tbsp (30 mL) rice vinegar

2 Tbsp (30 mL) honey

1 Tbsp (15 mL) canola oil

2 tsp (10 mL) toasted sesame oil (optional)

2 Tbsp (30 mL) sesame seeds (optional)

MEAT:

1 London broil (flank steak) (about 2 lb/1 kg)

TERIYAKI LONDON BROIL (continued)

- **Teriyaki sauce:** At the end of Step 6, dissolve 1 Tbsp (15 mL) cornstarch in 2 Tbsp (30 mL) cold water. Stir mixture into the boiling marinade and cook, stirring constantly, until smooth and thickened, about 2 minutes.

- **Leftovers?** Thinly sliced London broil is delicious cold in a salad or wrapped in whole grain tortillas.

DR. ED SAYS:

- **Sweet news:** Although juice and honey increase the sugar content, they do enhance the flavor, creating a tender and tasty dish.

- **Flank steak** has the common attributes of all beef recipes, with a high protein content of 57 g per serving, almost a full day's requirement. Beef is an excellent source of vitamin B12, which is difficult to source outside of red meat, and is an excellent source of vitamin B6, zinc, and choline; it also supplies reasonable levels of magnesium.

- **Don't spare the sesame seeds or sesame oil!** The oil is a rich source of phytosterols, which help reduce cholesterol, and sesame seeds are an excellent source of brain-healthy nutrients.

> **DID YOU KNOW?** Because of the heme iron in red meat, flank steak provides a high quantity of iron, which can be a pro-oxidant—this is one possible reason for the increased cancer risk that accompanies red meat.

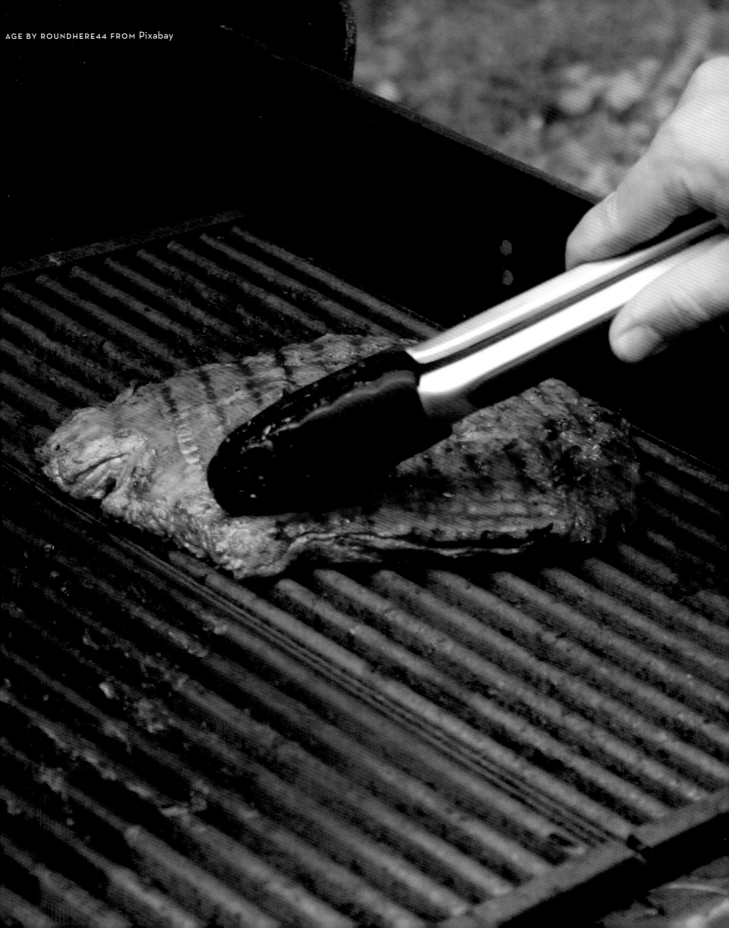

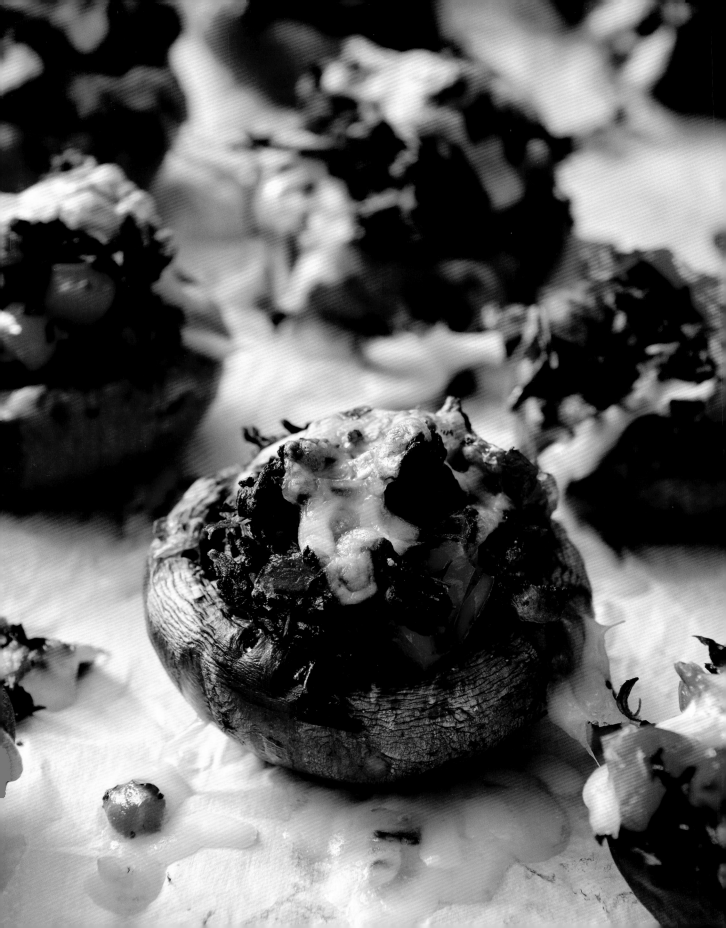

MAKE IT MEATLESS

THE GARDEN OF EATING: Eating a plant-based diet offers many brain-boosting benefits. Instead of focusing on meat and potatoes, make meatless side dishes the main part of your meal more often. Beans, grains, and vegetables can fill you up without filling you out.

PLANT POWER: Eating a plant-based diet of beans and legumes, soy products, grains, pasta, nuts, and seeds will provide you with plenty of protein. These items also contain magnesium, folate, potassium, antioxidants, and phytochemicals, are low in saturated fat, high in fiber, and are cholesterol free.

TOFU TIPS: The firmer the tofu, the more nutritious it is. Its firmness depends on the amount of water that has been pressed out of it. For stir-fries, use extra-firm tofu or it will break up during cooking. Silken tofu is fragile and better when puréed and used in salad dressings, desserts, and drinks.

TO SOY OR NOT TO SOY? Protein from soy foods (e.g., tofu and soy milk) is a good alternative to animal protein.

FULL OF BEANS: Explore the world of legumes, which includes beans, lentils, peanuts, and soybeans—you'll incorporate more fiber into your diet.

SNEAKY CUISINE: Add mashed beans, lentils, or chickpeas to meatloaf or spaghetti sauce—a good guideline is a third to a half legumes and the rest meat. Spread multigrain bread or pita with natural peanut butter or hummus. Add canned chickpeas, beans, or lentils to soups, salads, pasta, rice, or other grains.

BEAN ME UP! Beans and legumes are high in protein and fiber, low in fat, cholesterol-free, and gluten-free. They're also rich in B vitamins, calcium, iron, phosphorous, zinc, potassium, and magnesium. They are packed with folate, which helps reduce the risk of heart disease and Alzheimer's/dementia.

COMPLETE OR INCOMPLETE? Some proteins are complete, containing all the amino acids your body needs. Other proteins are incomplete and lack one or more essential amino acids. Meat, poultry, fish, and cheese are complete proteins, but contain saturated fat and cholesterol. Vegetable protein is often incomplete, so eat a mix of beans and legumes, nuts, whole grains, and vegetables to get your fair share of complete proteins, especially if you're vegetarian (e.g., combine beans with rice).

BEAN COUNTER: Beans, lentils, edamame, and peas contain about 5–8 g protein/½ cup (125 mL), which is approximately the same amount as in 1 oz (30 g) meat, poultry, or fish. Legumes also contain 75–125 calories, 18–20 g carbohydrates, and 6–8 g fiber/½ cup (125 mL).

FILL UP ON FIBER: Beans and other legumes are high in fiber, which your body can't digest. Fiber helps delay the absorption of sugars and fats into the body, reducing spikes in insulin and decreasing the risk of heart attack and diabetes. This is helpful for people concerned with insulin-resistance, diabetes, and GI, or for those who suffer from constipation, diverticulitis, or irritable bowel syndrome.

FILLING UP WITH GAS: Increase fiber slowly to avoid problems with bloating and gas when fiber is increased too quickly. Eventually your body will adapt. Like many of life's problems, this too shall pass. Good news—black beans are easier to digest than most beans.

WHAT'S THE DIFFERENCE? Soluble fibers (e.g., oat bran, legumes, nuts, seeds) produce gas because they are used by colon bacteria, whereas insoluble fibers (e.g., wheat bran, whole grains) are mainly bulking agents.

GO SLOW: Shift slowly to a higher-fiber diet by adding about 5 g more fiber each week. Keep adding fiber each week until you reach 25–35 g fiber daily.

TIME TO SOAK: Soaking beans for 24 hours shortens cooking time and also helps remove the indigestible sugars that cause gastric distress. It can also remove phytates in foods, which can reduce iron absorption. Soaking too long can lead to losing more essential vitamins and minerals, along with the phytates. Lentils don't usually require soaking—rinsing is enough.

OVERNIGHT SOAK METHOD: Soak a big batch of dried beans in triple the amount of cold water on the counter overnight. (In hot weather, soak them in the fridge.) Drain thoroughly, but do not cook—beans will double in volume. Refrigerate up to 2 days or freeze in airtight containers up to 6 months. When needed, add frozen beans (no thawing needed) to your favorite chili, soup, or stew.

QUICK SOAK METHOD: Rinse dried beans. Place in a saucepan and cover with triple the amount of cold water. Bring to a boil and cook for 5 minutes. Remove from heat and let stand for 1 hour. Drain and rinse well.

COOK IT RIGHT: Cook soaked beans in triple the amount of fresh cold water (not the soaking water). Bring to a boil, then cover and simmer until tender. If beans are very old or dry, they can take longer to cook. To add flavor and help reduce gas, add 2 or 3 cloves garlic or a slice of fresh ginger. (See Cooking Chart for Legumes, p. 348.)

LOVE ME TENDER: Don't add salt or acidic ingredients such as lemon juice or vinegar until near the end of cooking—they prevent the beans from softening. When almost tender, add salt or acidic ingredients; cook 10–15 minutes longer.

READY OR NOT? Beans are ready when you can crush them between your tongue and the roof of your mouth. For salads, cook just until firm or they'll be mushy.

SALT ALERT! To reduce the sodium in canned beans and legumes by half, place in a colander and rinse thoroughly under cold running water. Drain well. Choose no-salt-added versions or low-sodium brands. Rinsing canned beans also helps reduce gas. Beans can also be found in the frozen section with no preservatives.

CALCI-YUM! Dairy sources of calcium include milk, cheeses, and yogurt. Adults need 1000–1300 mg per day.

GOT MILK? An 8-oz (230 mL) glass of milk contains 300 mg calcium. Lactose-free milk and sour cream are available for those who are lactose intolerant. Yogurt with live cultures is usually tolerated by those who are lactose intolerant.

D-LICIOUS! Vitamin D is essential for calcium absorption. Milk contains vitamin D, and many other foods are now fortified with it. Vitamin D can also be found in limited amounts in salmon, sardines, herring, egg yolks, fortified cereal, fortified orange juice, almonds, beans, broccoli, figs, and breads.

CALCIUM WITHOUT THE COW: Many people are allergic to dairy products, while others may be lactose intolerant and cannot digest this natural sugar in milk. Calcium is found in leafy dark green vegetables (cooked broccoli, collards, kale, bok choy, spinach), beans, and legumes (chickpeas, black beans, kidney beans), soy products (fortified soy milk, tofu processed with calcium), nuts and seeds (almonds, peanuts, walnuts, hazelnuts), figs, raisins, oranges, and fortified orange juice. Eat canned salmon and sardines with the bones.

CHEESE PLEASE! Choose low-fat cheeses (<20% milk fat) when possible. Compare labels for fat and calorie content. Low-fat cheeses are sometimes rubbery, so you may have to experiment and try different brands. Use small amounts of strong cheeses, such as Parmesan or strong cheddar, rather than mild cheeses. This ensures maximum flavor and minimum calories. Just 1 Tbsp (15 mL) grated Parmesan contains 20 calories, so a little goes a long way.

A-PEELING: A quick way to grate a small amount of cheese is to use a vegetable peeler. Cheese will grate more easily if it's chilled.

MEASURE UP: When grating cheese, 4 oz (125 g) solid cheese yields 1 cup (250 mL) grated.

GRATE IDEA! A food processor grates cheese quickly. Use medium pressure on the pusher when putting the cheese through the feed tube while grating/shredding. Chilled cheese is easier to grate—freeze it first for 15 minutes.

IN THE BAG! Grate or shred cheese and freeze in heavy-duty resealable bags for 2–3 months. Press out excess air to prevent ice crystals from forming. No need to defrost it before using it in recipes. If cheese is lumpy and frozen into a clump, give it a few bangs on the counter to break it up.

Cooking Chart for Legumes

Use 3 cups (750 mL) unsalted water for each 1 cup (250 mL) of presoaked beans. Yields are for 1 cup (250 mL) dried beans or legumes. (Refer to Table 12, p. 78.)

Beans and Legumes	Cooking Time	Yield
Aduki beans	1–1½ hours	2 cups (500 mL)
Black (turtle) beans	1½–2 hours	2 cups (500 mL)
Black-eyed peas	1–1½ hours	2¼ cups (560 mL)
Cannellini (white kidney beans)	1–1½ hours	2 cups (500 mL)
Chickpeas (garbanzo beans)	2–3 hours	2½ cups (625 mL)
Fava beans	1½–2 hours	2 cups (500 mL)
Great northern beans	1–1½ hours	2¼ cups (560 mL)
Kidney beans	1½–2 hours	2 cups (500 mL)
Lentils (don't presoak)	30–45 minutes	2 cups (500 mL)
Lima beans (always cook with salt or they will get mushy)	¾–1½ hours	2 cups (500 mL)
Navy or pea (white) beans	1½–2 hours	2 cups (500 mL)
Pinto beans	1½–2 hours	2¼ cups (560 mL)
Romano (cranberry) beans	1½–2 hours	2¼ cups (560 mL)
Soybeans	3–4 hours	2¼ cups (560 mL)
Split peas (green/yellow—don't presoak)	45 minutes	2 cups (500 mL)

Equivalents for Beans and Legumes:

1 cup (250 mL) dried = 3 cups (750 mL) cooked
1 can (15 oz/425 g) = 1½ cups (375 mL) cooked
1 can (19 oz/540 g) = 2 cups (500 mL) cooked

CAULIFLOWER-CRUSTED PIZZA

DAIRY | GLUTEN-FREE OPTION | FREEZES/REHEATS WELL | KEEPS
2–3 DAYS IN REFRIGERATOR | MAKES 1 LARGE PIZZA (8 SLICES)

Most pizza crusts made with riced cauliflower don't taste great, and they definitely don't resemble pizza at all. Great news, the search is over! Carolyn Cohen, owner of Delicious Dish Cooking School in Toronto, shared her recipe for Cauliflower-Crusted Pizza, which I've adapted slightly.

1. Place an oven rack in the second lowest position and preheat oven to 425°F (220°C). Heat a large, rimmed baking sheet in the oven as it pre-heats (see Norene's Notes).

2. **CAULIFLOWER CRUST:** In a food processor fitted with the steel blade, pulse cauliflower florets for 25–30 seconds, until they resemble rice. Measure 4 cups (1 L) riced cauliflower into a microwave-safe bowl. Cover with a damp paper towel and microwave on high power for 4 minutes.

3. Transfer cauliflower to a clean kitchen towel and let cool. Wrap up cauliflower in the towel and squeeze out as much moisture as possible.

4. Transfer cauliflower to a large bowl. Add spelt flour, almond flour, salt, and garlic powder; stir well. Add egg and cheese and work dough with your hands so that everything is evenly distributed.

5. Remove hot baking sheet from oven and place on a heatproof surface. Line baking sheet with parchment paper and brush with olive oil—be careful, the baking sheet is very hot!

6. Spoon cauliflower mixture onto the parchment-lined sheet and carefully spread it out. (Tip: If you place another piece of parchment paper on top and press down it will help keep your hands clean!) Flatten crust into an oval or round shape, creating a nice, raised edge.

7. Bake crust for 12–15 minutes, until golden and set.

8. **TOPPINGS:** Remove pan from oven and add toppings, starting with cheese. Bake 10–12 minutes longer, or until cheese is melted and bubbly.

9. Remove from oven and let cool for a few minutes. Cut into wedges and enjoy.

RECIPE CONTINUED . . .

CAULIFLOWER CRUST:

1 medium cauliflower, florets only (4 cups/1 L finely riced cauliflower)

½ cup (125 mL) spelt flour (or any flour you like)

½ cup (125 mL) almond meal/flour

½ tsp (2 mL) kosher salt

½ tsp (2 mL) garlic powder

1 egg

½ cup (125 mL) finely grated reduced-fat mozzarella cheese

2 Tbsp (30 mL) olive oil, for brushing

TOPPINGS:

1 cup (250 mL) shredded smoked or reduced-fat mozzarella cheese (approx.)

12 cherry tomatoes, quartered (approx.)

Big handful of spinach (approx. ¾ cup/185 mL)

10 fresh basil leaves, roughly torn

CAULIFLOWER-CRUSTED PIZZA (continued)

201 calories per slice, 12 g carbohydrates, 3 g sugar, 3 g fiber, 11 g protein, 13 g fat (4 g saturated), 321 mg sodium, 287 mg potassium

NORENE'S NOTES:

- **Carolyn's tip:** Carolyn uses a cast iron flat top sheet and preheats the oven to 500°F (260°C), using this temperature throughout the recipe. Her baking times are slightly shorter, bake until golden and crispy. Never use parchment paper at temperatures over 425°F (220°C) as it will burn.

- **It's in the bag!** Riced cauliflower has gone mainstream. It is available at many supermarkets and specialty stores. No prep, easy cleanup!

- **Gluten-free option:** Replace spelt flour with gluten-free flour (e.g., chickpea flour, gluten-free oat flour, or all-purpose gluten-free flour).

- **Nut-free crust:** Omit almond meal and increase grated mozzarella to 1 cup (250 mL).

- **Top it up!** In Step 7, add a handful of broccoli florets, sundried tomatoes, roasted red peppers, zucchini, and/or diced red onion. Crumbled feta or goat cheese and/or grated Parmesan cheese also make tasty toppings.

DR. ED SAYS:

- **Cut the carbs:** This recipe is a wonderful way to cut back on the high digestible carbs in pizza by replacing a good part of the flour with cauliflower.

- **Cauliflower** is very low in carbs, fat, and sodium and rich in vitamin C, B vitamins, choline, and some important minerals and phytonutrients.

- **Overall,** this recipe is an excellent source of vitamin B12, vitamin C, and plant antioxidants, as well as a good source of B6, folate, and zinc.

EGGPLANT MOCK PIZZAS

DAIRY | PAREVE | GLUTEN-FREE | PASSOVER | REHEATS AND/OR
FREEZES WELL | MAKES 8–10 EGGPLANT PIZZAS

This makes a terrific low-carbohydrate vegetarian main dish. It's an excellent choice for people with diabetes. This recipe multiplies easily.

1 large eggplant, unpeeled

2 Tbsp (30 mL) olive oil

Salt and freshly ground
black pepper

Dried basil to taste

Dried oregano to taste

¾–1 cup (185–250 mL) tomato
sauce (preferably low-sodium or
no-salt-added)

1 cup (250 mL) grated low-fat
mozzarella cheese

---

1. Preheat oven to 400°F (200°C). Line a baking sheet with parchment paper or foil. If using foil, spray with cooking spray.

2. Cut off the top and bottom ends of the eggplant. Slice eggplant into rounds about ½ inch (1 cm) thick and arrange on the prepared baking sheet. Lightly brush both sides of the eggplant slices with oil. Sprinkle on both sides with salt, pepper, basil, and oregano.

3. Bake, uncovered, for 8–10 minutes, or until lightly browned. Remove pan from oven. Spread each eggplant slice with tomato sauce and top with cheese. (Can be prepared up to this point and stored in the refrigerator up to 24 hours.)

4. Bake 12–15 minutes longer, or until piping hot and cheese is melted and golden. Serve immediately.

110 calories per eggplant pizza, 7 g carbohydrates, 2 g fiber, 4 g sugar, 6 g protein, 7 g fat (2 g saturated fat), 59 mg sodium, 173 mg potassium

NORENE'S NOTES:

- **Eggplant info:** Eggplant comes in many varieties and shapes. The most common variety is pear-shaped. Asian eggplants are straight and narrow in shape, with a tender, slightly sweet flesh. Sicilian eggplant, which is like a round purple ball, is excellent for eggplant pizzas.

- **Store it right:** Eggplant keeps 7–10 days in the refrigerator.

- **To peel or not to peel:** The skin of older, tougher eggplants can be peeled, cut up, and simmered with other ingredients. However, if the skin is tender, peeling isn't necessary.

RECIPE CONTINUED . . .

EGGPLANT MOCK PIZZAS (continued)

DR. ED SAYS:

- **Eggplant,** although higher in sugar and somewhat lower in nutrient content than cauliflower, is an excellent substitute for reducing digestible carbs in pizza, as well as a good source of fiber. It is also an excellent source of one particular type of plant antioxidant called anthocyanidins.

- **Basil and oregano** provide high levels of other plant antioxidants.

> **DID YOU KNOW?** In one study listing the top fifty foods with the highest antioxidant contents per 100 g, both basil and oregano were in the top ten.

PORTOBELLO MUSHROOM PIZZAS

DAIRY | PAREVE | GLUTEN-FREE | PASSOVER | DO NOT FREEZE |
MAKES 6 MUSHROOM CAPS

Portobello mushroom caps make an excellent alternative to pizza crust if you are watching your carbohydrate intake. To remove excess moisture, broil or bake the mushrooms before adding the toppings. These make a luscious vegetarian main dish and are also excellent as a side dish or easy appetizer.

6 large portobello mushroom caps, stems removed

1 Tbsp (15 mL) olive oil

1 clove garlic (about 1 Tbsp/ 15 mL minced)

Salt and freshly ground black pepper

Dried basil

Dried Oregano

½ cup (125 mL) tomato sauce (preferably low-sodium or no-salt-added)

½ cup (125 mL) diced tomato

¾–1 cup (185–250 mL) grated low-fat mozzarella cheese

1. Preheat oven to 425°F (220°C). Rinse mushroom caps briefly and pat dry with paper towels. Lightly brush mushroom caps on all sides with oil, then sprinkle with garlic and seasonings. Arrange on a parchment-lined baking sheet, rounded side up. Bake, uncovered, for 5 minutes.

2. Remove sheet from oven and turn mushroom caps over. Fill each with a spoonful of tomato sauce and diced tomato. Sprinkle with cheese. Return mushrooms to the oven and bake 5 minutes longer.

3. Serve 2 or 3 pizzas per person, along with your favorite salad.

103 calories per mushroom cap pizza, 6 g carbohydrates, 2 g fiber, 4 g sugar, 7 g protein, 6 g fat (2 g saturated fat), 60 mg sodium, 352 mg potassium

NORENE'S NOTES:

- **Size counts:** Portobello mushrooms are just an oversized version of mushrooms. They can measure up to 6 inches (15 cm) in diameter and have a dense, meaty texture with a fabulous flavor.

- **Weighing in:** One portobello mushroom weighs about 3 oz (85 g), with just 27 calories, 4 g of carbohydrate, and 1 g of fiber.

- **What's in store:** Choose mushrooms that have firm, smooth caps—avoid those that are bruised, wrinkled, or have a broken surface.

- **Store it right:** Wrap unwashed mushrooms in paper towels or place them in a brown paper bag and refrigerate; they'll keep 7–10 days. Don't store them in plastic as they'll get wet and slimy.

RECIPE CONTINUED . . .

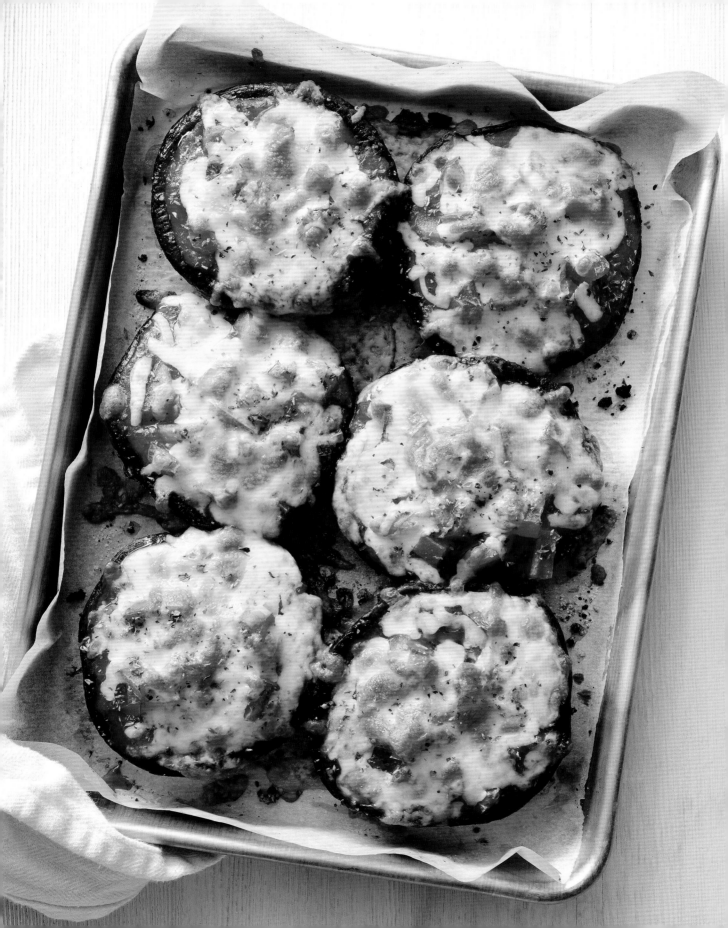

- **Cleaning mushrooms:** Clean mushrooms just before using. Rinse quickly in cold water, then pat dry with paper towels.

- **Save the stems:** The stems are very woody and should be removed. Don't throw them out—just chop them up and add them to soups and sauces. They add wonderful flavor.

- **Portobello cheese burgers:** Broiled or grilled portobellos are great served as a "burger" on a crusty multigrain roll and topped with sliced tomatoes, roasted red bell peppers, onions, and low-fat cheese.

DR. ED SAYS:

- **Mushrooms** are one of the few sources of the powerful antioxidants glutathione and ergothionine; they also contain other plant antioxidants, as well as the mineral selenium (which is also an antioxidant). Additionally, mushrooms are a good source of fiber and protein and are low in sodium, sugars, carbs, and fat. They also have reasonable amounts of important brain nutrients.

- **Overall,** this recipe is a good and varied source of plant antioxidants once we include the oregano, basil, tomatoes, and garlic.

> **DID YOU KNOW?** Mushrooms are the only fruit or vegetable capable of producing vitamin D when exposed to sunlight. In fact, some growers now produce mushrooms rich in vitamin D.

EASY VEGETARIAN CHILI

PAREVE | GLUTEN-FREE OPTION | REHEATS AND/OR FREEZES WELL | MAKES 10 CUPS (2.5 L)

1 Tbsp (15 mL) olive oil

2 medium onions, chopped

1 green bell pepper, chopped

1 red bell pepper, chopped

3 cloves garlic, crushed (about 1½ tsp/12 mL)

2 cups (500 mL) sliced mushrooms

1 can (19 oz/540 g) red kidney beans, rinsed and drained (preferably no-salt-added)

1 can (19 oz/540 g) chickpeas, rinsed and drained (preferably no-salt-added)

½ cup (125 mL) bulgur, couscous, or barley, rinsed (for a gluten-free option, see Norene's Notes)

1 can (28 oz/796 g) crushed tomatoes, including liquid (preferably no-salt-added)

1 cup (250 mL) bottled mild or medium salsa (preferably unsalted)

½ cup (125 mL) water

1 tsp (5 mL) salt (or to taste)

1 Tbsp (15 mL) chili powder

1 tsp (5 mL) dried basil

½ tsp (2 mL) pepper

½ tsp (2 mL) dried oregano

½ tsp (2 mL) cumin

¼ tsp (1 mL) cayenne

1 Tbsp (15 mL) unsweetened cocoa powder

Don't be deterred by the long list of ingredients—they're mostly herbs and spices. This delicious fiber-packed chili is quick to prepare and tastes even better the next day! Cocoa is the secret ingredient that deepens the color and rounds out the flavor. Best of all, leftovers keep about 1 week in the refrigerator!

---

1. Heat oil on medium in a large pot. Sauté onions, bell peppers, and garlic for 5 minutes. Add mushrooms and sauté for 4–5 minutes longer.

2. Stir in the remaining ingredients. Bring to a boil, then reduce heat and simmer, covered, for 25 minutes, stirring occasionally.

214 calories per 1-cup (250 mL) serving, 39 g carbohydrates, 13 g fiber, 6 g sugar, 11 g protein, 2 g fat (trace saturated fat), 363 mg sodium, 545 mg potassium

NORENE'S NOTES:

- **Variation:** Add 2 cups (500 mL) coarsely chopped fresh spinach during the last 5 minutes of cooking as a brain booster.

- **Gluten-free option:** Use kasha (buckwheat groats) or gluten-free couscous instead of the bulgur, couscous, or barley.

- **Use your noodle:** As a low-carbohydrate alternative, serve chili over Spaghetti Squash Noodles (p. 478) instead of pasta or rice. If you have a spiralizer, serve chili over lightly steamed zucchini noodles, or buy them ready-made.

DR. ED SAYS:

- **Mushrooms:** This is another recipe that includes the benefits of mushrooms, as described in Portobello Mushroom Pizzas (p. 353). Rehydrated dried mushrooms are also an excellent choice.

RECIPE CONTINUED . . .

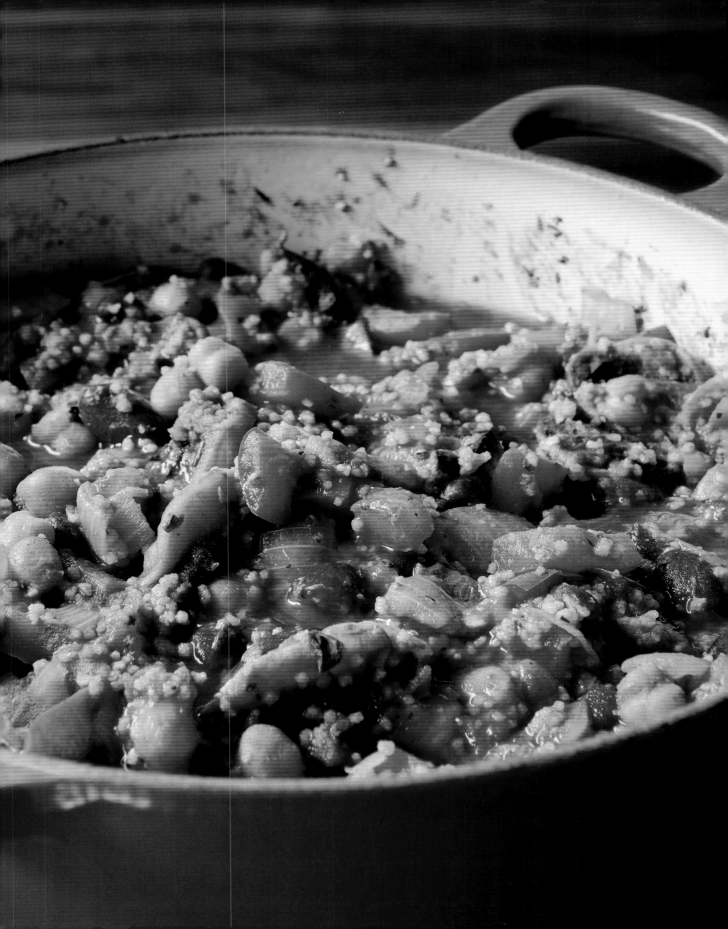

- **Red kidney beans and chickpeas** are members of the legume family, which has been shown to reduce the risk of developing AD/dementia. Both are rich in antioxidants and zinc, very high in fiber, and have good amounts of magnesium plus vitamins B6 and folate (especially chickpeas). These legumes have no saturated fat and are low in available sugar. Regular canned versions can contain about a quarter of the daily sodium limit per serving, so unsalted versions are recommended.

- **Spinach:** If you add spinach as recommended (see Norene's Notes), you will significantly improve the brain health benefits of this recipe. Spinach has the most evidence among leafy greens for reducing the risk of AD/dementia.

- **Cocoa powder, oregano, basil, and cumin** are excellent antioxidant sources.

- **Crushed tomatoes and garlic** are components of the Mediterranean diet.

- **Overall,** this hearty vegetarian chili is fortified with a variety of spices and antioxidant-rich vegetables. It contains high levels of fiber, vitamins C and B6, and folate. It provides good amounts of magnesium and zinc, as well as Omega-3 fats (though they are of a lesser quality than fish-source Omega-3 fats). Use either salt-free canned legumes or dried legumes to minimize sodium intake.

> DID YOU KNOW? In a list of the top 50 foods with the highest content of plant antioxidants, spices occupy 8 of the top 10 places.

LENTIL VEGETABLE MEDLEY

PAREVE | GLUTEN-FREE | REHEATS AND/OR FREEZES WELL |
MAKES 10 CUPS (2.5 L)

Don't be turned off by the long list of ingredients—just turn on your processor and give it a whirl! This fiber-packed brain-boosting dish is delicious over bulgur, farro, freekeh, quinoa, or zucchini noodles.

---

1. In a food processor fitted with the steel blade, process garlic, onions, and celery until chopped, using 2 or 3 quick on/off pulses. Transfer to a bowl.

2. Add carrots and mushrooms to the food processor and process with several on/off pulses, until chopped. Add them to the bowl.

3. In a large pot, heat oil on medium. Add chopped vegetables and sauté for about 8 minutes, or until tender, stirring occasionally.

4. Add tomatoes, water, lentils, bay leaf, and Italian seasoning; bring to a boil. Reduce heat to low. Simmer, partially covered, for 25–30 minutes, or until vegetables are tender, stirring occasionally. Add a little extra water if needed.

5. Add salt, pepper, lemon juice, and maple syrup; simmer 10 minutes longer. Remove bay leaf and stir in parsley. Adjust seasonings to taste.

360 calories per 1-cup (250 mL) serving, 63 g carbohydrates, 11 g fiber, 7 g sugar, 22 g protein, 4 g fat (<1 g saturated fat), 32 mg sodium, 863 mg potassium

NORENE'S NOTES:

- **Protein boost:** In Step 5, add one 14-oz (398 g) package extra-firm tofu, drained and diced.

- **Leftovers?** Transform them into soup! In a large saucepan, combine 4 cups (1 L) cooked lentil mixture with 3 cups (750 mL) vegetable broth. Season with salt and pepper and bring to a boil. Reduce heat to low and simmer, partially covered, for 20 minutes. Makes 6 servings.

RECIPE CONTINUED . . .

3 cloves garlic (about 1 Tbsp/ 15 mL minced)

2 medium onions, cut into chunks

2 stalks celery, cut into chunks

3 medium carrots, cut into chunks

1½ cups (375 mL) mushrooms

2 Tbsp (30 mL) olive oil

1 can (28 oz/796 mL) diced tomatoes (including liquid)

1½ cups (375 mL) water

2 cans (15 oz/425 g each) lentils, rinsed and drained

1 bay leaf

1 tsp (5 mL) Italian seasoning (or a mixture of oregano, basil, and thyme)

Salt and freshly ground black pepper

2 Tbsp (30 mL) lemon juice (preferably fresh)

1 Tbsp (15 mL) maple syrup or honey

¼ cup (60 mL) minced fresh parsley

LENTIL VEGETABLE MEDLEY (continued)

DR. ED SAYS:

- **Lentils** belong to the legume family, which tends to be high in digestible carbohydrates, so they should be eaten in moderation. However, they are also very high in fiber, protein, manganese, folate, and zinc, and therefore have a role in a brain-healthy diet.

- **Tomatoes, mushrooms, onions, carrots, and celery** add a good variety of different sourced antioxidants. And remember, onions have a special antioxidant called quercetin, which helps in the absorption of other antioxidants.

- **Overall,** this recipe provides excellent levels of vitamin C, vitamin B6, folate, zinc, fiber, and protein, though it is somewhat high in digestible carbs.

DID YOU KNOW? The legume family, to which lentils belong, contains significant amounts of a soluble fiber called oligosaccharides that can cause gas formation and bloating in the body. There are enzyme pills that can be purchased to help prevent this.

HEARTY VEGETABLE STEW

PAREVE | GLUTEN-FREE | DO NOT FREEZE | MAKES 7–8 CUPS
(1.75–2 L)

This updated version of my cousin Carol Teichman's fiber-packed vegetable stew is sure to warm you up on a cold winter day. Don't stew over the long list of ingredients—this dish comes together quite quickly. Chop the vegetables in batches in your food processor and add them to the pot as they are ready. This would make a great lunchbox addition.

1. Heat oil in a large, heavy-bottomed pot over medium heat. Add onions and celery; sauté for 6–8 minutes, or until golden.

2. Stir in garlic, carrots, parsnips, and green beans; mix well. Cook for 2–3 minutes. Add bell pepper and mushrooms and cook for 2 minutes. Add dill, oregano, and broth; bring to a boil.

3. Reduce heat to low and stir in mustard and maple syrup. Simmer, uncovered, for 10–12 minutes, or until vegetables are tender. Season with salt and pepper to taste.

151 calories per 1-cup (250 mL) serving, 25 g carbohydrates, 6 g fiber, 11 g sugar, 3 g protein, 5 g fat (<1 g saturated fat), 155 mg sodium, 602 mg potassium

NORENE'S NOTES:

- **Protein power:** Add 1½–2 cups (375–500 mL) black, navy, or red kidney beans (canned are fine, but drain and rinse well) in Step 2, along with the bell pepper and mushrooms. You can add 2 cups (500 mL) diced extra-firm tofu during the last 5 minutes of cooking.

- **Variation:** Add 2 cups (500 mL) butternut squash or sweet potato chunks along with the bell peppers and mushrooms in Step 2. Increase cooking time to 15–18 minutes.

RECIPE CONTINUED . . .

2 Tbsp (30 mL) olive oil

2 large onions, chopped

2 stalks celery, chopped

2 cloves garlic (about 2 tsp/10 mL minced)

2 medium carrots, chopped

2 parsnips, peeled and chopped

2 cups (500 mL) green beans, trimmed and sliced into 1-inch (2.5 cm) pieces

1 red or yellow bell pepper, coarsely chopped

2 cups (500 mL) sliced mushrooms

1–2 Tbsp (15–30 mL) chopped fresh dill

1 tsp (5 mL) dried oregano

2½ cups (625 mL) vegetable broth (preferably low-sodium or no-salt-added)

1 Tbsp (15 mL) Dijon mustard

1 Tbsp (15 mL) maple syrup or desired sweetener

Salt and freshly ground black pepper

DR. ED SAYS:

- **Green beans and parsnips** are not powerhouses of brain-friendly nutrients as they tend to be somewhat high in digestible carbs, but they are good sources of vitamin C, fiber, potassium, folate, zinc, manganese, and carotenoid antioxidants. The other vegetables compensate for the weaknesses of the parsnip and green beans. It's good to see oregano again, which was rated number 2 on the top 50 foods with the highest antioxidant content.

- **Overall,** although somewhat high in carbs and sugar, this recipe is an excellent source of fiber, vitamin E, vitamin C, folate, and magnesium; it is also low in sodium and high in potassium. The variety of vegetables offers different types of antioxidants for maximum effect.

VEGETARIAN CHOLENT

PAREVE | REHEATS AND/OR FREEZES WELL | MAKES ABOUT 20–24 CUPS (5–6 L)

This recipe from Susie Fishbein's bestselling cookbook, *Kosher by Design*, was originally adapted for *Norene's Healthy Kitchen*. It comes from her friend who is famous in his Upper West Side neighborhood for his vegetarian version of cholent. If you make this heart-healthy dish, you'll be famous in your neighborhood, too!

½ cup (125 mL) dried red kidney beans

½ cup (125 mL) dried white navy beans

1 cup (250 mL) dried brown lentils

2 large sweet potatoes, peeled and cut into chunks (about 4 cups/1 L)

2 medium potatoes, peeled and cut into chunks (about 2 cups/500 mL)

1 large or 2 medium onions, chopped

3–4 cloves garlic (about 1 Tbsp/15 mL minced)

3 medium carrots, peeled and cut into chunks (or 1½ cups/375 mL baby carrots)

8 cups (2 L) water (approx.)

1 cup (250 mL) old-fashioned oats

½ cup (125 mL) pot or pearl barley, rinsed and drained

2 tsp (10 mL) kosher or coarse salt (or to taste)

1. Place kidney beans, navy beans, and lentils in a large pot. Cover with 6 cups (1.5 L) water and bring to a boil; cover pot and continue boiling for 5 minutes. Turn off the heat and let the bean mixture sit, covered, for 1 hour. Rinse thoroughly and drain.

2. Transfer bean mixture to a 6-quart slow cooker that has been sprayed with nonstick cooking spray. Add sweet potatoes, potatoes, onions, garlic, and carrots. Pour in enough water to come to the top of the pot. Cover and cook on high for 1 hour.

3. After 1 hour, remove lid, add oats, and mix well. Add barley, using a wooden spoon to push it just below the surface but not all the way to the bottom. If necessary, add more water so that it fills the slow cooker to the top. Sprinkle with salt.

4. Cover, reduce heat to low, and cook overnight. Serve for Shabbat lunch, hot from the pot.

151 calories per 1-cup (250 mL) serving, 31 g carbohydrates, 7 g fiber, 4 g sugar, 7 g protein, 1 g fat (0 g saturated fat), 260 mg sodium, 516 mg potassium

NORENE'S NOTES:

- **It's in the bag!** Liners, which save on cleanup, are available to fit slow cookers in a variety of sizes. For a 6-quart slow cooker, use either a 16- × 17½-inch (40 × 44 cm) liner or a heatproof cooking bag. Add ingredients and close the bag or liner—make several slits in the top to allow steam to escape. Don't add any water to the bottom of the slow cooker, or your cooking bag or liner will bob up and down.

RECIPE CONTINUED . . .

VEGETARIAN CHOLENT (continued)

- **Leftovers?** Turn your leftover cholent into a scrumptious soup. Spray a large saucepan with cooking spray. Add leftover cholent and an equal amount of vegetable broth; mix well. Slowly simmer over medium-low heat for 15 minutes, stirring occasionally. Freezes well up to 3 months.

DR. ED SAYS:

- **Benefits:** Although this recipe is somewhat high in carbs, primarily due to the potatoes, it does contain significant fiber and protein from the beans and significant antioxidants from the carrots, onions, and garlic.

- **Overall,** this recipe is a good source of vitamin C, vitamin B6, folate, magnesium, and zinc.

> DID YOU KNOW? Any food containing starches, sugar, and protein that is cooked at high temperatures for a long period of time can produce a carcinogen and gene disruptor called acrylamide. However, as long as the cholent is kept below 250°F (120°C) and is not too dry, this should not be a cause for concern. The onions and other vegetable antioxidants will also help prevent formation of acrylamide.

ELANA'S VEGETABLE BOLOGNESE

PAREVE | GLUTEN-FREE | REHEATS AND/OR FREEZES WELL |
MAKES ABOUT 19 CUPS (4.75 L)

Elana Abramovitch, sister of our dietician Sharona, created this fiber-packed, heart-healthy dish as a way to use up all the vegetables in her refrigerator. Don't worry about exact measurements—just use what you have on hand. The recipe makes a big batch, so fill your freezer for future meals. Tastes so good, and it's good for you too!

---

1. Drizzle olive oil into a large deep soup pot with a wide base.

2. Sauté onions over medium heat for a good 10 minutes, stirring occasionally, until golden and translucent.

3. Add celery and sauté for another 10 minutes.

4. Add bell peppers and grape tomatoes and sauté for another 10 minutes.

5. Stir in garlic, broccoli, and kale.

6. Add tomato paste, crushed tomatoes, and diced tomatoes; mix well. Simmer, uncovered, for about 10 minutes.

7. Add water, lentils, and oregano, and stir to combine. Bring to a boil. Reduce heat and simmer, partially covered, about 30 minutes, stirring occasionally.

8. Add salt and pepper. Test lentils for doneness (see Norene's Notes). Sauce should be thick and chunky when ready.

149 calories per 1-cup (250 mL) serving, 27 g carbohydrates, 7 g sugar, 6 g fiber, 7 g protein, 2 g fat (trace saturated), 410 mg sodium, 545 mg potassium

ELANA'S NOTES:

- **Vegetable time!** The onions, celery, peppers, and tomatoes benefit from the long cooking process, enhancing the taste. Onions become sweet when cooked, rounding out the flavor of the sauce. It's okay if the vegetables brown a bit—just don't let them burn! Stir frequently and adjust heat accordingly.

RECIPE CONTINUED . . .

2 Tbsp (30 mL) olive oil

2 medium–large sweet onions, diced

6 stalks celery, diced

2 large orange, yellow, or red bell peppers, diced

6 cups (1.5 L) grape tomatoes, quartered

6 cloves garlic, minced

2 large broccoli crowns, finely chopped

1 cup (250 mL) kale (approx.), shredded into bite-sized pieces

1 can (5½ oz/156 g) tomato paste

1 can (28 oz/796 g) crushed tomatoes, including liquid (preferably no-salt-added)

1 can (28 oz/796 g) diced tomatoes, including liquid (preferably no-salt-added)

3½ cups (875 mL) water

1 cup (250 mL) dried green lentils

1 cup (250 mL) dried red lentils

1 Tbsp (15 mL) dried oregano

Sweetener equivalent to ½ cup (125 mL) sugar (e.g., granulated Splenda)

1 Tbsp (15 mL) sea salt (or to taste)

1 tsp (5 mL) freshly ground black pepper (or to taste)

- **Lentils** should be tender but al dente—don't let them get mushy. It takes about 30 minutes to get to this point, but simmer longer if you think they are too hard. Lentils are high in protein and fiber and are inexpensive. Use dried red or green lentils, or both, whatever you have.

- **Sweet news:** Granulated Splenda adds a bit of sweetness to rich sauces—add a little and taste as you go. The sweetness reminds Elana of her late Bubbie's cooking and her Eastern European roots!

- **Serving tip:** Serve with a mix of zucchini noodles and whole grain spaghetti, and top with a little bit of light goat cheese.

DR. ED SAYS:

- **Eat your veggies:** This recipe contains many of the same vegetables as the previous recipes for meatless dishes. The distinguishing feature here is the inclusion of kale and broccoli. Both are excellent for cognition, and both belong to the cruciferous vegetable family.

- **Kale** is very high in fiber and very low in digestible carbs, unlike some other vegetables with high fiber and correspondingly high digestible carbs. It is also noted for its very high carotenoid antioxidant content, especially lutein and zeaxanthin, which are both beneficial to brain health. It is also a rich source of flavonol antioxidants, and kaempferol. vitamin C, manganese, folate, and B6 are all found in high amounts. Altogether, this is a powerhouse of brain-directed antioxidants.

- **Broccoli** has similar features to kale but is not quite as good.

- **Overall,** this recipe is an excellent source of vitamin C, plant antioxidants, folate, B6, and zinc, and a good source of vitamin E and magnesium.

> DID YOU KNOW? The kaempferol antioxidant is being considered for cancer treatment.

"SPAGHETTI" WITH OVEN-ROASTED VEGETABLES

PAREVE | GLUTEN-FREE | PASSOVER | REHEATS WELL (DO NOT FREEZE) | MAKES 6 SERVINGS

Spaghetti squash "noodles" are low in calories and high in fiber, making this is an excellent alternative to traditional pasta. Enjoy this nutrition-packed delight for dinner tonight.

Oven-Roasted Vegetable Medley (p. 488)

1 large spaghetti squash (about 3–4 lb/1.5–1.8 kg)

Salt and freshly ground black pepper

3 cups (750 mL) tomato sauce (preferably low-sodium or no-salt-added; see Norene's Notes)

Grated Parmesan or mozzarella cheese (optional)

1. Roast vegetables as directed.

2. Meanwhile, pierce spaghetti squash all over with the point of a sharp knife. Microwave, uncovered, on high power, allowing about 5 minutes per pound. Turn squash over halfway through cooking process. An average squash cooks in about 15–18 minutes in the microwave. Let stand 5–10 minutes.

3. Cut squash in half. Using a spoon or melon baller, scrape out and discard seeds and stringy fibers. Use a fork to gently separate cooked squash into short, spaghetti-like strands. Place strands into a large microwavable baking dish and discard skins.

4. Season squash strands with salt and pepper. Toss with tomato sauce and top with roasted vegetables. Sprinkle with cheese, if desired. Reheat briefly in the microwave before serving.

298 calories per serving, 41 g carbohydrates, 20 g sugar, 10 g fiber, 10 g protein, 14 g fat (2 g saturated), 271 mg sodium, 919 mg potassium

NORENE'S NOTES:

- **Long strand variation:** For long, spaghetti-like strands, see Spaghetti Squash Noodles (p. 478).

- **Switch it up:** Instead of squash noodles, serve roasted vegetables over quinoa, cauliflower rice, or zucchini noodles.

- **Saucy secret:** Instead of jarred tomato sauce, use Oven-Roasted Tomato Sauce (p. 490), which has almost half the sodium and no added sugars.

RECIPE CONTINUED . . .

"SPAGHETTI" WITH OVEN-ROASTED VEGETABLES (continued)

DR. ED SAYS:

- **Spaghetti squash noodles** are a good way to reduce the carb content of regular pasta noodles. However, be aware that on a dry weight basis, carbs represent 82% of the total weight, with fiber representing only 18% of this amount. Although it is a better alternative than pasta, with more antioxidants, low sodium, and high potassium, it should still be eaten in moderation.

- **Overall,** this potassium-packed recipe provides an excellent source of vitamin E, vitamin C, vitamin B6, folate, magnesium, and zinc, but at 20 g sugar per serving it should be eaten in moderation.

INDIVIDUAL EGGPLANT LASAGNAS

DAIRY | GLUTEN-FREE | PASSOVER | REHEATS AND/OR FREEZES
WELL | MAKES 4 EGGPLANT LASAGNAS

These individual lasagnas make an excellent vegetarian main dish. Guests for dinner? Just double the recipe! If you don't like spinach, omit it.

1. Preheat oven to 400°F (200°C). Line a large, rimmed baking sheet with parchment paper.

2. Slice eggplant lengthwise into eight ½-inch (1 cm) thick slices. Discard end pieces that are mostly skin. Arrange slices in a single layer on the prepared baking sheet; sprinkle with salt and pepper. Bake, uncovered, for 15–20 minutes, or until tender. Cool slightly.

3. In a food processor fitted with the steel blade, combine spinach, green onions, cottage cheese, Parmesan cheese, and Italian seasoning. Sprinkle with salt and pepper and process until combined, about 10 seconds.

4. Spread spinach mixture on 4 of the eggplant slices. Top with the remaining eggplant slices to make 4 "sandwiches." Top each eggplant sandwich with tomato sauce and sprinkle with cheese. (Can be prepared up to this point, covered, and refrigerated up to 24 hours.)

5. Bake, uncovered, for about 20 minutes, or until tops are golden and eggplant is piping hot.

204 calories per eggplant lasagna, 18 g carbohydrates, 6 g fiber, 10 g sugar, 20 g protein, 8 g fat (4 g saturated fat), 268 mg sodium, 696 mg potassium

NORENE'S NOTES:

- **Meal deal:** Serve with a mixed green salad tossed with Italian dressing, and a side of whole grain pasta topped with low-sodium tomato sauce and grated Parmesan cheese.

- **Use your noodle:** For a low-carb option, serve with lightly steamed zucchini noodles or Spaghetti Squash Noodles (p. 478).

RECIPE CONTINUED . . .

1 large eggplant, unpeeled

Salt and freshly ground black pepper

Half of a 10-oz (300 g) pkg frozen chopped spinach, cooked, drained, and squeezed dry

2 green onions

1¼ cups (310 mL) pressed cottage cheese (skim or 1%) or low-fat ricotta cheese

2 Tbsp (30 mL) grated Parmesan cheese

½ tsp (2 mL) Italian seasoning

1 cup (250 mL) tomato sauce (preferably low-sodium or no-salt-added)

1 cup (250 mL) grated low-fat mozzarella cheese

DR. ED SAYS:

- **Eggplant** provides some fiber and a significant amount of antioxidants from a group called anthocyanadins (they also give the eggplant its color).

- **Spinach** is a great source of brain-supporting nutrients, and it's an excellent source of vitamin C, magnesium, manganese, vitamin E, and folate. Additionally, it is a very rich source of fat-soluble carotenoid antioxidants, including the brain-important nutrients lutein and zeaxanthin.

- **Tomato sauce** also provides a good source of lycopene carotenoid.

- **Overall,** although this recipe is somewhat high in sugar, it provides an excellent amount of protein and fiber, as well as vitamin B12, folate, magnesium, and zinc. It also provides good amounts of vitamin C and B6.

> DID YOU KNOW? By serving the eggplant with a salad tossed with an acidic, fat-containing dressing (see Norene's Notes), the absorption of the fat-soluble carotenoids and the eggplant anthocyanidins is improved. The fat helps solubilize the carotenoids and the acid of the dressing helps solubilize and stabilize the eggplant anthocyanidins.

PASTA PRIMAVERA

DAIRY-FREE OPTION | GLUTEN-FREE OPTION | PASSOVER OPTION |
DO NOT FREEZE | MAKES 6 SERVINGS

Use this nutritious vegetable-packed recipe as a springboard for your favorite vegetables. Spring forward to good health!

---

1. Bring a large pot of lightly salted water to a boil.

2. **SAUCE:** Meanwhile, heat oil in a large nonstick wok or deep skillet over medium heat. Add onion, bell pepper, and garlic; sauté for 3–4 minutes, or until tender-crisp. Add tomatoes and mix well. Season with salt and pepper. Reduce heat and simmer, uncovered, for 10 minutes, stirring occasionally.

3. Add asparagus and cook 5 minutes more. Stir in spinach and fresh basil and cook 2 minutes longer.

4. **PASTA:** While sauce is simmering, cook pasta in boiling water according to package directions, until al dente. Drain pasta and combine with sauce.

5. Divide pasta among 6 bowls and top with cheese. Serve immediately.

212 calories per serving, 31 g carbohydrates, 7 g fiber, 5 g sugar, 9 g protein, 7 g fat (2 g saturated fat), 141 mg sodium, 443 mg potassium

NORENE'S NOTES:

- **Veggie power:** Add 1–2 cups (250–500 mL) sliced mushrooms with the onions and bell pepper; use yellow, orange, or purple bell peppers as well as red. Instead of asparagus, use green beans or snow peas. Sun-dried tomatoes and/or roasted red bell peppers also make tasty additions.

- **Say cheese!** Instead of Parmesan, top pasta with ¾–1 cup (185–250 mL) crumbled goat cheese or grated low-fat mozzarella cheese.

- **Pesto power:** In Step 3, omit basil and add ½ cup (125 mL) Power Pesto (p. 492) to the sauce along with the spinach.

- **Dairy-free option:** Omit Parmesan. Add flaked canned tuna to the pasta and sauce.

- **Lighter option (gluten-free/passover):** Instead of pasta, use steamed vegetable zucchini noodles or Spaghetti Squash Noodles (p. 478).

SAUCE:

2 Tbsp (30 mL) olive oil

1 medium red onion, halved and thinly sliced

1 red bell pepper, halved and thinly sliced

3 cloves garlic (about 1 Tbsp/ 15 mL minced)

6 plum (Roma) tomatoes, coarsely chopped

Salt and freshly ground black pepper

1 lb (500 g) asparagus, trimmed and cut into 1-inch (2.5 cm) pieces

4 cups (1 L) lightly packed fresh baby spinach

½ cup (125 mL) chopped fresh basil

PASTA:

4 cups (1 L) whole grain pasta (e.g., rotini, penne, bow ties, or macaroni)

½–¾ cup (125–185 mL) grated Parmesan cheese

RECIPE CONTINUED . . .

PASTA PRIMAVERA (continued)

DR. ED SAYS:

- **Although pasta** primarily contributes to the high digestible carb content, this recipe without the pasta is a poster child for brain-healthy nutrients.

- **Spinach,** the main component, is a fount of brain-healthy nutrients as described in previous recipes. This is fortified by the powerful antioxidants found in the relatively large quantity of basil.

- **Tomatoes, bell peppers, and onions,** the stand-by vegetables used in many of our recipes, as well as olive oil and garlic, are all known for their brain-supporting nutrients. If you take into account the other nutrients provided in this recipe, a moderate serving, even with the pasta, is justified.

- **Overall,** this recipe is an excellent source of vitamin C, folate, and magnesium, and is a good source of vitamin E, vitamin B6, and vitamin B12. Without the pasta, many of the "good" source nutrients could be pushed into the "excellent" source category. So "use your noodle" and serve the sauce over vegetable noodles (e.g., zucchini noodles) instead of pasta!

BAKED VEGGIE "BURGERS"

PAREVE | GLUTEN-FREE OPTION | PASSOVER | REHEATS AND/OR
FREEZES WELL | MAKES 20–24 BURGERS

These colorful, nutritious "burgers" are packed with goodness. Minis make great hors d'oeuvres and maxis are an excellent vegetarian main course. Vegetarians and meat-eaters alike will ask for seconds!

3 large sweet potatoes

1 pkg (10 oz/300 g) frozen chopped spinach, thawed and squeezed dry

2 cloves garlic

2 Tbsp (30 mL) fresh dill

2 Tbsp (30 mL) fresh parsley

2 medium onions, cut into chunks

1 red bell pepper, cut into chunks

1 Tbsp (15 mL) olive oil + extra 1 Tbsp (15 mL), for coating

2 medium carrots, peeled

2 medium zucchini (no need to peel)

2 eggs

1 cup (250 mL) whole wheat matzo meal (use almond meal or gluten-free matzo meal for Passover)

Salt and freshly ground black pepper

1. Pierce sweet potatoes in several places with the point of a knife. Either microwave until tender, about 8–10 minutes, or bake in a pre-heated 400°F (200°C) oven for 1 hour, until tender. Let cool. Cut in half and scoop out the pulp. Place in a large mixing bowl along with spinach.

2. In a food processor fitted with the steel blade, drop garlic through the feed tube and process until minced. Add dill and parsley and process until minced. Add to the sweet potato mixture and stir to combine.

3. Process onions and bell pepper with quick on/off pulses, until coarsely chopped.

4. Heat oil in a large nonstick skillet over medium heat. Sauté onions and bell pepper for 5 minutes, until tender.

5. Insert grater in the food processor. Grate carrots and zucchini, using medium pressure. Add to onions and red pepper and cook 3–4 minutes longer. Cool slightly. Add to the sweet potato mixture.

6. Stir in eggs, matzo meal, salt, and pepper; mix well. (Can be prepared in advance up to this point and refrigerated overnight.)

7. Preheat oven to 375°F (190°C). Line a large baking sheet (or sheets) with parchment paper.

8. Shape vegetable mixture into 20–24 burgers and place on the prepared baking sheet(s). Oil your fingertips, then lightly oil the top of each one, flattening them slightly.

9. Bake, uncovered, for 10 minutes. Turn burgers over and bake 10–12 minutes longer, until golden.

79 calories per burger, 13 g carbohydrates, 3 g fiber, 3 g sugar, 3 g protein, 2 g fat (trace saturated fat), 37 mg sodium, 236 mg potassium

RECIPE CONTINUED . . .

NORENE'S NOTES:

- **Gluten-free options:** Although sweet potatoes are gluten-free, some tasty options are to replace them with 2 cups (500 mL) leftover cooked quinoa, buckwheat groats (kasha), or brown rice. You can also substitute 2 cups (500 mL) canned lentils, chickpeas, or green peas, rinsed and drained (however, most of these options can't be used for Passover, except the quinoa version).

- **Mini burgers:** In Step 8, form mixture into small burgers and oil the tops. Bake 15–20 minutes, flipping them over halfway through baking. Makes about 60 minis.

DR. ED SAYS:

- **Carb info:** This recipe tends to be on the high side of digestible carbs, primarily due to the potatoes and the whole wheat matzo meal. Using almond flour instead of wheat flour (not just for Passover) may be a way to partially reduce the carbs and increase the amount of brain-friendly nutrients (e.g., vitamin E).

- **Eggs** provide a good wallop of vitamin D, vitamin B12, and choline, which tend to be in low amounts in non-animal sources. Eggs also provide an excellent source of protein.

- **Overall,** the combination of ingredients in this recipe brings up the brain-relevant nutrient content to reasonable levels for vitamin E, vitamin C, vitamin B6, folate, magnesium, and zinc.

> **DID YOU KNOW?** Egg protein is considered the highest-quality protein of any food protein. This means you need less of it for the body than a poorer-quality protein such as bean protein.

VEGETARIAN SHEPHERD'S PIE

PAREVE | GLUTEN-FREE | REHEATS/FREEZES WELL | 6 SERVINGS

The shepherd will be out of work if too many people discover this meat-less version of shepherd's pie! This fiber-packed dish looks and tastes as if it was made with meat. We've reduced the carbs from my original recipe by replacing half the potatoes with cauliflower. Can you pull the wool over everyone's eyes?

1. **TOPPING:** Place potatoes and cauliflower in a medium saucepan. Add enough water to cover by 1 inch (2.5 cm) and bring to a boil. Reduce heat and simmer, covered, for about 15 minutes, until tender. Transfer to a colander and drain well. Return potatoes and cauliflower florets to the saucepan and mash with a potato masher. Add broth, olive oil, salt, and pepper; mix well and set aside.

2. **FILLING:** Heat oil in a large, deep nonstick skillet on medium-high. Add onion, red pepper, mushrooms, and garlic; sauté for 5 minutes, or until golden. Stir in ground beef substitute and tomato sauce. Cook, uncovered, for 3–4 minutes on medium-high, until heated through.

3. **ASSEMBLY:** Spread filling mixture evenly in a sprayed, 2-quart rect-angular casserole dish. Spoon frozen mixed vegetables evenly over the filling (no need to thaw). Top with the potato mixture and sprinkle with paprika. (Can be assembled in advance up to this point and refrigerated overnight.)

4. Bake, uncovered, in a 350°F (175°C) oven for 25–35 minutes, or until the layers are heated through and the top is golden.

295 calories per serving, 39 g carbohydrates, 11 g fiber, 8 g sugar, 23 g protein, 6 g fat (1 g saturated fat), 575 mg sodium, 1306 mg potassium

NORENE'S NOTES:

- **Variation:** Use the topping from Sweet Potato Shepherd's Pie (p. 331).

RECIPE CONTINUED . . .

TOPPING:

3 medium Yukon Gold potatoes, peeled and cut into 1-inch (2.5 cm) chunks

4 cups (1 L) cauliflower florets

½ cup (125 mL) low-sodium vegetable broth (approx.)

1 Tbsp (15 mL) extra virgin olive oil

Salt and freshly ground black pepper

Paprika (for garnish)

FILLING:

1 Tbsp (15 mL) olive oil

1 medium onion, chopped

1 red bell pepper, chopped

2 cups (500 mL) chopped mushrooms

2–3 cloves garlic (about 2 tsp/ 10 mL minced)

2 pkgs (12 oz/340 g each) vege-tarian ground beef substitute

⅓ cup (80 mL) tomato sauce (preferably low-sodium or no-salt-added)

1 cup (250 mL) frozen mixed vegetables (e.g., corn, peas, carrots, and green beans)

VEGETARIAN SHEPHERD'S PIE (continued)

DR. ED SAYS:

- **Cauliflower** helps reduce the digestible carb content per serving while increasing the concentration of brain-promoting nutrients and fiber.

- **Mushrooms** also help lower carb content and provide the unique plant antioxidants glutathione and ergothioneine, as well as protein, fiber, and brain-friendly nutrients.

- **Bell peppers and tomato paste** round out the antioxidant and nutrient contributions to the recipe.

- **Overall,** this recipe provides an excellent source of fiber, protein, vitamin C, vitamin B6, vitamin B12, folate, magnesium, and zinc.

CONFETTI VEGETABLE STRUDEL

DAIRY-FREE OPTION | REHEATS AND/OR FREEZES WELL | MAKES
6 STRUDELS

This elegant vegetarian main dish is also fabulous as an appetizer or side dish. To speed up preparation time, chop the vegetables in batches in a food processor. This recipe is quite flexible, so choose whatever vegetables you like.

1. Spray a large skillet with nonstick cooking spray and heat on high. Add spinach and stir-fry for 1 minute, until slightly wilted. Transfer to a large bowl.

2. Heat 1 Tbsp (15 mL) oil in the same skillet on medium-high. Add onion, zucchini, and asparagus. Stir-fry for 4–5 minutes, until tender-crisp. Add to the spinach.

3. Heat the remaining 1 Tbsp (15 mL) oil in the skillet. Stir-fry peppers, mushrooms, and garlic for 3–4 minutes, until tender-crisp. Stir in the spinach/onion mixture; season with dill, salt, and pepper. Remove from heat and let cool, draining any excess liquid. (Can be prepared up to this point and refrigerated, covered, for 24 hours.)

4. Preheat oven to 400°F (200°C). Line a large, rimmed baking sheet with parchment paper.

5. Place 1 sheet of phyllo dough on a dry work surface, with the short side facing you. Top with a second layer of dough. Lightly brush the top of the second dough layer with olive oil. Top with 2 more sheets of dough and brush lightly once again. You will have 4 layers of dough. (Keep the remaining dough covered with plastic wrap to prevent it from drying out.)

6. **ASSEMBLY:** Spoon half the vegetable mixture in a narrow band along the short end of the phyllo, leaving a 1½-inch (4 cm) border around the bottom and sides. Sprinkle with half the cheese. Fold the short edge of the phyllo over the filling, then fold in the long edges. Roll up the dough, starting from the bottom, forming a roll. Place seam side down on the prepared baking sheet. Repeat with the remaining dough, filling, and cheese.

RECIPE CONTINUED . . .

3 cups (750 mL) lightly packed
fresh baby spinach leaves

2 Tbsp (30 mL) olive oil, divided +
extra, for brushing

1 medium onion, chopped

1 medium zucchini (about
1 cup/250 mL chopped)

1 cup (250 mL) asparagus, sliced
in 1-inch (2.5 cm) pieces

1 red bell pepper, chopped

1 yellow bell pepper, chopped

2 cups (500 mL) chopped
mushrooms

3 cloves garlic (about 1 Tbsp/
15 mL minced)

¼ cup (60 mL) chopped fresh
dill or basil

½ tsp (2 mL) salt

¼ tsp (1 mL) freshly ground
black pepper

8 sheets phyllo dough, thawed

1 cup (250 mL) grated
low-fat mozzarella, cheddar,
or Swiss cheese

1–2 Tbsp (15–30 mL)
sesame seeds

7. Lightly brush the top of each roll with oil and sprinkle with sesame seeds. Using a sharp knife, partially cut through the top of the phyllo—but not through the filling—marking where you will slice it once it's baked. (You will get 6 main dish slices or 12 appetizer slices from each roll.)

8. Bake for 25–30 minutes, until crisp and golden. Remove from oven, slice, and serve warm.

276 calories per ½ strudel, 24 g carbohydrates, 3 g fiber, 4 g sugar, 10 g protein, 16 g fat (4 g saturated fat), 491 mg sodium, 449 mg potassium

NORENE'S NOTES:

- **Freeze with ease:** Reduce baking time by 10 minutes if you plan to freeze this strudel. Cool completely, then slice with a sharp knife. Transfer slices carefully to a deep foil baking pan, wrap well with heavy-duty foil, and freeze. When needed, don't thaw—just bake, uncovered, at 350°F (175°C), for about 20 minutes, until heated through. Strudel will taste just-baked and won't be soggy.

- **Phyllo facts:** For more tips on phyllo dough, see Spanakopita Roll-Ups (p. 195).

- **Dairy-free option:** Omit mozzarella cheese.

DR. ED SAYS:

- **Spinach** is the star of this recipe because of its high concentration of brain-supporting nutrients.

- **Olive oil** helps with the absorption of the fat-soluble antioxidants from the spinach and other vegetables.

- **Basil,** in its dry form, ranks 7th of the top 50 foods with the highest antioxidant content.

- **Asparagus** itself is not an insignificant player in the brain nutrition field. It is low in carbs and sugar, with good amounts of carotenoid and quercetin antioxidants. In addition, it has a reasonably full complement of other important vitamins and minerals for the brain.

- **Overall,** this recipe is an excellent source of vitamin C, vitamin B12, folate, and zinc, as well as a good source of vitamin E, vitamin B6, and magnesium. It is somewhat high in digestible carbs.

DID YOU KNOW? Asparagus contains a sulfur-containing chemical called asparagusic acid that breaks down in the body and causes a smell in urine. However, only 40% of people can detect this smell. It is not harmful.

CRUSTLESS ZUCCHINI QUICHE

DAIRY | REHEATS AND/OR FREEZES WELL | MAKES 8 SERVINGS

3–4 medium zucchini
(about 1½ lb/750 g)

2 medium onions, cut
into chunks

2 cloves garlic (about 2 tsp/
10 mL minced)

4 large eggs

½ cup (125 mL) canola oil

¾ cup (185 mL) whole wheat flour

¾ tsp (4 mL) baking powder

½ tsp (2 mL) salt

½ tsp (2 mL) dried oregano

½ tsp (2 mL) dried basil

½ tsp (2 mL) dried thyme

1 cup (250 mL) grated low-fat
mozzarella cheese

This treasured family recipe comes with "hugs and quiches" from Shani Bitan of Hong Kong. Her late grandmother, Ray Goldin, made this quiche for her family, and now her two granddaughters make it for their families in Hong Kong and Lyon, France.

---

1. Preheat oven to 375°F (190°C). Spray a 10-inch (25 cm) ceramic quiche dish with nonstick cooking spray.

2. In a food processor fitted with the grater, grate zucchini, using medium pressure. Transfer to a large bowl.

3. Insert the steel blade in the food processor. Add onions and garlic and process with quick on/off pulses, until chopped. Add eggs and oil and process briefly to combine. Add flour, baking powder, salt, oregano, basil, and thyme; process just until blended.

4. Add flour mixture along with cheese to the reserved zucchini. Stir with a wooden spoon to combine.

5. Pour mixture into the prepared dish and spread evenly. Bake, uncovered, for 45–50 minutes, or until golden brown.

272 calories per serving, 15 g carbohydrates, 2 g fiber, 3 g sugar, 10 g protein, 20 g fat (4 g saturated fat), 299 mg sodium, 392 mg potassium

NORENE'S NOTES:

- **Herbal magic:** Grandma Ray used dried parsley, her granddaughters use herbes de Provence, but I use basil and thyme because I always have them in my kitchen.

- **Say cheese!** Shani uses 1½ cups (375 mL) cheese and likes a mixture (Swiss, cheddar, havarti, etc.).

DR. ED SAYS:

- **Zucchini,** which is the main ingredient here, is just average in brain-healthy nutrients but is low-carb and low-fat, with some fiber. Its main claim to fame is that it is a good source of the important brain antioxidants lutein and zeaxanthin.

- **Added benefits:** It's also good to see the powerful antioxidant-containing spices oregano and basil, and the inclusion of eggs, which provide the needed animal-source nutrients vitamin B12, vitamin D, and choline, as well as high-quality protein.

- **Overall,** this recipe is an excellent source of vitamin E, vitamin B12, and plant Omega-3 fat (from the canola oil). It is also a good source of vitamin C, vitamin D, vitamin B6, folate, magnesium, and zinc. All in all, a comprehensive supply of many brain-benefitting nutrients.

DID YOU KNOW? Lutein's and zeaxanthin's original claim to fame was their use to prevent macular degeneration and cataract formation in the eyes. Since the eyes are directly connected to the brain, this led to promising research on their benefits to the brain.

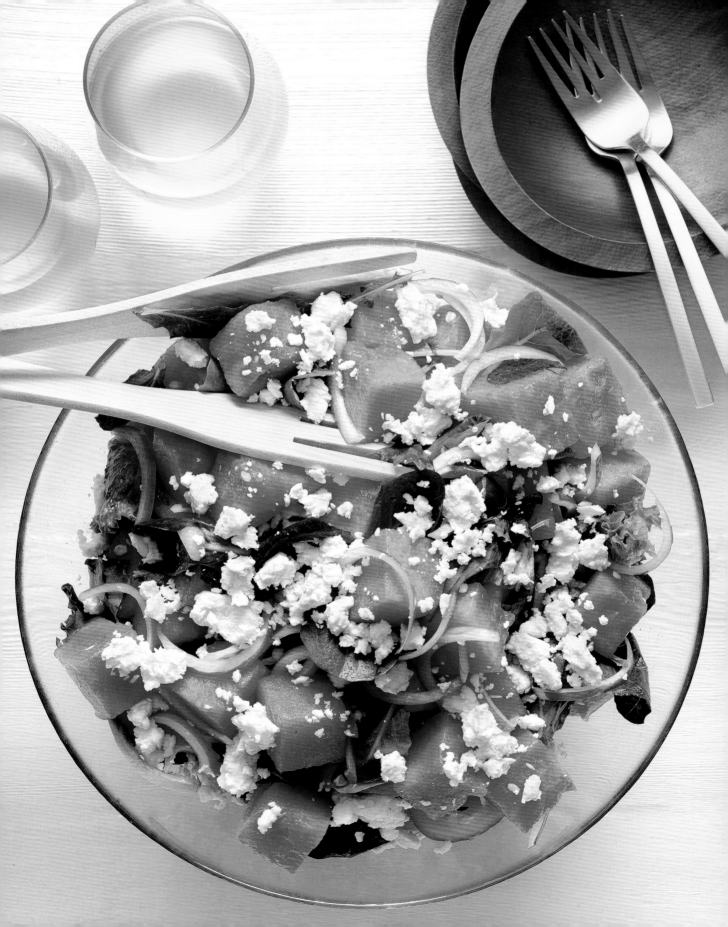

SAVVY SALADS, DRESSINGS, AND MARINADES

I BE LEAF! The darker the greens, the better. There's life beyond iceberg lettuce, so experiment with different leafy greens! Try arugula, Bibb, Boston, endive, kale, mâche, mixed greens, radicchio, romaine, spinach, or watercress—so many choices! Consider using kale or spinach instead of other salad greens to obtain a larger quantity of brain-healthy nutrients (e.g., potassium, folate, magnesium, vitamin K, vitamin C, vitamin A, and riboflavin).

IT'S IN THE BAG! Although the instructions on prewashed packaged salad greens state that they don't need to be washed, it's still best to wash them in cold water and dry well in a lettuce spinner. Wrap them in paper towels in a resealable plastic bag, squeeze out the air, and seal well. They keep in the refrigerator for a few days.

COLOR YOUR WORLD: Insert splashes of color into your salad greens by adding brightly colored vegetables. Try avocado, beets, bell peppers, broccoli, red or green cabbage, carrots, cauliflower, celery, corn, cucumbers, olives, red/green/sweet onions, sugar snap peas, radishes, and tomatoes.

BUY READY-TO-GO VEGETABLES: If you have no time to cut up your own vegetables or know that you won't eat as many if they are not already prepared, buy them cut up. They are not much more expensive and are often on sale. Salad bars and frozen vegetables are another easy alternative.

TUTTI FRUITI: Add some fresh and/or dried fruits to your salad. Try apples, assorted berries, figs, grapefruit, grapes, kiwi, mangoes, nectarines, oranges, pears, plums, pomegranate seeds, star fruit, and watermelon. Or include dried fruits such as apricots, cranberries, mangoes, or raisins. Add fruit, seeds, or nuts to your salad instead of croutons, which provide limited nutrition and are usually made from white flour.

BEAN ME UP: For a fiber boost, include canned or cooked legumes in your salads. Experiment with black, kidney, or shelled edamame beans, or add green or black lentils. If using canned beans, drain and rinse well to reduce the sodium content.

GRAIN POWER: Leftover cooked grains make an excellent base for salads. Try barley, buckwheat groats (kasha), bulgur, couscous, farro, quinoa, rice, wheat berries, or whole grain pasta.

HERB-ALICIOUS! Enhance the flavor of salads with the addition of herbs—fresh, frozen, or dried. Purchase dried herbs in small amounts for maximum flavor and freshness. As a general guideline, substitute 1 tsp (5 mL) dried herbs for 1 Tbsp (15 mL) fresh herbs. If fresh herbs are not available, chop together equal parts fresh parsley and your desired dried herb. Try basil, cilantro, dill, mint, oregano, parsley, rosemary, sage, and thyme.

PROTEIN POWER: Transform your salads into a main dish with the addition of protein. No-cook options include canned salmon, tuna, sardines, chickpeas, edamame, lentils, or cheeses such as goat, feta, or reduced-fat cheddar or mozzarella. Add leftover cooked/grilled salmon or tofu. Meat options include chicken or turkey.

NUTS AND SEEDS: Tasty toppers include almonds, hazelnuts, peanuts, pecans, pine nuts, pistachios, and walnuts. Toast them first in the oven or a skillet for a flavor boost. Experiment with different seeds such as hemp, pumpkin, sesame, or sunflower seeds.

PREPARED VS HOMEMADE SALAD DRESSINGS: Many salad dressings can surprisingly add 350–400 calories to a typical salad plate. When eating out, consider asking for your salad dressing on the side. First, dip your fork into the dressing, then into your salad. You will still get the taste of the dressing but will use much less. You can also ask for your salad to be lightly dressed (e.g., adding only half the dressing). At the supermarket, try choosing a dressing that is equal to or less than 45 calories per 1 Tbsp (15 mL)—no need to choose the lower-fat option. Also, choose lower-sugar dressings over higher-sugar options. Or, make your own dressing, which is often the best choice. That way you know exactly what is in it!

WELL DRESSED! When you make your own salad dressings, you control what goes into them—and what goes into you. As a basic guideline, use two parts of oil to one part acid, such as different vinegars or citrus juices. A drizzle of honey, maple syrup, or your favorite sweetener will round out the flavor. Mustard also adds a nice punch. Add your favorite fresh or dried herbs.

OIL STORAGE: Store oils in a sealed container away from heat and light. Although pure olive oil retains its freshness when refrigerated, it does thicken and become cloudy. No problem—just bring it back to room temperature and it will become liquid again. Also read "Oil About Fats!" (p. 387) for information on various oils.

DRESS RIGHT AT THE LAST MINUTE: Toss salads together with dressing just before serving. Make sure that salad greens are dry or the dressing won't cling to them. Serve salad on chilled plates to preserve crispness.

TOSS THE DRESSING? Homemade dressings keep in the refrigerator for about 1–2 weeks, especially those that contain fresh garlic.

WHAT'S IN STORE? Commercial dressings can often last for months in the refrigerator once they have been opened, as they contain preservatives. Choose a store-bought brand that doesn't contain high-fructose corn syrup, hydrogenated oils, or trans-fats. Dressings should contain less than 4 g saturated fat and less than 4 g sugar per serving.

GLUTEN-FREE SOY OPTION: Did you know that most brands of soy sauce contain wheat? You can substitute gluten-free soy sauce or reduced-sodium tamari in salad dressings, marinades, or other recipes.

DOUBLE-DUTY: Many dressings can be used as a marinade—double your pleasure!

MARIN-AIDES: Marinades enhance flavor and increase the tenderness of meats, poultry, and fish. Marinating foods also protects them from forming harmful carcinogens (HCAs) during grilling or broiling. Good news—HCAs don't form on grilled vegetables or fruit!

BAG IT! Marinating foods in a heavy-duty resealable plastic bag allows for a more-thorough coating—you'll also use less marinade! Shake the bag or massage the food so it will be evenly coated.

TIME TO MARINATE: Marinate meats or poultry at room temperature for 30–60 minutes, or in the refrigerator for a day or two. Don't marinate fish for more than an hour before cooking or it will affect the texture.

FROZEN ASSETS: You can freeze most marinades with the chicken or meat up to 2 months. Thaw overnight in the refrigerator, then cook as directed.

LEFTOVER MARINADE? To use it for basting or as a sauce, bring leftover marinades to a boil, then simmer for 5 minutes before drizzling over cooked food. Marinade that is used for raw meat, poultry, or fish should be either discarded after draining or boiled for 5 minutes to kill harmful bacteria.

BRUSH UP! Use separate brushes to baste raw and cooked meats, poultry, or fish. Silicone brushes are easy to clean and are dishwasher safe.

OIL ABOUT FATS! Remember that oils are just fats that happen to be liquid at room temperature—they are referred to as unsaturated fats. This property distinguishes them as healthy for the brain and heart, as opposed to saturated fats. Saturated fats, such as those found in meat and dairy, are solid at room temperature and considered unhealthy by many health professionals.

BRAIN BENEFITS: The brain needs fats, but the right kind of fats. To provide benefits for the brain and heart, choose from the following oils, listed in order of efficacy:

- Fish oils from fish (Omega-3 fats) such as salmon, sardines, and anchovies. These are best consumed with the fish rather than as a supplement.
- Polyunsaturated alpha-linoleic acid oils such as flaxseed, hemp, chia, and walnut oil. These are another form of Omega-3 fats, but less effective than fish oils.
- Other polyunsaturated oils such as grapeseed, safflower, sunflower, and soybean oil.
- Monounsaturated oils such as avocado, olive, canola, and high-oleic sunflower oil.

WHAT'S THE DIFFERENCE? Polyunsaturated and monounsaturated oils are equally healthy for the brain (and the heart), but be aware that polyunsaturated oils are less stable and go rancid more quickly.

OIL RIGHT! Although the list of oils above is given in order of efficacy, any of these oils is healthy enough to be part of a brain-healthy diet. This is because most oils will contain a mixture of polyunsaturated and monounsaturated fats, as well as alpha-linolenic acid.

COCONUT OIL is currently being studied for its effect on brain function. However, the American Heart Association considers it unhealthy because of its high level of saturated fats.

MEDITERRANEAN BEAN SALAD

DAIRY OPTION | PAREVE | GLUTEN-FREE | KEEPS ABOUT 3 DAYS IN
THE REFRIGERATOR | MAKES 4 SERVINGS

1 can (19 oz/540 g) red
kidney beans, drained and rinsed
(preferably unsalted)

3 green onions, trimmed and
thinly sliced

2 cloves garlic (about 2 tsp/
10 mL minced)

½ cup (125 mL) minced
fresh parsley

1 yellow, orange, or red bell
pepper, chopped

1 cup (250 mL) grape or cherry
tomatoes, halved

2 Tbsp (30 mL) extra virgin
olive oil

2 Tbsp (30 mL) lemon juice
(preferably fresh)

Salt and freshly ground
black pepper

½ tsp (2 mL) dried oregano, basil,
thyme, or rosemary (or 2 tsp/
10 mL minced fresh)

This Mediterranean delight is packed with fiber and is a good source of protein. It also works well with chickpeas or black beans. This satisfying, nutritious salad makes a delicious addition to your lunch box.

1. Combine beans, green onions, garlic, parsley, bell pepper, and tomatoes in a large bowl. Add oil, lemon juice, and seasonings. Mix well.

2. Marinate at room temperature for 15 minutes, or overnight, covered, in the refrigerator. Best served chilled.

204 calories per serving, 27 g carbohydrates, 3 g sugar, 13 g fiber, 11 g protein, 7 g fat (1 g saturated), 26 mg sodium, 778 mg potassium

NORENE'S NOTES:

- **Dairy option:** Sprinkle ½ cup (125 mL) crumbled goat or feta cheese overtop.

- **Mediterranean mixed bean salad:** Expecting a crowd? Double or triple the recipe, using a mixture of red or white kidney beans, black beans, and chickpeas. If desired, add a handful of black olives and 2 Tbsp (30 mL) chopped sundried tomatoes.

- **Lauren's black bean salad, greek-style:** Use black beans instead of kidney beans. Use ½ cup (125 mL) chopped red onion instead of green onions. Replace lemon juice with balsamic vinegar. Sprinkle ½ cup (125 mL) crumbled feta or goat cheese overtop.

- **Beans, bell pepper, and tomatoes** are the key ingredients. When combined with the other ingredients, they provide almost 50% of the daily value for fiber (which is deficient in the North American diet) as recommended by government health authorities, as well as a number of important complex plant antioxidants and vitamin C. The important brain minerals magnesium and zinc are also in good supply here.

- **The fat** is mostly healthy monounsaturated fats, and olive oil is probably the best oil for the brain.

- **Bonus!** Researchers have found that oleocanthal, a chemical in olive oil, is a potent anti-cancer agent.

MARINATED VEGETABLE SALAD

PAREVE | GLUTEN-FREE | PASSOVER | KEEPS ABOUT 10 DAYS IN THE REFRIGERATOR | MAKES 12 SERVINGS

SALAD:

1 small head cauliflower, broken into florets

1 small head broccoli, broken into florets (cut stems into 1-inch/ 2.5-cm pieces)

1 red bell pepper, cut into 1-inch (2.5 cm) pieces

1 yellow bell pepper, cut into 1-inch (2.5 cm) pieces

2 large sweet onions, cut into 1-inch (2.5 cm) pieces

1 stalk celery, cut into ¼-inch (0.5 cm) pieces

4 medium carrots, sliced into ¼-inch (0.5 cm) coins

1 can (12 oz/340 g) pitted black olives, drained and rinsed (see Norene's Notes)

½ small head red or green cabbage, shredded (optional)

MARINADE:

2 cloves garlic, minced

1 cup (250 mL) white vinegar

¼ cup (60 mL) vegetable oil

Sweetener equivalent to ⅓ cup (80 mL) sugar (or to taste)

½ tsp (2 mL) kosher salt (or to taste)

Mimi Markofsky, a kosher caterer in West Bloomfield, MI, modified the marinated fresh vegetable salad recipe in my food processor cookbook and made it Passover-friendly. In her words: "This salad is a staple throughout the spring and summer in my house because it's easy to make, light, and a great snack during the before-dinner munchie time." My original recipe called for beans, but Mimi converted the ingredients to Passover-friendly vegetables.

---

1. **SALAD:** Prepare all vegetables as directed above and place them into a large mixing bowl.

2. **MARINADE:** Combine marinade ingredients in a saucepan and bring to a rolling boil, stirring occasionally.

3. Pour hot marinade over vegetables and mix well.

4. Cover and refrigerate for at least 1 hour, or overnight, to blend the flavors. Serve chilled.

148 calories per serving, 12 g carbohydrates, 5 g sugar, 2 g fiber, 2 g protein, 10 g fat (1 g saturated), 336 mg sodium, 293 mg potassium

NORENE'S NOTES:

- **Olive info:** Green olives are picked when they have reached full size, but before the ripening process has begun. Black olives are picked at maturity, when they are fully ripe, and range in color from purple to brown to black. Kalamata olives are larger, meatier, and saltier than most olives. They are native to Greece and although they are considered a black olive, they are actually purple-black in color.

DR. ED SAYS:

- **Cauliflower, broccoli, and cabbage,** the main cruciferous vegetables, are all featured in this salad. Broccoli provides good quantities of lutein and zeaxanthin, which have been shown to be beneficial to the brain as well as the eyes. As a bonus, the cruciferous vegetables also supply sulforaphane, which helps reduce the risk of cancer.

- **Olives** generally provide good levels of fiber, the brain antioxidants vitamin C and vitamin E, as well as other carotenoids (much of which also comes from carrots). They supply necessary monounsaturated fats and unique brain-healthy compounds.

- **Celery** has a chemical constituent called luteolin, which has been shown to reduce inflammation in the brain.

- **Overall,** this salad is low in sugar and carbs, and high in magnesium, zinc, and folate. Consider replacing the vegetable oil with olive or avocado oil.

RED CABBAGE COLESLAW

PAREVE | GLUTEN-FREE | PASSOVER | KEEPS ABOUT 1 WEEK IN THE REFRIGERATOR | MAKES 7½–8 CUPS (1.85–2 L)

COLESLAW:

1 large head red cabbage, thinly sliced (about 8 cups/2 L)

2 medium carrots, shredded (about 1 cup/250 mL)

¾ cup (185 mL) chopped red onion or green onions

1 red bell pepper, chopped

2 cloves garlic (about 2 tsp/ 10 mL minced)

2 Tbsp (30 mL) minced fresh dill

Salt and freshly ground black pepper to taste

Toasted slivered almonds (optional, for garnish)

DRESSING:

¼ cup (60 mL) balsamic vinegar

¼ cup (60 mL) extra virgin olive oil

Sweetener equivalent to ¼ cup (60 mL) sugar

It's culinary magic—pour this hot dressing over the slaw and the red cabbage will turn a brilliant magenta color! If you prefer green cabbage, try Asian coleslaw (below). Double your pleasure!

---

1. **COLESLAW:** Combine cabbage, carrots, onion, red pepper, and garlic in a large mixing bowl.

2. **DRESSING:** In a small saucepan, combine vinegar and oil; heat until almost boiling. (Alternatively, combine vinegar and oil in a 2-cup/ 500-mL glass measure and microwave on high for 45 seconds). Add sweetener and stir to dissolve.

3. Pour hot dressing over the vegetables and toss well. Add dill, salt, and pepper, and toss again.

4. Cover and refrigerate for at least 1 hour, or overnight, to blend the flavors.

5. Adjust seasonings before serving. Top with almonds, if using.

86 calories per ¾-cup (185 mL) serving, 9 g carbohydrates, 5 g sugar, 2 g fiber, 1 g protein, 6 g fat (1 g saturated), 23 mg sodium, 85 mg potassium

NORENE'S NOTES:

- **Processor power:** Slice cabbage quickly in the food processor, using the slicing blade. Cut cabbage into wedges small enough to fit through the feed tube and discard the core. Slice cabbage wedges, using extremely light pressure on the pusher.

- **Quick coleslaw:** Substitute 2 bags (16 oz/454 g each) shredded red cabbage.

- **Asian coleslaw:** Use green or Napa cabbage instead of red cabbage and omit the dill. Add ⅓ cup (80 mL) unsweetened dried cranberries and 1 well-drained can (11 oz/312 g) mandarin orange segments. Instead of using the dressing above, use Asian Dressing/Marinade (p. 422); no need to boil it first.

- **Cabbage, carrots, and bell pepper** are the main components of this salad. Cabbage represents the cruciferous vegetable group we talked about in Marinated Vegetable Salad (p. 390), with high magnesium, reasonable sugar levels, and good amounts of zinc, vitamin C, and folate for the brain. Contributions of the bell pepper and carrots were discussed in previous recipes.

- **Olive oil,** an important component of the Mediterranean diet, rounds out the recipe, as well as almonds, which supply some needed vitamin E.

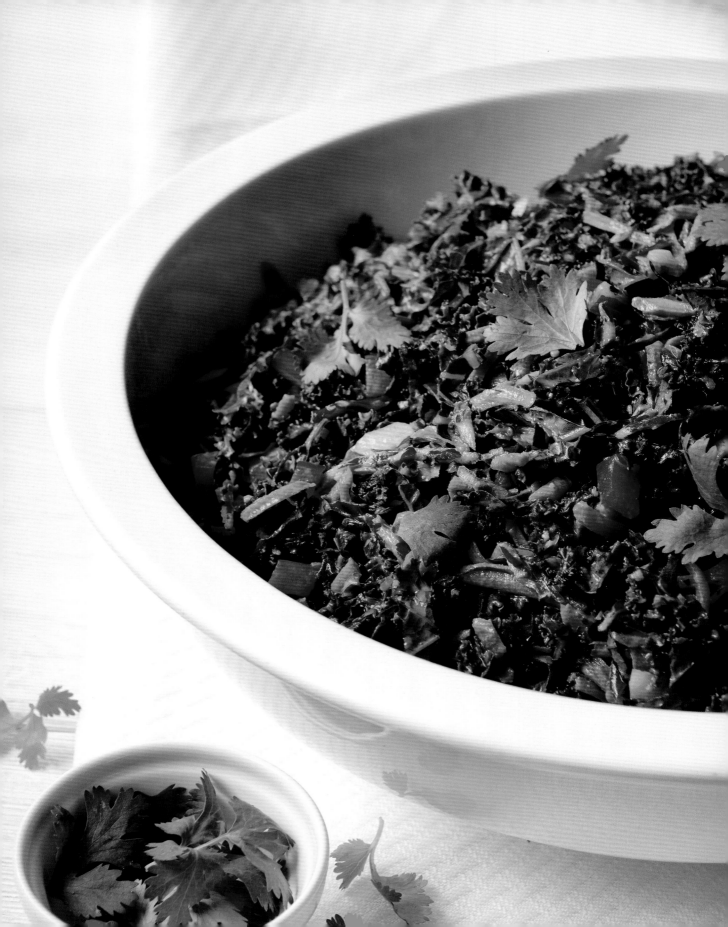

KALE SLAW WITH PEANUT DRESSING

PAREVE | GLUTEN-FREE OPTION | KEEPS ABOUT 3 DAYS IN THE REFRIGERATOR | MAKES 8 SERVINGS

The creamy peanut dressing tempers the bitterness of the kale. For a gluten-free option, substitute tamari for soy sauce in the dressing. Everyone will go nuts for this recipe!

Peanut Dressing/Marinade (p. 427)

KALE SLAW:

1 medium bunch kale (about 1 lb/500 g)

1 Tbsp (15 mL) canola oil

4 cups (1 L) shredded red cabbage (or one 16-oz/500-g pkg)

2 cups (500 mL) shredded carrots (about 4 medium carrots)

1 red bell pepper, diced

½ cup (125 mL) diced red onion

½ cup (125 mL) chopped fresh parsley or cilantro

½ cup (125 mL) toasted slivered almonds (for garnish)

1. Prepare Peanut Dressing/Marinade as directed and refrigerate until needed.

2. **KALE SLAW:** Wash kale and dry thoroughly. Remove and discard tough stalks and center veins. Chop kale into bite-sized pieces and place in a large bowl. Using your fingertips, massage kale with oil for 2–3 minutes to break down the tough fibers.

3. Add cabbage, carrots, red pepper, onion, and parsley. Drizzle with dressing and toss to combine. Refrigerate, covered, to blend flavors.

4. At serving time, place salad into 8 individual salad bowls and top with almonds. Serve chilled.

201 calories per serving, 22 g carbohydrates, 12 g sugar, 5 g fiber, 7 g protein, 11 g fat (1 g saturated), 394 mg sodium, 351 mg potassium

NORENE'S NOTES:

- **Switch it up!** Replace half the kale with 2 cups (500 mL) shredded broccoli slaw. Add 1 tsp (5 mL) minced fresh ginger, if desired. Instead of almonds, top with coarsely chopped roasted peanuts or pine nuts.

DR. ED SAYS:

- **Kale and cabbage,** members of the cruciferous vegetable family, are rich in brain and heart benefits. Kale is very rich in the anti-inflammatory flavonoid antioxidants quercetin and kaempferol, as well as the carotenoid antioxidants lutein and zeaxanthin (good for the eyes as well as the brain). These add to the antioxidants from the carrots (carotenes) and other ingredients. Getting a variety of antioxidants from different sources is important to ensure maximum efficacy. Kale is also rich in vitamin C and contains good amounts of vitamin B6, folate, and magnesium—all good for the brain.

RECIPE CONTINUED . . .

- **Canola oil, almonds, and the Peanut Dressing/Marinade** (p. 427) provide good amounts of monounsaturated fats. Almonds offer a good amount of natural vitamin E in all its varied forms, which is better than taking single-form vitamin E capsules.

- **Overall,** this recipe provides an excellent 20% of recommended dietary fiber intake per serving, and is relatively low in digestible carbs.

COLORFUL KALE SALAD

PAREVE | MEAT OPTION | GLUTEN-FREE | PASSOVER OPTION |
MAKES 6 SERVINGS

When you massage kale's fibrous leaves, they become tender and are more easily digestible. Other leafy greens will work well in this recipe (see Norene's Notes).

---

1. **DRESSING:** Combine dressing ingredients in a jar, cover tightly, and shake well. Store in the refrigerator until ready to use.

2. **SALAD:** Wash kale and dry thoroughly. Remove and discard tough stalks and center veins. Chop kale into bite-sized pieces and place in a large bowl.

3. Using your fingertips, massage kale with oil for 2–3 minutes to break down the tough fibers (kale reduces a lot after being massaged). Add onion, red pepper, and cranberries, if using, but do not toss. Cover and chill.

4. Shortly before serving, peel, pit, and dice avocado and mango. Add to salad, drizzle with dressing, and toss gently to combine. Sprinkle sunflower seeds overtop.

305 calories per serving, 27 g carbohydrates, 12 g sugar, 6 g fiber, 6 g protein, 23 g fat (3 g saturated), 45 mg sodium, 218 mg potassium

NORENE'S NOTES:

- **Green power:** Kale is nutrient-packed and an excellent source of fiber and iron. This colorful salad also works well with spinach, leafy mixed greens, or your favorite salad greens—and there's no need to massage them with oil, as described in Step 3.

- **Make it a meal:** Add sliced cooked chicken or turkey, or chunks of poached salmon.

- **Passover option:** Instead of rice vinegar, use white wine vinegar or lemon juice. Omit mustard. Replace sunflower seeds with toasted walnuts, pecans, pistachios, or slivered almonds.

RECIPE CONTINUED . . .

DRESSING:

¼ cup (60 mL) extra virgin olive oil

2 Tbsp (30 mL) rice or apple cider vinegar

2 Tbsp (30 mL) lemon, mango, or orange juice

1 Tbsp (15 mL) honey

½ tsp (2 mL) Dijon mustard

Salt and freshly ground black pepper to taste

SALAD:

1 medium bunch kale (about 1 lb/500 g)

1 Tbsp (15 mL) extra virgin olive oil

½ cup (125 mL) diced red onion

1 red bell pepper, diced

½ cup (125 mL) unsweetened dried cranberries (optional)

1 ripe Hass avocado

1 firm ripe mango

½ cup (125 mL) toasted sunflower seeds (for garnish)

DR. ED SAYS:

- **Avocado,** which is very low in harmful sugars, digestible carbs, and sodium, is a great complement to this kale salad. Avocado has a fair amount of fat (about 15%, which is mostly monounsaturated). It is also one of the few vegetables that contains significant saturated fats (about 15% of the total fat), but since the actual amount of saturated fat consumed is relatively small, and since it provides a good source of brain-benefiting vitamin B6, folate, magnesium, choline, powerful proanthocyanidine antioxidants (in the flavonoid group), and fiber, its advantages far outweigh the disadvantages.

- **Mango** provides soluble fiber, high vitamin C, good B vitamin levels, and alternate sources of mixed antioxidants. Go easy on the mango, however, as it is relatively high in sugars.

- **Olive oil and sunflower seeds** are the source of good fats in this recipe, and sunflower seeds are the next best source of wide-spectrum natural vitamin E after the almonds.

MIXED GREENS WITH MANDARINS, BERRIES, AND PEARS

DAIRY OPTION | PAREVE | MEAT OPTION | PASSOVER OPTION |
MAKES 8 SERVINGS

This scrumptious salad, with its crunchy nut topping, is a perfect pairing of fruits and salad greens. The fat is mainly heart-healthy monounsaturated. It's a culinary trifecta!

Raspberry Vinaigrette (p. 431)

SALAD:

4 cups (1 L) packed baby spinach or mixed salad greens

1 head romaine, torn into bite-sized pieces (about 6 cups/1.5 L)

½ red onion, thinly sliced

1 can (11 oz/312 g) mandarin orange segments, drained (about 1 cup/250 mL)

1 cup (250 mL) fresh strawberries, hulled and halved

1 cup (250 mL) fresh raspberries

2 firm ripe pears, peeled and sliced

2 tsp (10 mL) lemon juice (preferably fresh)

½ cup (125 mL) toasted pistachios, walnuts, or slivered almonds (for garnish)

1. Prepare Raspberry Vinaigrette as directed and chill until serving time.

2. **SALAD:** Combine spinach, romaine, onion, orange segments, strawberries, and raspberries in a large salad bowl, but don't toss. (Salad can be prepared in advance up to this point and refrigerated for several hours or overnight.)

3. To serve, sprinkle pears with lemon juice to prevent discoloration and add to the salad. Drizzle chilled vinaigrette overtop and toss gently. Garnish with nuts and serve immediately.

118 calories per serving, 20 g carbohydrates, 10 g sugar, 5 g fiber, 4 g protein, 4 g fat (0 g saturated), 29 mg sodium, 220 mg potassium

NORENE'S NOTES:

- **Fruitful thinking:** Instead of pears, use sliced mangoes or apples. Instead of mandarin oranges, add 1 cup (250 mL) grapefruit segments.

- **Nut-free option:** Use pumpkin or sunflower seeds instead of nuts (but not during Passover).

- **Meal deal:** To turn this into a main dish, top salad with sliced grilled chicken or turkey, salmon (canned or cooked), or crumbled goat or feta cheese.

- **Salad for one:** Prepare dressing as directed in Step 1. Combine ingredients as directed in Step 2. Cover salad with a paper towel (or towels) to absorb extra moisture, and refrigerate. To serve, transfer the desired quantity of salad to a plate or bowl. Top with pears and drizzle with dressing, using 2 Tbsp (30 mL) dressing per serving. Garnish with pistachios.

RECIPE CONTINUED . . .

MIXED GREENS WITH MANDARINS, BERRIES, AND PEARS (continued)

- **Passover option:** Use Balsamic Vinaigrette/Marinade (p. 423) instead of Raspberry Vinaigrette.

DR. ED SAYS:

- **Leafy green vegetables,** especially spinach, have repeatedly been shown to be beneficial for preventing AD/dementia. This is probably because spinach contains very high levels of the brain antioxidants lutein and zeaxanthin, carotenoid antioxidants, vitamin C, and folate, in addition to good levels of natural vitamin E, vitamin B6, and magnesium.

- **Berries** are great sources of fiber and antioxidants, while being relatively low in sugar (especially raspberries) and high in vitamin C.

- **Nuts** have been shown to be an important staple of the Mediterranean diet. Almonds and walnuts are probably at the top of the list—almonds for their high natural vitamin E, and walnuts because they also contain significant quantities of Omega-3 fats in addition to vitamin E.

- **Overall,** this excellent recipe contains three of the most documented foods for reducing the risk of AD/dementia.

ROMAINE, AVOCADO, AND MANGO SALAD

DAIRY OPTION | PAREVE | GLUTEN-FREE | MEAT OPTION | PASS-
OVER OPTION | MAKES 6 SERVINGS

I love to serve this elegant salad on a large platter—it's perfect for a crowd and pretty as a picture.

Citrus Dressing (p. 425)

SALAD:

1 large romaine lettuce, trimmed and torn into bite-sized pieces (about 6 cups/1.5 L)

1 mango, peeled and diced

2 mini cucumbers, halved and thinly sliced (no need to peel)

¼ red onion, thinly sliced (about ½ cup/125 mL chopped)

¼ cup (60 mL) thinly sliced radishes

½ red bell pepper, thinly sliced

1 ripe medium avocado

¼ cup (60 mL) chopped fresh basil or parsley

½ cup (125 mL) toasted slivered almonds

1. Prepare Citrus Dressing as directed and chill until serving time.

2. **SALAD:** Arrange lettuce on a large oval platter or in a bowl. Scatter mango, cucumbers, onion, radishes, and red pepper over the lettuce. (Can be prepared a day in advance and refrigerated.)

3. Just before serving, pit, peel, and dice avocado. Scatter avocado, basil, and almonds overtop. Drizzle with dressing.

236 calories per serving, 19 g carbohydrates, 12 g sugar, 4 g fiber, 5 g protein, 18 g fat (2 g saturated), 17 mg sodium, 409 mg potassium

NORENE'S NOTES:

- **Green power!** Other greens, such as baby spinach, arugula, mesclun mix, Boston lettuce, or baby kale can be substituted.

- **Meal deal:** To turn this salad into a main dish, top with sliced grilled chicken, turkey, salmon, or crumbled goat or feta cheese.

- **Salad for one:** Prepare dressing as directed in Step 1 and refrigerate. Combine ingredients as directed in Step 2. Cover salad with a paper towel (or towels) to absorb extra moisture and refrigerate. To serve, transfer the desired quantity of salad to a plate and scatter avocado, basil, and almonds overtop. Use 2 Tbsp (30 mL) dressing per serving.

- **Passover option:** Replace Dijon mustard in the salad dressing with ½ tsp (2 mL) white horseradish (or just omit the mustard).

- **Switch it up!** Instead of mango, use orange or clementine segments. Instead of almonds, use pecans or pistachios. Add dried cranberries for a colorful touch.

RECIPE CONTINUED . . .

ROMAINE, AVOCADO, AND MANGO SALAD (continued)

DR. ED SAYS:

- **Romaine lettuce,** the main component of this salad, is beneficial as a leafy green (though not as good as spinach). It contains a high amount of folate and reasonable fiber and carotenoid antioxidants, such as lutein and zeaxanthin, as well as the flavonol antioxidant quercetin.

- **Mango** is high in sugar, so don't overdo it.

- **Red bell pepper and avocado** balance out the nutrients with the flavonoid proanthocyanidin antioxidants from the avocado, as well as good amounts of vitamins C, E, B6, and folate. Red bell pepper contains a very level of high vitamin C (contributing, along with the other ingredients, about 50% of the daily vitamin C requirement), good amounts of vitamin B6 and folate, and reasonable amounts of natural vitamin E.

- **Almonds** also add significantly to the vitamin E, resulting in almost 10% of the daily vitamin E requirement.

- **Parsley and basil** are powerful antioxidant sources.

- **Radishes** are primarily known for their relatively high flavonoid anthocyanin antioxidant level.

WATERMELON & FETA SALAD

DAIRY | GLUTEN-FREE | PASSOVER OPTION | MAKES 8 SERVINGS

This refreshing summer salad will be a "feta'" in your cap! The recipe was inspired by my friend, the late Monty Joffin, who was interested in my opinion on this unusual combination of ingredients. I explained that the combination of sweet watermelon and salty feta cheese is a perfect pairing. In Middle Eastern countries, eating watermelon with salt is quite common.

1. Prepare Raspberry Vinaigrette as directed and refrigerate.

2. **SALAD:** Wash salad greens and dry thoroughly. Place in a shallow, round bowl, or on an oval platter. Tuck watermelon cubes among the greens. Scatter sliced onion on top and sprinkle with crumbled feta cheese.

3. Cover and refrigerate until serving time. (Can be prepared in advance up to this point and refrigerated for several hours or overnight.)

4. To serve, drizzle dressing over salad, but don't toss. Serve immediately.

105 calories per serving, 13 g carbohydrates, 8 g sugar, 2 g fiber, 5 g protein, 3 g fat (2 g saturated), 267 mg sodium, 143 mg potassium

NORENE'S NOTES:

- **Green power:** Mâche (pronounced "mah-sh"), also known as field salad or lamb's lettuce, has a mild, nutty flavor. You can also use Boston, Bibb, red leaf, or butter lettuce.

- **Here's the scoop:** If you have time and patience, use a mini ice-cream scoop or melon baller and make small watermelon balls.

- **Dress swap:** Instead of Raspberry Vinaigrette, use Shake-It-Up Vinaigrette/Marinade (p. 432).

- **Dress it up:** For an elegant presentation, serve salad in individual butter lettuce cups. (You'll need 2 large heads of butter lettuce to give you 16 leaves.) Arrange 1 large lettuce cup and 1 small lettuce cup on each plate, overlapping slightly. Spoon some salad into each lettuce cup, drizzle with dressing, and garnish with a few black olives.

RECIPE CONTINUED . . .

⅓ cup (80 mL) Raspberry Vinaigrette (p. 431)

SALAD:

6 cups (1.5 L) mixed salad greens, mâche, or baby spinach

6 cups (1.5 L) cubed seedless watermelon (about ¼ small watermelon cut into 1-inch/ 2.5-cm cubes)

½ cup (125 mL) thinly sliced red onion

¾ cup (185 mL) crumbled low-fat feta cheese

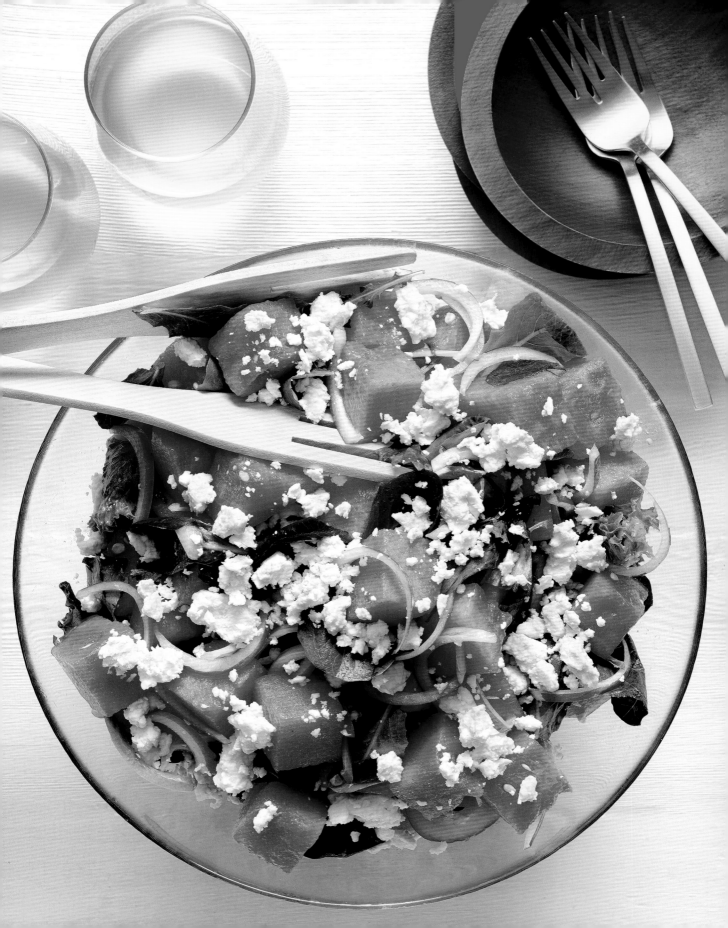

- **Add-ins:** In Step 1, tuck 1 cup (250 mL) halved grape tomatoes and/or diced mini cucumbers between watermelon cubes. In Step 4, sprinkle salad with 3 Tbsp (45 mL) assorted chopped fresh herbs (e.g., dill, basil, or mint). If desired, garnish with ½ cup (125 mL) toasted slivered or sliced almonds or toasted chopped pistachios.

- **Passover option:** Either omit the mustard from the dressing or replace it with white horseradish.

DR. ED SAYS:

- **Leafy greens, watermelon, and feta cheese** are featured in this healthy, colorful salad. Choose spinach as a leafy green whenever possible because of its correlation with reduced AD/dementia risk, as described in Mixed Greens with Mandarins, Berries, and Pears (p. 399).

- **Watermelon** doesn't have a lot of nutrients and is relatively high in sugar, but its claim to fame is its high level of a carotenoid antioxidant called lycopene, which has been shown to be effective against many diseases including AD/dementia and heart disease—and watermelon is so refreshing!

- **Feta cheese** adds a wallop of protein (about 14% by weight of the cheese), and is a rich source of the important brain vitamin B12, which tends to be found primarily in animal sources. Its weakness is that it is very high in saturated fat (two-thirds of the daily limit in 100 g) and sodium (almost half the daily limit in 100 g), so be aware of how much you add.

BARLEY VEGETABLE SALAD

PAREVE | GLUTEN-FREE OPTION | KEEPS ABOUT 3 DAYS IN THE
REFRIGERATOR | MAKES 6 SERVINGS

3 cups (750 mL) lightly salted
water or vegetable broth

1 cup (250 mL) hulled, pot, or
pearl barley (see Norene's Notes)

SALAD:

1 English cucumber (or 4 mini
seedless cucumbers), chopped
(no need to peel)

1 red or yellow bell pepper,
chopped

1 medium onion, chopped
(or 3 green onions, thinly sliced)

3 cups (750 mL) baby
spinach, chopped

2 stalks celery, chopped

½ cup (125 mL) minced
fresh parsley

¼ cup (60 mL) minced fresh basil,
dill, or mint

¼ cup (60 mL) extra virgin
olive oil

¼ cup (60 mL) lemon juice
(preferably fresh)

1 tsp (5 mL) Dijon mustard

Salt and freshly ground
black pepper

Barley, with its chewy texture and nutty flavor, is fabulous in salads. This grain-based salad is great for vegans, vegetarians, and meat-eaters alike. Pearl and pot barley are the most popular varieties on the market, but hulled barley, which is a whole grain, is more nutritious. They are all interchangeable in this recipe.

1. Boil water in a large saucepan and add barley. Reduce heat to medium and cook, covered, without stirring, until barley is soft yet chewy and tripled in volume. Hulled barley takes about 1 hour to cook (start checking it at 45 minutes). Pot and pearl barley take 35–45 minutes (start checking at 30 minutes).

2. Remove saucepan from heat, uncover, and cool completely. Fluff with a fork. You'll have 3–4 cups (1 L) cooked barley. (Can be made in advance and refrigerated, covered, up to 2 days.)

3. **SALAD:** In a large bowl, combine cooked barley with cucumber, bell pepper, onion, spinach, celery, parsley, and basil.

4. Add oil, lemon juice, mustard, salt, and pepper, and toss to combine. Serve chilled.

226 calories per serving, 29 g carbohydrates, 3 g sugar, 8 g fiber, 6 g protein, 10 g fat (1 g saturated), 105 mg sodium, 218 mg potassium

NORENE'S NOTES:

- **Barley basics:** Hulled barley, which is the natural unpolished whole grain, is light golden brown in color. Hulled barley is nuttier, chewier, and more nutritious than pearl or pot barley. Pearl and pot barley have been put through a pearling machine, which removes the inedible hull and polishes the kernel. Pot barley has been pearled for a shorter amount of time, so it still has most of the barley bran intact. Hulled, pot, and pearl barley are interchangeable in recipes, so use what you have on hand, adjusting the cooking time accordingly.

- **Go with the grain!** Other cooked grains excel in this simple salad. Try bulgur (cracked wheat), couscous, farro, millet, orzo, wheat berries, or whole grain pasta.

- **Gluten-free option:** Since barley contains gluten, substitute 3–4 cups (750–1000 mL) cooked quinoa, buckwheat groats (kasha), basmati, brown, black, or wild rice. Cook according to package directions.

- **Switch it up!** Instead of red pepper, use 1 cup (250 mL) halved grape tomatoes. Omit the spinach. Increase parsley to 1 cup (250 mL).

- **Dress it right:** Instead of oil and lemon juice, use your favorite salad dressing (homemade or store-bought). Choose a store-bought brand that doesn't contain high-fructose corn syrup, hydrogenated oils, or trans-fats. It should contain less than 4 g saturated fat and less than 4 g sugar per serving.

DR. ED SAYS:

- **Hulled barley,** a high-fiber whole grain cereal, is featured in this grain-based salad. Because barley only contains about 10% water, it is more nutrient-dense than fruits or vegetables and contains high quantities of protein, fiber, magnesium, potassium, and a group of flavonoid antioxidants called proanthocyanidins. It also contains good levels of vitamin B6 and zinc. At the same time, barley is low in fat, sugar, and sodium, which is a good thing.

- **Onions** are used in many of our salad recipes, primarily as a flavor booster. Although they are relatively weak in brain-healthy nutrients, they do have one of the largest concentrations of a flavonoid antioxidant called quercetin, which enhances the effectiveness of other antioxidants that you consume from tea or fruits.

- **Overall,** the one weakness that barley shares with other cereals and grains is its high digestible carb level, but combined with the other ingredients, especially the spinach, this recipe is healthy.

JEWELED BLACK RICE SALAD

PAREVE | GLUTEN-FREE | KEEPS ABOUT 3 DAYS IN THE REFRIGERATOR | MAKES 8 SERVINGS

2 cups (500 mL) lightly salted water

1 cup (250 mL) black rice, rinsed and drained

SALAD:

1 red bell pepper, diced

1 medium red onion, diced (about 1 cup/250 mL)

½ cup (125 mL) dried mango, diced

½ cup (125 mL) dried apricots, diced

½ cup (125 mL) minced fresh parsley

¼ cup (60 mL) minced fresh basil or mint

1 can (11 oz/312 g) mandarin orange segments, drained and patted dry

1 firm ripe avocado

DRESSING:

¼ cup (60 mL) extra virgin olive oil or avocado oil

¼ cup (60 mL) orange juice (preferably fresh)

2 Tbsp (30 mL) honey

1 tsp (5 mL) Dijon mustard

Salt and freshly ground black pepper

Black rice was often referred to as "forbidden rice" because it was only served to the royal family. When cooked, it becomes a deep purple color. When you combine black rice with dried mango, apricots, red bell pepper, and red onion, it looks like tiny jewels. For a different twist, substitute black lentils (see Norene's Notes).

1. In a medium saucepan over high heat, bring water to a boil. Stir in rice, cover, and simmer for 35–40 minutes. Rice should be tender but slightly chewy. Remove from heat and let stand, covered, for 10 minutes. Fluff with a fork, transfer to a large bowl, and cool completely. (Can be prepared a day in advance, covered, and refrigerated.)

2. **SALAD:** Add red pepper, onion, mango, apricots, parsley, and basil to the cooled rice. (A food processor or mini prep minces the dried fruits and herbs in moments.) Top with mandarin orange segments.

3. **DRESSING:** Combine dressing ingredients in a jar, seal tightly, and shake well. Drizzle dressing over salad and toss to combine. Cover and refrigerate.

4. Just before serving, dice avocado and add to the salad. Toss gently to combine. Adjust seasonings to taste. Serve chilled.

283 calories per serving, 45 g carbohydrates, 19 g sugar, 5 g fiber, 4 g protein, 10 g fat (1 g saturated fat), 34 mg sodium, 243 mg potassium

NORENE'S NOTES:

- **Jeweled black lentil salad:** Instead of black rice, use dried black lentils (beluga lentils). Rinse thoroughly. Bring 2 cups (500 mL) water to a boil. Add 1 cup (250 mL) lentils and simmer, covered, for 25–30 minutes, until tender but not mushy. Continue as directed above in Steps 2–4.

- **Switch it up!** Substitute other gluten-free grains such as quinoa, brown rice, or buckwheat (kasha). Use fresh mango rather than dried. Diced peaches and/or nectarines are excellent options when fresh fruit is in season. Add a handful of pomegranate seeds or dried cranberries for a splash of color. For a flavor boost, add 1 tsp (5 mL) minced fresh ginger to the dressing.

DR. ED SAYS:

- **Black rice** is unique because it contains the highest levels of antioxidants and fiber of any variety of rice. The dark purple or black color makes it comparable to blueberries in antioxidant power. It also contains reasonable levels of vitamin B6 and magnesium.

- **Dried black lentils** are also high in antioxidants. See "jeweled black lentil salad" (above).

- **Onion,** along with the added fruit, contributes some vitamin C to this recipe. Onion also adds fiber and contains one of the highest levels of the important antioxidant quercetin of all fruits and vegetables.

- **Avocado** also provides the same beneficial brain nutrients as an onion, but has significantly higher levels of fiber and vitamin C. Avocado is very low in harmful sugars.

- **Dried cranberries, pomegranate seeds, and ginger** are excellent additions because of their antioxidant brain benefits.

- **Overall,** this grain-based salad is a wonderful source of varied antioxidants. Low in sodium and a good source of fiber, this dish contains the important vitamins B6 and folate. Although the rice contains high available sugars, the other beneficial ingredients in this recipe compensate for it, making it an ideal brain-boosting dish.

ASIAN QUINOA SALAD

PAREVE | GLUTEN-FREE | KEEPS ABOUT 3 DAYS IN THE REFRIGERATOR | MAKES 6 SERVINGS

¼–⅓ cup (60–80 mL) Asian Dressing/Marinade (p. 422)

2 cups (500 mL) water

1 cup (250 mL) quinoa, rinsed and drained

SALAD:

1 pkg (12 oz/340 g) frozen shelled edamame

6 green onions, chopped

1 red bell pepper, diced

½ cup (125 mL) shredded carrots

½ cup (125 mL) thinly sliced celery

½ cup (125 mL) fresh flat-leaf parsley, finely chopped

½ cup (125 mL) sesame seeds (for garnish)

This scrumptious salad comes together quickly once you prepare the dressing and cook the quinoa. Leftovers make an excellent lunch option, especially with the addition of salmon or chicken.

1. Prepare Asian Dressing/Marinade as directed and refrigerate.

2. Bring water to a boil in a medium saucepan over high heat. Add quinoa and reduce heat. Simmer, covered, for 15 minutes, until tender. Remove from heat and let stand for 5 minutes. Fluff with a fork. Transfer to a large serving bowl, cover, and refrigerate.

3. **SALAD:** Bring another medium saucepan of lightly salted water to a boil. Add edamame and boil for 3–4 minutes, until tender-crisp. Drain, rinse well under cold running water, and drain again. Pat dry with paper towels.

4. **ASSEMBLY:** Add edamame, green onions, red pepper, carrots, celery, and parsley to the chilled quinoa. Add dressing and toss to combine. Garnish with sesame seeds. Serve chilled.

301 calories per serving, 37 g carbohydrates, 7 g sugar, 7 g fiber, 13 g protein, 11 g fat (trace saturated), 275 mg sodium, 134 mg potassium

NORENE'S NOTES:

- **Switch it up!** Use tri-colored quinoa for a pretty presentation. Instead of edamame, use ½ lb (250 g) green beans or snow peas, trimmed and cut diagonally into 1-inch (2.5 cm) pieces. Instead of sesame seeds, top salad with pumpkin seeds, slivered almonds, or chopped pistachios.

DR. ED SAYS:

- **Quinoa,** like all cereals and grains, is high in digestible carbs but has good protein levels, folate, and magnesium, and is low in sodium.

- **Edamame beans,** from which soy protein is made, are rich in protein, fiber, potassium, and folate, while being low in sugar, digestible carbs, and sodium. They also have good levels of the brain-friendly antioxidants lutein and zeaxanthin. The main attraction of these legumes is their high natural vitamin E content (over 50% of the daily value per 100 g) in the forms of gamma and delta tocopherols. These are not usually found in supplements and seem to have a positive effect on AD/dementia risk reduction.

- **Sesame seeds** are very low in moisture (about 3%) and, because of this, are very nutrient-dense. They have a whopping 17% protein by weight and very high magnesium, zinc, potassium, folate, and vitamin B6 levels. They are also high in fat, but over 85% of the fat is the good, unsaturated kind, and they are low in digestible carbs. Don't spare the sesame seeds!

> **DID YOU KNOW?** There is a lot of controversy about the phytoestrogens that legumes contain. Some evidence says they could increase the risk of certain types of breast cancer, while other evidence says they reduce the risk. The jury is still out.

QUINOA CHICKPEA SALAD

DAIRY | GLUTEN-FREE | KEEPS ABOUT 3 DAYS IN THE REFRIGERATOR | MAKES 6 SERVINGS

2 cups (500 mL) water

1 cup (250 mL) quinoa (white, red, or tri-colored), rinsed and drained

DRESSING:

¼ cup (60 mL) balsamic vinegar

¼ cup (60 mL) extra virgin olive oil

1 Tbsp (15 mL) honey

2 cloves garlic (about 2 tsp/10 mL minced)

Salt and freshly ground black pepper

SALAD:

3 mini cucumbers, chopped (no need to peel)

1½ cups (375 mL) grape tomatoes, halved

1 orange or yellow bell pepper, chopped

5 or 6 green onions, chopped

1 cup (250 mL) fresh flat-leaf parsley, finely chopped

¼ cup (60 mL) fresh dill or basil, finely chopped

1 can (19 oz/540 g) chickpeas, drained and rinsed (about 2 cups/500 mL)

1 cup (250 mL) pitted black olives (optional)

1½ cups (375 mL) crumbled feta or goat cheese, divided

This scrumptious brain-boosting salad is ideal for a hot summer day, or any time at all. It's so versatile—check out the variations below. It's a winner!

---

1. Bring water to a boil in a medium saucepan over high heat. Add quinoa and reduce heat. Simmer, covered, for 15 minutes, until tender. Remove from heat and let stand for 5 minutes. Fluff with a fork. Transfer to a large bowl, cover, and refrigerate.

2. **DRESSING:** Combine balsamic vinegar, olive oil, honey, and garlic in a glass jar. Add a dash of salt and pepper, cover tightly, and shake well. Refrigerate.

3. **SALAD:** Add cucumbers, tomatoes, bell pepper, green onions, parsley, and dill to the chilled quinoa. Add chickpeas, olives (if using), and 1 cup (250 mL) feta cheese.

4. Pour dressing over the salad and toss to combine. Sprinkle the remaining ½ cup (125 mL) feta on top as garnish. Serve chilled.

407 calories per serving, 37 g carbohydrates, 9 g sugar, 6 g fiber, 18 g protein, 17 g fat (6 g saturated), 720 mg sodium, 509 mg potassium

NORENE'S NOTES:

- **Salt sensitivity?** Either use no-salt-added canned chickpeas or cook your own. Use goat cheese instead of feta, and omit the olives.

- **Couscous chickpea salad:** No cooking required! Substitute whole wheat or regular couscous for quinoa. Combine 1 cup (250 mL) couscous with 1½ cups (375 mL) boiling water in a large bowl. Cover and let stand for 10 minutes, until liquid is absorbed. Fluff with a fork. Continue as directed above in Steps 2–4. (If using gluten-free couscous, prepare according to package directions.)

- **Brain-friendly grains:** Instead of quinoa, use 3 cups (750 mL) cooked buckwheat (kasha), which is gluten-free. You can also use barley, farro, or wheat berries (which are not gluten-free). Cook according to package directions.

- **Switch it up!** Instead of chickpeas, substitute red or white kidney beans, black beans, or cooked shelled edamame. Omit feta and top with grilled salmon.

DR. ED SAYS:

- **Between the olives and the olive oil,** we're making sure you get all the aspects of this important component of the Mediterranean diet. Olives provide the fiber and some antioxidants that olive oil alone does not provide, though both supply the healthy monounsaturated fats that are good for the heart and brain. The only downside is that olives are very high in sodium—try to limit your olive intake to 1–2 servings per day (see Norene's Notes).

- **Chickpeas,** which belong to the legume family and are the major component of hummus, have very high fiber levels as well as high protein and good quantities of magnesium and folate.

- **Feta cheese** provides vitamin B12, which is difficult to get from non-animal sources, as well as high quantities of vitamin B6. It also has a good chunk of protein, but is very high in sodium and saturated fat, so consider it as part of the weekly cheese allocation outlined in the menu plan in the first part of this book.

- **Suggestion:** Substitute salmon for feta (see Norene's Notes). It's an even better choice since you then get the bonus of fish Omega-3 fats, protein, and less saturated fat.

QUINOA TABBOULEH

PAREVE | GLUTEN-FREE | PASSOVER | KEEPS ABOUT 3 DAYS IN THE
REFRIGERATOR | MAKES ABOUT 6 CUPS (1.5 L)

2 cups (500 mL) water

1 cup (250 mL) quinoa, rinsed
and drained

SALAD:

3 cups (750 mL) tightly packed
flat-leaf parsley (washed and well
dried, stems discarded)

2 cloves garlic (about 2 tsp/10 mL
minced)

2 or 3 ripe, firm plum (Italian)
tomatoes, coarsely chopped

½ cup (125 mL) chopped
red onion

2 tsp (10 mL) dried mint
(or 2 Tbsp/30 mL minced
fresh mint)

3 Tbsp (45 mL) extra virgin
olive oil

3 Tbsp (45 mL) lemon juice
(preferably fresh)

½ tsp (2 mL) salt (or to taste)

Freshly ground black pepper

This heart-healthy tabbouleh is packed with brain-boosting greens and whole grains. You can make half the recipe for a smaller family or double it up for a crowd. Leftover cooked quinoa is perfect as a breakfast cereal and can be added to salads, or transformed into a pilaf, so why not make extra?

1. Bring water to a boil in a medium saucepan over high heat. Add quinoa and reduce heat. Simmer, covered, for 15 minutes, until tender. Remove from heat and let stand for 5 minutes. Fluff with a fork. Transfer to a large bowl and let cool.

2. **SALAD:** In a mini prep or food processor fitted with the steel blade, process parsley and garlic until minced. Add to the quinoa. Add tomatoes, onion, and mint, and stir to combine. Add oil, lemon juice, salt, and pepper. Mix well.

3. Cover and refrigerate for at least an hour. Serve chilled.

99 calories per ½-cup (125 mL) serving, 14 g carbohydrates, 2 g sugar, 2 g fiber, 3 g protein, 4 g fat (<1 g saturated), 110 mg sodium, 126 mg potassium

NORENE'S NOTES:

- **To rinse or not?** Some brands of quinoa do not require rinsing. Otherwise, place quinoa in a fine-mesh strainer and rinse under cold running water for 1 minute to remove the bitter coating (saponin). If your strainer is not fine-meshed, line it with a large paper coffee filter or cheesecloth.

- **Confetti tabbouleh:** For a more colorful salad, add any of the following: ½ cup (125 mL) chopped cucumber, ½ cup (125 mL) chopped red bell pepper, ½–1 cup (125–250 mL) corn kernels or baby green peas. Reduce parsley to 2½ cups (625 mL) and add ¼ cup (60 mL) tightly packed fresh cilantro or basil.

- **Variation:** Replace cooked quinoa with 3 cups (750 mL) riced cauliflower (see p. 463).

- **Parsley,** the main ingredient in tabbouleh, belongs to the leafy green family that is so good for the brain. Parsley contains large quantities of two antioxidant families—it has high levels of carotenoid antioxidants, including lutein and zeaxanthin, which have been shown to be beneficial for both the brain and eyes (the eyes are considered an extension of the brain), and large quantities of a flavonoid antioxidant called apigenin, which, among other functions, reduces anxiety (important since anxiety can lead to worsening dementia symptoms). As a bonus, this compound is also a potent anti-cancer agent. Parsley is also very high in vitamin C and folate, as well as being a good source of magnesium.

- **Olive oil,** a staple of a brain-healthy diet, is also included.

- **Mint and garlic** round out both the antioxidant profile and the taste.

GRILLED CORN, RED PEPPER, AND SNAP PEA SALAD

PAREVE | DAIRY OPTION | GLUTEN-FREE | KEEPS ABOUT 3 DAYS IN
THE REFRIGERATOR | MAKES 6 SERVINGS

4 ears corn on the cob, husked

2 red bell peppers, halved and seeded

Oil, for brushing

1 pkg (8 oz/227 g) sugar snap peas (1½ cups/500 mL)

1 can (19 oz/540 g) red kidney beans, drained and rinsed (preferably no-salt-added)

¼ cup (60 mL) extra virgin olive oil

2 Tbsp (30 mL) rice or apple cider vinegar

1 Tbsp (15 mL) maple syrup or honey

Salt and freshly ground black pepper to taste

¼ cup (60 mL) minced fresh basil

Easy-peasy! Daniella Silver, my co-author for *The Silver Platter: Simple to Spectacular*, introduced me to this spectacular presentation of sugar snap peas in their pods. They add a simple, elegant look to this gorgeous summer salad when corn is in season.

1. Preheat barbecue or grill. Brush corn and red peppers with oil. Grill on all sides, about 10–15 minutes. Let cool.

2. Cut corn kernels off the cobs with a sharp knife. Cut bell peppers into long, narrow strips. Cut snap peas in half lengthwise along the straight edge of seam so that peas are exposed.

3. Combine corn, peppers, snap peas, and kidney beans in a large salad bowl. Add oil, vinegar, maple syrup, salt, pepper, and basil. Toss together. Serve chilled.

248 calories per serving, 32 g carbohydrates, 9 g sugar, 8 g fiber, 8 g protein, 11 g fat (1 g saturated), 116 mg sodium, 491 mg potassium

NORENE'S NOTES:

- **Israeli-style corn salad:** Instead of kidney beans, add halved grape tomatoes. If desired, add ½ cup (125 mL) thinly sliced red onion. Instead of peas, add 3 or 4 sliced, unpeeled baby cucumbers.

- **Greek-style corn salad:** Substitute lemon juice for vinegar and use dill instead of basil. For a dairy option, top with 1 cup (250 mL) crumbled feta cheese for an extra protein punch.

- **Switch it up!** If snap peas aren't available, substitute cooked shelled edamame.

- **No barbecue?** No problem! Boil the corn and sauté the peppers.

DR. ED SAYS:

- **Corn kernels, snap peas, kidney beans, and bell peppers** are the main components of this eye-catching salad, but most of the brain-healthy nutrients come from the latter three.

- **Corn** is relatively moderate in nutrients (though it does have reasonable fiber, choline, and carotenoid antioxidants) and, as a cereal grain, has high digestible carbs and moderately high sugar.

- **Snap peas** are a part of the brain-healthy legume family, providing fiber, reasonable levels of folate, vitamin B6, and carotenoid antioxidants. They also have relatively moderate amounts of sugars and digestible carbs.

- **Kidney beans** provide fiber and protein, typical of legumes, but these beans also contain reasonable levels of magnesium and good quantities of folate. Kidney beans have been shown to help reduce the risk of other diseases besides AD/dementia because of their phytonutrients and antioxidants. Please note that dried beans contain a toxin called phytohemagglutinin, so they must be soaked and boiled first.

- **Bell peppers,** used extensively in our recipes, provide antioxidants, fiber, vitamin C, folate, vitamin B6, and some natural vitamin E, all of which have been linked to improved brain function.

- **Overall,** this protein-packed salad provides an excellent source of vitamin C, fiber, and folate. It is also a good source of vitamin B6, magnesium, antioxidants, and vegetable-based Omega-3 fats.

GRILLED CHICKEN, RED PEPPER, AND MANGO SALAD

MEAT | GLUTEN-FREE | PASSOVER OPTION | CHICKEN FREEZES WELL | MAKES 6 SERVINGS

Double-Duty Vinaigrette/ Marinade (p. 422)

6 boneless, skinless single chicken breasts

Garlic powder, onion powder, pepper, and basil to taste

SALAD:

6 cups (1.5 L) mixed salad greens

1 firm ripe mango, peeled and sliced

1 red or yellow bell pepper, thinly sliced

1 medium red onion, halved and thinly sliced

1 medium carrot, grated

12 grape tomatoes, halved

Grilled chicken breasts make a wonderful addition to this scrumptious salad. Cook an extra batch or two of chicken breasts the next time you grill. Freeze or refrigerate extras in a single layer in resealable freezer bags. Cook once, enjoy twice!

1. Prepare Double-Duty Vinaigrette/Marinade as directed and refrigerate.

2. Season chicken breasts lightly on both sides.

3. Preheat barbecue or grill. Grill chicken 4–6 minutes per side, depending on thickness. Chicken is done if it springs back when lightly touched. Once cooled, cover and refrigerate.

4. **SALAD:** Wash salad greens and dry thoroughly. Place greens on individual dinner plates. Top with mango, bell pepper, onion, carrot, and tomatoes. (If preparing salad in advance, cover and refrigerate until serving time.)

5. Slice chicken into long, narrow strips and arrange in an attractive design on top of the salad. Drizzle with dressing and serve.

359 calories per serving, 29 g carbohydrates, 22 g sugar, 4 g fiber, 29 g protein, 14 g fat (2 g saturated), 78 mg sodium, 700 mg potassium

NORENE'S NOTES:

- **Double up:** Make a double batch of dressing/marinade. Use half to marinate the chicken and the rest as a dressing for the salad. Marinate chicken for at least 30 minutes, or up to 24 hours in the refrigerator. (Note: Discard any leftover marinade from chicken as it contains bacteria.)

- **Switch it up:** Substitute different salad dressings (e.g., Asian Dressing/Marinade, p. 422). Instead of mango slices, use orange segments or pineapple chunks.

- **Passover option:** Substitute Balsamic Vinaigrette/Marinade (p. 423).

- **Time-saver tip:** Wash and dry salad greens in advance. Wrap in paper towels or a clean kitchen towel. Store in a large resealable bag and refrigerate until needed.

DR. ED SAYS:

- **Chicken** provides important brain nutrients that are difficult to obtain from non-meat sources, such as high-quality protein, vitamin B12, and choline. Primarily because of the nutrient density and quantity of the chicken, this recipe is highly enriched in choline, folate, vitamin B6, magnesium, and protein. It also provides a good level of natural vitamin E and is low in carbs.

- **Leafy greens,** which are so important to a brain-healthy diet (or to any diet), balance the nutrients deficient in the chicken by providing fiber and antioxidants.

GRILLED CHICKEN SALAD WITH ROSEMARY VINAIGRETTE

MEAT | GLUTEN-FREE | PASSOVER | CHICKEN FREEZES WELL |
MAKES 6 SERVINGS

ROSEMARY VINAIGRETTE:

½ cup (125 mL) extra virgin olive oil

3 Tbsp (45 mL) balsamic vinegar

2 cloves garlic (about 2 tsp/10 mL minced)

1 Tbsp (15 mL) minced fresh rosemary (or 1 tsp/5 mL dried)

½ tsp (2 mL) salt

Freshly ground black pepper

CHICKEN AND VEGETABLES:

6 boneless, skinless single chicken breasts

3 red bell peppers, quartered

6 large portobello mushrooms, stems discarded

SALAD:

1 pkg (10 oz/300 g) baby spinach or mixed salad greens

1 medium red onion, quartered and thinly sliced

Salt and freshly ground black pepper

6 Tbsp (90 mL) toasted sliced almonds (for garnish)

This scrumptious meal-in-one salad is packed with vitamins, minerals, and phytonutrients. It's excellent for entertaining as it multiplies easily and can be prepared in advance. Not in the mood for chicken? See the variations for beef or salmon below.

1. **ROSEMARY VINAIGRETTE:** In a 2-cup (500 mL) glass measure, whisk together oil, vinegar, garlic, rosemary, salt, and pepper. You'll have about ¾ cup (185 mL) dressing.

2. **CHICKEN AND VEGETABLES:** Place chicken breasts in a resealable plastic bag and add ¼ cup (60 mL) of the dressing. Refrigerate the remaining dressing. Marinate chicken for at least 30 minutes, or up to 24 hours in the refrigerator.

3. Preheat grill. Brush peppers and mushrooms with 3 Tbsp (45 mL) of the reserved dressing.

4. Grill vegetables and chicken over indirect medium-high heat, turning once, about 4–6 minutes per side. Chicken is done when it is no longer pink in the center and juices run clear.

5. Transfer chicken, peppers, and mushrooms to a cutting board and cut into ½-inch (1 cm) wide strips. (Can be prepared up to a day in advance, covered, and refrigerated.)

6. **SALAD:** Combine spinach and onion in a large bowl. Drizzle with the remaining salad dressing and toss well. Season with salt and pepper.

7. **ASSEMBLY:** Transfer spinach mixture to a large serving platter (or individual plates). Top with peppers, mushrooms, and chicken strips. Sprinkle with almonds. Serve chilled.

423 calories per serving, 16 g carbohydrates, 7 g sugar, 5 g fiber, 32 g protein, 26 g fat (4 g saturated), 294 mg sodium, 959 mg potassium

NORENE'S NOTES:

• **Double-duty:** Use Rosemary Vinaigrette in other salad recipes or as a marinade.

- **Switch it up!** If you don't like rosemary, substitute other fresh or dried herbs such as basil, oregano, dill, or thyme.

- **Marin-aides:** Discard any leftover marinade used for chicken as it contains bacteria (see "Marin-aides," p. 386).

- **Tuscan London broil salad:** Substitute London broil (about 2 lb/1 kg) for chicken. Marinate for at least 30 minutes, or up to 24 hours in the refrigerator. Grill meat for 7–8 minutes per side, then let rest for 5–10 minutes. Slice diagonally against the grain into thin slices. Assemble as directed above.

- **Tuscan salmon salad:** Substitute salmon fillets for chicken. Marinate salmon for 30–60 minutes. Grill 3–4 minutes per side (do not overcook or fish will be dry). Let cool. Assemble as directed above, topping each salad with a salmon fillet (no need to slice or flake it).

DR. ED SAYS:

- **Portobello mushrooms** provide extra quantities of choline, protein, and fiber, are also very low in saturated fat and sodium, and possess reasonable quantities of magnesium, folate, and vitamin B6.

- **Almonds and rosemary** round out the recipe, with the almonds contributing a wide spectrum of natural vitamin E, and the rosemary contributing one of the more powerful antioxidants.

- **Spinach** provides all the brain goodness previously described in Mixed Greens with Mandarins, Berries, and Pears (p. 399).

- **Fishful thinking:** Substituting salmon for chicken (see Norene's Notes) is an excellent idea as salmon contains higher levels of vitamins B12 and D, which need to be obtained from animal sources. In addition, salmon provides a high level of fish Omega-3 fats, the best kind that you can obtain for the brain.

- **Overall,** this recipe contains very healthy contributions of natural vitamin E, B vitamins, magnesium, zinc, and 150% of the daily requirement of vitamin C.

> **DID YOU KNOW?** Rosemary is such a good antioxidant that it is often used in processed foods to prevent oxygen deterioration.

ASIAN DRESSING/MARINADE

PAREVE | GLUTEN-FREE OPTION | KEEPS ABOUT 2 WEEKS IN THE
REFRIGERATOR | MAKES ¾ CUP (185 ML)

2 tsp (10 mL) minced garlic

1 tsp (5 mL) minced ginger
(optional)

¼ cup (60 mL) soy sauce or
tamari (preferably low-sodium)

¼ cup (60 mL) rice vinegar

¼ cup (60 mL) canola oil

2 Tbsp (30 mL) honey (or to taste)

2 Tbsp (30 mL) sesame seeds

1 tsp (5 mL) toasted sesame oil

This Asian-inspired dressing is scrumptious on baby spinach leaves,
leafy greens, cabbage, grains, or cooked veggies (e.g., green beans, broccoli, bok choy). It also makes a terrific marinade for fish, chicken, beef,
and tofu.

1. Combine all ingredients in a jar, cover tightly, and shake well.

2. Store in the refrigerator until ready to use. Shake well before using.

63 calories per 1 Tbsp (15 mL), 3 g carbohydrates, 3 g sugar, 0 g fiber, 1 g
protein, 5 g fat (0 g saturated), 186 mg sodium, 2 mg potassium

NORENE'S NOTES:

• **Sodi-yum!** Make your own low-sodium soy sauce by combining 3 Tbsp
(45 mL) soy sauce with 1 Tbsp (15 mL) water.

• **Gluten-free soy option:** Most brands of soy sauce contain wheat, so
substitute gluten-free soy sauce or reduced-sodium tamari.

DR. ED SAYS:

• **Salad dressings and marinades** don't provide big brain nutrition
boosts because they are used in relatively small quantities in salads.
One exception may be the herbs and spices in the dressings, as these
tend to be powerhouses of antioxidants.

• **Sesame seeds** are an example of a good nutrient-dense ingredient.
As a low-moisture food, they do add some nutrition because they are
packed with nutrients. However, it is a small contribution compared
to the salad.

• **Overall,** try to limit components such as added sugars and salt; in
this marinade/dressing, they are concentrated in the honey and soy
sauce, respectively.

BALSAMIC VINAIGRETTE/MARINADE

PAREVE | GLUTEN-FREE | PASSOVER | KEEPS ABOUT 2 WEEKS IN
THE REFRIGERATOR | MAKES ¾ CUP (185 ML)

This simple, versatile dressing is super on salads. It's also ideal as a marinade for chicken, fish, or roasted vegetables. It's better to make your own salad dressing/marinade, as you can control the sodium content and choose heart-healthy fats.

2 cloves garlic (about 2 tsp/10 mL minced)

½ cup (125 mL) extra virgin olive oil

¼ cup (60 mL) balsamic vinegar

2 tsp (10 mL) honey

¼ tsp (1 mL) salt

Freshly ground black pepper

¼ tsp (1 mL) dried basil

¼ tsp (1 mL) thyme

1. Combine all ingredients in a jar, cover tightly, and shake well.

2. Store in the refrigerator until ready to use. Shake well before using.

87 calories per 1 Tbsp (15 mL), 3 g carbohydrates, 3 g sugar, 0 g fiber, 0 g protein, 9 g fat (1 g saturated), 47 mg sodium, 3 mg potassium

DR. ED SAYS:

- **This homemade dressing** is lower in sodium than most commercial salad dressings, which pack as much as 300–500 mg sodium in a 2-Tbsp (30 mL) serving.

- **Olive oil** contributes some good monounsaturated fat to the recipe.

- **Overall,** this dressing will not make much nutritional difference to the salad other than perhaps its antioxidants; however, it does boost the flavor.

MAPLE BALSAMIC DRIZZLE

PAREVE | GLUTEN-FREE | PASSOVER OPTION | KEEPS ABOUT 10 DAYS IN THE REFRIGERATOR | MAKES ABOUT ¾ CUP (185 ML)

¼ cup (60 mL) balsamic vinegar

¼ cup (60 mL) orange or mango juice

¼ cup (60 mL) maple syrup

2 Tbsp (30 mL) extra virgin olive oil

1 clove garlic (about 1 tsp/5 mL minced)

1 tsp (5 mL) minced fresh ginger (optional)

This dressing pairs perfectly with mixed salad greens, romaine hearts, baby spinach, or kale. A drizzle goes a long way!

1. Combine all ingredients in a jar, cover tightly, and shake well.

2. Store in the refrigerator until ready to use. Shake well before using.

46 calories per 1 Tbsp (15 mL), 7 g carbohydrates, 6 g sugar, 0 g fiber, 0 g protein, 2 g fat (0 g saturated), 1 mg sodium, 24 mg potassium

NORENE'S NOTES:

- **Color your world!** For a splash of color, combine leafy greens with sliced strawberries, mangoes, pineapple pieces, and/or orange segments. Drizzle with the dressing. For added crunch, scatter toasted slivered almonds, walnut halves, or chopped pistachios overtop.

- **Passover option:** Use a brand of maple syrup that has been certified for Passover. Alternatively, substitute honey or a sugar substitute for maple syrup.

DR. ED SAYS:

- **Fruit juice and maple syrup** are high in sugar, but you only need to add a drizzle of dressing to your salad. Consider using a non-nutritive sweetener, such as stevia or sucralose. You may also want to consider using a reduced-sugar or sugar-free syrup. This dressing can be enjoyed by those who follow a low-fat diet.

CITRUS DRESSING

PAREVE | GLUTEN-FREE | PASSOVER OPTION | KEEPS ABOUT
10 DAYS IN THE REFRIGERATOR | MAKES ½ CUP (125 ML)

Although this refreshing dressing tastes best using fresh citrus juices, use bottled juices if you're in a tight squeeze! It's wonderful on the Romaine, Avocado, and Mango Salad (p. 401).

2 Tbsp (30 mL) lemon or lime juice (preferably fresh)

2 Tbsp (30 mL) orange juice (preferably fresh)

¼ cup (60 mL) extra virgin olive oil or avocado oil

1 clove garlic (about 1 tsp/5 mL minced)

1 tsp (5 mL) Dijon mustard (omit for Passover)

½ tsp (2 mL) honey

Salt and freshly ground black pepper

1. Combine all ingredients in a jar, cover tightly, and shake well.

2. Store in the refrigerator until ready to use. Shake well before using.

65 calories per 1 Tbsp (15 mL), 1 g carbohydrates, 1 g sugar, 0 g fiber, 0 g protein, 7 g fat (1 g saturated), 15 mg sodium, 13 mg potassium

NORENE'S NOTES:

- **Marin-aides:** Use this easy dressing as a marinade for chicken, fish, or grilled vegetables. See "Marin-Aides" (p. 386).

DR. ED SAYS:

- **Sweet news:** This recipe is a better choice than many of the other dressings/marinades because less sugars are added and the sodium content is very low. Also, we get a fair slug of natural vitamin C from the fruit juices, as well as the usual antioxidant hit.

- **Olive oil** adds a good amount of beneficial monounsaturated fat.

DOUBLE-DUTY VINAIGRETTE/MARINADE

PAREVE | GLUTEN-FREE | PASSOVER OPTION | KEEPS ABOUT
2 WEEKS IN THE REFRIGERATOR | MAKES ½ CUP (125 ML)

3 Tbsp (45 mL) balsamic or
rice vinegar

2 Tbsp (30 mL) extra virgin
olive oil

1 tsp (5 mL) toasted sesame oil
(omit for Passover)

2 Tbsp (30 mL) orange juice

1 Tbsp (15 mL) honey or
maple syrup

2 cloves garlic (about 2 tsp/10 mL
minced)

Salt and freshly ground black
pepper to taste

Why not double your pleasure? Make a double batch of dressing—use some on your favorite salad and the rest as a marinade for chicken, fish, or vegetables.

1. Combine all ingredients in a jar, cover tightly, and shake well.

2. Store in the refrigerator until ready to use. Shake well before using.

53 calories per 1 Tbsp (15 mL), 5 g carbohydrates, 4 g sugar, 0 g fiber, 0 g protein, 4 g fat (<1 g saturated), trace sodium, 11 mg potassium

DR. ED SAYS:

- **Olive oil and sesame oil** provide a significant amount of monounsaturated fat, and we also get the phytonutrients that come with these oils.

- **Sweet option:** Use reduced-sugar syrups with natural or synthetic intense sweetener (e.g., stevia or sucralose).

PEANUT DRESSING/MARINADE

PAREVE | GLUTEN-FREE OPTION | KEEPS ABOUT 10 DAYS IN THE REFRIGERATOR | MAKES ABOUT ¾ CUP (185 ML)

This Szechuan-inspired dressing can be made in advance and refrigerated. It makes a marvelous marinade for fish, chicken, tofu, or roasted vegetables.

2 cloves garlic

¼ cup (60 mL) peanut butter (preferably natural with no added sugar)

2 Tbsp (30 mL) rice vinegar

2 Tbsp (30 mL) soy sauce or tamari (preferably low-sodium)

2 Tbsp (30 mL) honey

1 tsp (5 mL) toasted sesame oil

3–4 Tbsp (45–60 mL) orange juice (preferably fresh)

Pinch red pepper flakes

1. Mince garlic in a mini prep or food processor fitted with the steel blade. Add peanut butter, vinegar, soy sauce, honey, sesame oil, orange juice, and red pepper flakes. Process until blended, about 30 seconds. Scrape down the sides of the bowl as needed. If too thick, drizzle in a little more orange juice.

2. Store in a jar in the refrigerator until ready to use. Shake well before using.

55 calories per 1 Tbsp (15 mL), 5 g carbohydrates, 4 g sugar, 0 g fiber, 1 g protein, 3 g fat (1 g saturated), 176 mg sodium, 11 mg potassium

NORENE'S NOTES:

• **Peanut butter:** Store natural peanut butter in the refrigerator. When needed, stir well, measure desired quantity, and bring to room temperature for easier blending. Alternatively, microwave on medium for 30 seconds, then stir well.

• **Variation:** Use almond butter (homemade or store-bought) instead of peanut butter. If you are allergic to peanuts (or any nuts!), use a peanut butter substitute.

DR. ED SAYS:

• **Peanut butter** is a double-edged sword. On one hand, it is nutrient-dense and provides good amounts of protein, magnesium, zinc, vitamin B6, and folate, as well as vitamin E. (The majority of the vitamin E is in the form of gamma tocopherol, which the brain likes.) On the other hand, peanut butter comes with added salt and sugar—so look for natural, no-sugar peanut butter. If regular peanut butter is all you have on hand, it won't make as much difference in a dressing since the quantity used is rather minimal.

RECIPE CONTINUED . . .

PEANUT DRESSING/MARINADE (continued)

- **Instead of honey,** consider using a non-nutritive sweetener syrup.

- **Soy sauce tends** to be loaded with sodium, so use a low-sodium version.

- **Overall,** this salad dressing contains ingredients that make some contribution to the nutritional profile of any salad.

POMEGRANATE HONEY SPLASH

PAREVE | GLUTEN-FREE | PASSOVER OPTION | KEEPS ABOUT
10 DAYS IN THE REFRIGERATOR | MAKES ABOUT ¾ CUP (185 ML)

This is the perfect salad dressing for the Jewish High Holidays as it combines pomegranate juice and honey, two traditional holiday foods.

¼ cup (60 mL) balsamic vinegar

¼ cup (60 mL) pomegranate juice

¼ cup (60 mL) honey

2 Tbsp (30 mL) extra virgin olive oil or avocado oil

1 tsp (5 mL) Worcestershire sauce (optional; omit for Passover)

1 clove garlic (about 1 tsp/5 mL minced)

1. Combine all ingredients in a jar, cover tightly, and shake well.

2. Store in the refrigerator until ready to use. Shake well before using.

47 calories per 1 Tbsp (15 mL), 7 g carbohydrates, 7 g sugar, 0 g fiber, 0 g protein, 2 g fat (0 g saturated), 2 mg sodium, 21 mg potassium

NORENE'S NOTES:

- **Vegan/passover alert!** Did you know that some brands of Worcestershire sauce contain anchovies? If this is a concern, choose a brand that is anchovy-free. Alternatively, you can also substitute soy sauce or tamari, or just omit it from the recipe.

DR. ED SAYS:

- **Pomegranate juice and honey** add an additional 7 g of sugar per 1 Tbsp (15 mL) to a salad, in addition to any sugar provided by the salad itself. Try to source pomegranate juice with no added sugar as well as a non-nutritive sweetener syrup to reduce the sugar load.

POPPY SEED DRESSING

PAREVE | GLUTEN-FREE | KEEPS ABOUT 10 DAYS IN THE REFRIGER-
ATOR | MAKES ABOUT 1 CUP (250 ML)

¼ cup (60 mL) canola oil

¼ cup (60 mL) rice vinegar

2 Tbsp (30 mL) orange juice
(preferably fresh)

2 Tbsp (30 mL) lemon juice
(preferably fresh)

2 Tbsp (30 mL) honey (or to taste)

1 Tbsp (15 mL) poppy seeds

1 tsp (5 mL) Dijon mustard

Salt and freshly ground black
pepper to taste

This light dressing is lovely on mixed salad greens or baby spinach leaves. Scatter orange segments, sliced mangoes, kiwis, radishes, and/or thinly sliced red onions overtop.

1. Combine all ingredients in a jar, cover tightly, and shake well.

2. Store in the refrigerator until ready to use. Shake well before using.

41 calories per 1 Tbsp (15 mL), 3 g carbohydrates, 2 g sugar, 0 g fiber, 0 g protein, 4 g fat (0 g saturated), 7 mg sodium, 11 mg potassium

NORENE'S NOTES:

· **Variation:** Add 2 Tbsp (30 mL) light mayonnaise for a creamier version.

· **The seedy truth!** Poppy seeds are high in calcium, iron and zinc—but, believe it or not, research shows that eating a significant amount of seeds can also make you "high," as they contain trace amounts of morphine! This poppy seed dressing gets "high" marks for flavor.

DR. ED SAYS:

· **Poppy seeds** are a nutrient powerhouse, with very high fiber, vitamin E, unsaturated fats, magnesium, potassium, folate, and B6 vitamins. They contain natural phytosterols, which help to control cholesterol. To top it off, poppy seeds are very low in sugar, digestible carbs, and sodium. The quantity of poppy seeds used here is relatively small, but don't be afraid to use more.

· **Canola oil** provides good unsaturated fats and natural vitamin E (with a high concentration of brain-friendly gamma tocopherol), and the spices provide various antioxidants.

RASPBERRY VINAIGRETTE

PAREVE | GLUTEN-FREE | PASSOVER OPTION | KEEPS ABOUT
10 DAYS IN THE REFRIGERATOR | MAKES ABOUT ⅔ CUP (160 ML)

If you keep frozen raspberries on hand, you can whip up this fruity dressing in about 30 seconds. It's great over whole grains or greens. For a real taste sensation, drizzle it over grilled asparagus.

⅓ cup (80 mL) fresh or frozen raspberries (no need to defrost)

⅓ cup (80 mL) extra virgin olive oil

1 tsp (5 mL) Dijon mustard (omit for Passover)

2 Tbsp (30 mL) balsamic vinegar

1 Tbsp (15 mL) honey

Pinch of salt

Freshly ground black pepper

1. In a mini prep or food processor fitted with the steel blade, process raspberries for 8–10 seconds, until puréed.

2. Add the remaining ingredients and process 10 seconds longer to combine.

3. Transfer to a jar, cover, and store in the refrigerator until ready to use. Shake well before using.

69 calories per 1 Tbsp (15 mL), 3 g carbohydrates, 3 g sugar, 0 g fiber, 0 g protein, 7 g fat (1 g saturated), 11 mg sodium, 7 mg potassium

DR. ED SAYS:

- **Overall,** because the serving size of this salad dressing (and most dressings) is so small, the contribution of beneficial nutrients is negligible, except for unsaturated fat and antioxidants. Sugar content is moderately high at 3 g per 1 Tbsp (15 mL), but when used with a low-carb salad, it should be acceptable.

SHAKE-IT-UP VINAIGRETTE/MARINADE

PAREVE | GLUTEN-FREE | PASSOVER OPTION | KEEPS ABOUT
10 DAYS IN THE REFRIGERATOR | MAKES ABOUT 1 CUP (250 ML)

⅓ cup (80 mL) extra virgin olive oil

⅓ cup (80 mL) red wine vinegar

⅓ cup (80 mL) orange juice (preferably fresh)

1½ tsp (7 mL) Dijon mustard (omit for Passover)

1 Tbsp (15 mL) honey

2 cloves garlic (about 2 tsp/10 mL minced)

½ tsp (2 mL) salt

¼ tsp (1 mL) freshly ground black pepper

This luscious, low-calorie dressing also does double-duty as a quick marinade for chicken, beef, fish, tofu, or vegetables. Dress it up, dress it down, it's a winner all around!

1. Combine all the ingredients in a jar, cover tightly, and shake very well. Mixture will thicken as you shake it. Store in the refrigerator.

2. Remove from refrigerator a few minutes before you need it. Shake well.

46 calories per 1 Tbsp (15 mL), 2 g carbohydrates, 1 g sugar, 0 g fiber, 0 g protein, 4 g fat (1 g saturated), 68 mg sodium, 14 mg potassium

NORENE'S NOTES:

- **Measure up:** Instead of combining dressing ingredients in a jar, add oil, vinegar, and then orange juice to a 2-cup (500 mL) glass measure. No need to empty between additions! You'll have 1 cup (250 mL) liquid. Add the remaining ingredients and whisk well, using a mini whisk or fork.

- **Oil right:** Use canola, walnut, avocado, or grapeseed oil instead of olive oil.

- **Switch it up!** Substitute rice, balsamic, white wine, or apple cider vinegar for red wine vinegar. Instead of orange juice, use mango or pineapple juice, or try a combination of equal parts orange and lemon juice. Use maple syrup or your favorite sweetener instead of honey.

- **Hooray for herbs!** Add ½ tsp (2 mL) dried thyme, basil, oregano, or rosemary for an herb-flavored version. If desired, add 2 Tbsp (30 mL) minced fresh parsley or cilantro. Add 1 minced shallot as a flavor booster.

DR. ED SAYS:

- **Overall,** like most salad dressings, the contribution of beneficial nutrients is negligible because of the small serving size, yet they enhance the flavor, making brain-boosting salads much more appetizing.

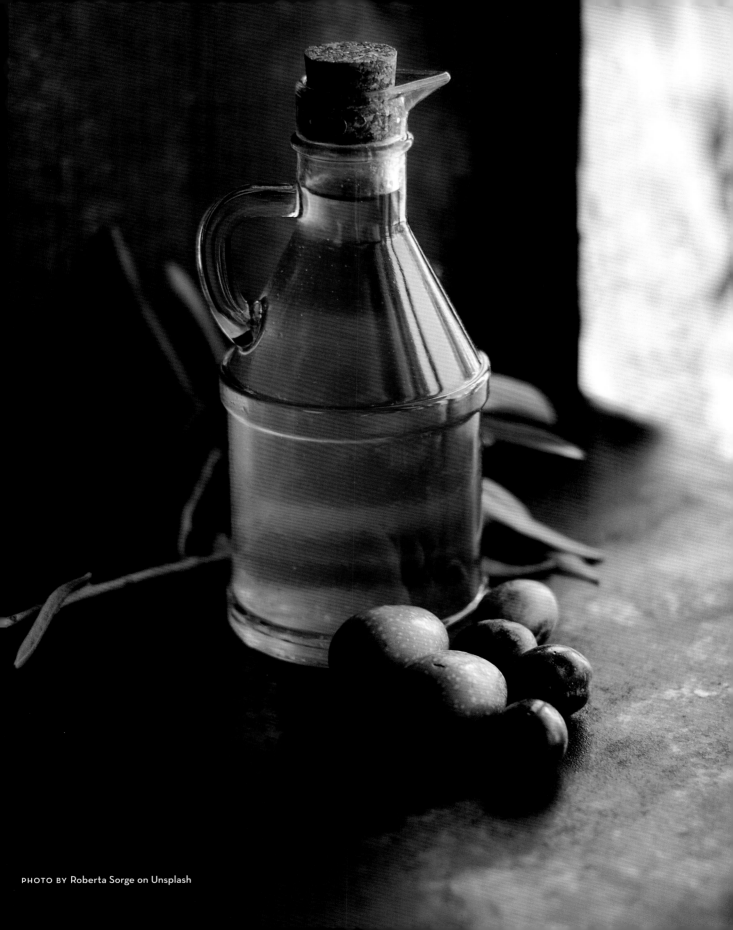

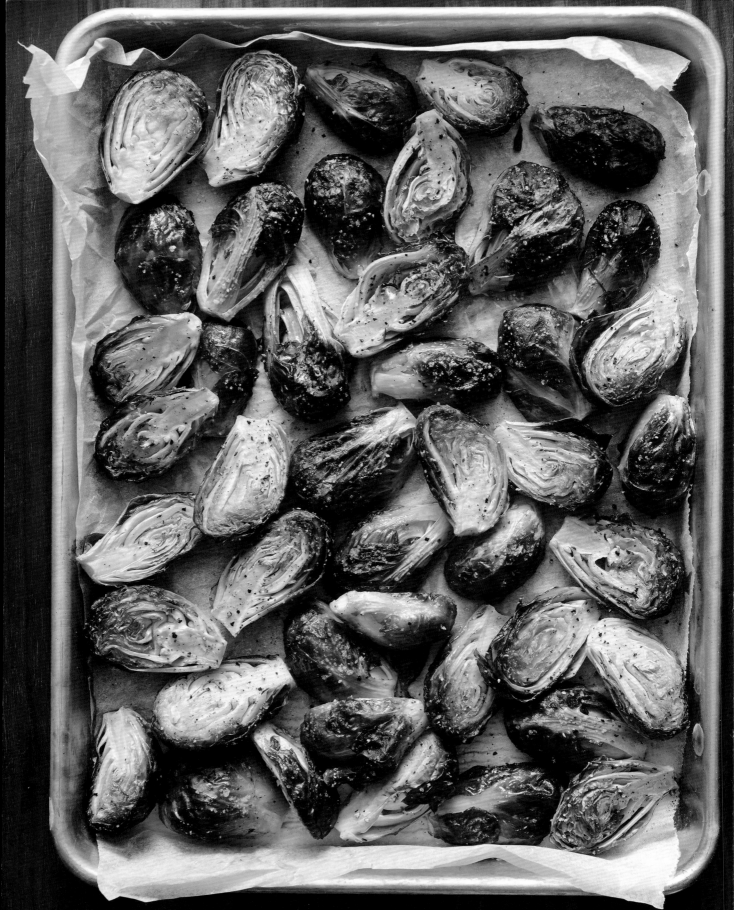

VERSATILE VEGETABLES & SIDES

THE GARDEN OF EATING: From asparagus to zucchini, vegetables provide a variety of nutrients for optimal health. They're low in calories and high in vitamins, minerals, fiber, antioxidants, and phytonutrients.

ARE YOU GETTING ENOUGH? A good starting goal is a minimum of 2 cups (500 mL) vegetables and 2–3 fruits per day. Aim for 5–7 servings of vegetables and fruits a day. Adults need more than children, and men need more than women. A serving is about 1 cup (250 mL) raw (the size of a baseball) or ½ cup (125 mL) cooked (the size of a tennis ball).

"BENEFITS!" Vegetables and fruits can help reduce your risk of Alzheimer's and dementia, heart disease, stroke, diabetes, cancer, cataracts, and macular degeneration. Their colorful pigments give them their disease-fighting antioxidant power, so fill your plate with a kaleidoscope of color and health.

HIGH SATIETY: Vegetables contain about 80–95% water, so they help fill you up and control hunger. Vegetables provide a large volume of food for less calories. By replacing especially calorie-dense foods with less-calorie-dense vegetables, you can eat bigger portions for the same number of calories.

WHAT IS THE GLYCEMIC INDEX (GI)? The GI is a ranking of carbohydrates on a scale from 0 to 100 according to the extent to which they raise blood sugar (glucose) levels after eating. Foods with a high GI are those which are rapidly digested, absorbed, and metabolized, and result in marked fluctuations in blood sugar (glucose) levels. Low-GI carbohydrates produce smaller fluctuations in your blood glucose and insulin levels.

GI GO! Most vegetables have a low glycemic index, especially if they are green. Some vegetables, such as asparagus, broccoli, cauliflower, and dark leafy greens, contain little or no carbohydrates. Here's a quick overview as a guide:

- **LOW GI (GI 55 OR LESS):** Green vegetables include asparagus, green beans, bok choy, broccoli, Brussels sprouts, cabbage, celery, collard greens, cucumber, kale, lettuce, peas, salad greens, snow peas, and Swiss chard. Other vegetables with a low GI are bell peppers, carrots, cauliflower, eggplant, fennel, garlic, jicama, leeks, mushrooms, onions, radishes, radicchio, tomatoes, yellow beans, sweet potato, butternut squash, and zucchini. Eat these in abundance. For a brain-healthy diet, Dr. Ed recommends focusing on foods with a GI of 45 or less.

- **MEDIUM GI (GI FROM 56 TO 69):** These vegetables include beets, corn, and Yukon gold potatoes. Eat these in moderation.
- **HIGH GI (GI OF 70 OR MORE):** These vegetables include acorn squash, broad beans, parsnips, pumpkin, rutabaga, and turnips. Most spuds are duds when it comes to GI. Russets and other white potatoes (boiled, baked, or mashed) score high on the GI scale, whereas new potatoes have a medium GI. Enjoy these occasionally.

THE NUMBERS GAME: Although starchier vegetables such as corn and beets have a medium GI, they are rich in nutrients and also boost your fiber intake. It's best to combine them with lower-GI foods.

CALLING ALL CRUCIFEROUS VEGGIES! Broccoli, cauliflower, cabbage, kale, and Brussels sprouts contain brain-boosting nutrients that help reduce the risk of Alzheimer's and dementia. They are also rich in sulphur-containing compounds, folate, calcium, iron, and vitamin K. Aim for 3–4 servings a week.

THE ALLURE OF ALLIUM: Garlic, onions, leeks, and chives belong to the allium family. They provide similar benefits to cruciferous veggies due to their powerful phytonutrients. Garlic, onions, and leeks stimulate the immune system, fight cancer, and boost flavor. Did you know that garlic acts as a natural antibiotic and an antifungal medication? To optimize garlic's benefits, let it sit for 10–15 minutes after it is cut. It's worth the wait!

GO FOR GREEN: Dark leafy greens include spinach, Swiss chard, kale, and collard greens. Spinach and Swiss chard are interchangeable in most recipes and their cooking time is similar. The darker the green, the higher the nutritional value and disease-fighting potential. Brain-boosting greens are high in folate and rich in lutein and zeaxanthin, which help reduce the risk of cataracts and macular degeneration.

PEPPER POWER: Bell peppers add color, fiber, and flavor to recipes. They are high in vitamins A and C, as well as lycopene. (Red peppers are higher in vitamin C than green and are easier to digest.) Peppers contain powerful antioxidants and promote heart and eye health.

STEP UP TO THE PLATE: The American Institute of Cancer Research recommends that your plate should contain two vegetables, one serving of whole grains, and a smaller portion of protein. Our dietician, Sharona Abramovitch, recommends covering half your plate with vegetables, which adds up to approximately two ½-cup (125 mL) portions of vegetables twice a day.

SNEAKY CUISINE: Sneak vegetables into puréed soups, smoothies, casseroles, whole grains, meatloaf, and burgers. Add them to stir-fries, dips, and spreads. Use your food processor to mince carrots, celery, onions, and garlic and add them to chicken, salmon, tuna salad, or even burgers.

A-PEELING SHORTCUTS: There are so many vegetables that require minimal effort to get to the table, with no cutting or peeling required. Try baby carrots, grape tomatoes, baby spinach, broccoli, cauliflower florets, coleslaw mix, jarred roasted peppers, sun-dried tomatoes, minced garlic, ginger, basil, and various herbs. Try precut vegetables (broccoli and cauliflower florets, sliced peppers, stir-fry mix, etc.). Although they are a bit more expensive, you can buy just the amount you need—no waste.

USE YOUR NOODLE: All sorts of vegetables are now available in "noodle" form including beets, carrots, squash, and zucchini. Look for them in the refrigerated section of the produce department or make your own using a spiralizer.

COOL TOOLS: You need a good vegetable peeler, a paring knife, a chef's knife, several cutting boards (color-coded if possible), a rimmed baking sheet (also known as a half sheet pan), and a salad spinner. A food processor makes chopping, mincing, puréeing, slicing, and shredding a breeze. A mini processor is helpful for mincing herbs and small quantities of foods. For cooking I use a steamer, wok, nonstick skillet, indoor and outdoor grills, and my microwave and conventional ovens.

COOK IT RIGHT: Vegetables can be blanched, boiled, steamed, sautéed, stir-fried, roasted, grilled, or microwaved to preserve flavor and texture. Sharona recommends limiting boiled vegetables as their nutrients tend to go into the water—steaming is better.

TIME TO COOK: The nutritional value of vegetables is affected by the cooking time and method. Cooking time depends on the type of vegetable and whether it is whole, sliced, chopped, or grated. For most methods (except roasting or grilling), estimate 3–4 minutes for grated vegetables, 5–6 minutes for chopped or sliced vegetables, and 10–15 minutes for whole veggies. Limit overcooking vegetables to help preserve nutritional value.

LESS-THAN-SEVEN RULE: Cook green vegetables no longer than 7 minutes to preserve their bright green color and texture. If necessary cut them into smaller pieces. Some veggies take longer to become tender, so if you cook them longer than 7 minutes their color won't be as bright.

QUICK CUISINE! Prepare vegetables ahead of time. Wash, trim, and cut them up, then plunge them into a large pot of boiling salted water. Cook uncovered until nearly tender, about 2 minutes; drain and rinse with cold water. Let cool, then refrigerate in resealable bags for 3–4 days. When needed, just sauté or stir-fry quickly in olive oil and garlic—or microwave them.

ROAST AND BOAST: Roasting vegetables concentrates their flavor and brings out their natural sweetness. They're delicious hot, cold, or at room temperature. Add them to whole grains such as quinoa, bulgur, or black rice. Try them in salads, wraps, casseroles, omelets, and frittatas, or enjoy them as a snack.

THE SPICE IS RIGHT: Kosher or sea salt and freshly ground black pepper add terrific flavor. Fresh herbs are best, but dried will do in a pinch. Citrus juices such as orange, lemon, or lime should be fresh, if possible. A little Parmesan, feta, or goat cheese will add calcium and flavor. Nuts add healthy fats and crunch.

COLD STORAGE: Most vegetables should be stored in the vegetable crisper in a loosely sealed plastic bag. This helps prevent moisture from being trapped, which causes softening or spoilage. Wrap unwashed leafy greens in paper towels and store them in a resealable plastic bag.

STORE IT RIGHT: Store root vegetables in a cool, well-ventilated pantry, away from light. Good keepers are onions, potatoes, sweet potatoes, and winter squash. Store potatoes and onions separately to avoid spoilage. Store garlic, uncovered, in a small basket for easy access.

MEAL PREP TIP: Be prepared! Slice raw vegetables in advance for an easy side dish or snack option. Cucumbers, celery, carrots, and bell peppers are some of the vegetables that will last up to a week in a good-quality storage container in the refrigerator.

FROZEN ASSETS: Frozen vegetables are handy and economical. The nutrient content is usually as good as if they were fresh—and sometimes it's even better. Although the texture of fresh veggies is better, frozen vegetables are convenient.

MICROWAVE MAGIC: Microwaving 1 lb (500 g) fresh vegetables (about 2 cups/500 mL) takes about 5 minutes on high, depending on the vegetable. A 10-oz (300 g) package (about 1½ cups/375 mL) of frozen vegetables cooks in 5 minutes on high. It's not necessary to add water, as the ice crystals will create enough steam to cook the vegetables. It takes 2–3 minutes on high to defrost.

GOT YOU COVERED! If your casserole doesn't have a lid, mold a sheet of wet parchment paper around it, tucking it underneath to secure it.

BABY BONUS: Baby carrots are regular carrots that have been machine-cut into minis. It takes 1 medium carrot to make 4–5 baby carrots. No peeling required!

MYTH-INFORMATION: Many people who follow a low-carb diet are afraid to eat carrots. However, their GI is 41, which makes them a low-GI food. The GI is based on eating 55 g of carbohydrates, about 9 carrots, or 1½ lb (750 g). One medium carrot contains 6 g carbs, 2 g fiber, and just 25 calories.

OVEN-ROASTED ASPARAGUS

DAIRY OPTION | PAREVE | GLUTEN-FREE | PASSOVER | DO NOT
FREEZE | MAKES 6–8 SERVINGS

This fiber-packed dish is a snap to prepare. Roasting concentrates the flavor of the asparagus and the tips will get very crispy. Warning—this dish is addictive. Leftovers are great in salads and wraps. Smaller family? Make half the recipe!

2 lb (900 g) asparagus spears

2 Tbsp (30 mL) extra virgin olive oil

3 cloves garlic (about 2 tsp/10 mL minced)

2 tsp (10 mL) freshly grated lemon zest

Salt and freshly ground black pepper

1. Preheat oven to 425°F (220°C). Line a rimmed baking sheet with foil; spray with nonstick spray.

2. Soak asparagus thoroughly in cold water and drain well. Bend asparagus and snap off the tough ends where they break off naturally. Place asparagus in a single layer on the prepared baking sheet.

3. In a small bowl, whisk together olive oil, garlic, and lemon zest. Brush asparagus evenly with the oil mixture. Season with salt and pepper.

4. Roast, uncovered, in the lower third of the oven for 10–12 minutes, or until spears are tender-crisp and lightly browned. Using tongs, turn asparagus once or twice during roasting for even browning.

5. Transfer to a serving platter. Serve hot, at room temperature, or chilled.

73 calories per serving, 6 g carbohydrates, 3 g fiber, 3 g sugar, 3 g protein, 5 g fat (1 g saturated fat), 3 mg sodium, 310 mg potassium

NORENE'S NOTES:

- **Grilled asparagus:** Preheat grill or BBQ. Prepare asparagus as directed in Steps 2–3. Transfer to the hot grill, laying spears crosswise so they won't fall through the grates (or place in a grill basket). Grill over medium-high for 8–10 minutes, or until spears are lightly browned and tender-crisp.

- **Herb-roasted asparagus:** Add 1 tsp (5 mL) minced fresh rosemary, thyme, tarragon, or ½ tsp (2 mL) dried Italian seasoning to the olive oil mixture. Roast or grill asparagus.

RECIPE CONTINUED . . .

OVEN-ROASTED ASPARAGUS (continued)

- **Dairy option:** Omit oil, lemon zest, and garlic. Coat asparagus with ¼ cup (60 mL) low-calorie Caesar dressing. Sprinkle with 2 Tbsp (30 mL) sesame seeds and 2 Tbsp (30 mL) grated Parmesan cheese. Roast as directed in Step 4.

- **Juicy secret:** Lemon zest adds a fresh flavor to asparagus without discoloring it.

- **Size counts:** Try to buy spears that are all the same thickness for even cooking. One bunch of asparagus weighs about 1 lb (500 g) and contains 16–20 spears. Calculate 4–6 spears per person as a serving.

DR. ED SAYS:

- **Asparagus and olive oil,** the two major ingredients in this recipe, are both significant contributors to a brain-healthy diet. Although asparagus is only about 7% dry solids (the rest being water), its fiber content is 54% of the dry solids and, surprisingly, 33% of the dry weight is protein. It is a good source of carotenoid and flavonol antioxidants, both of which are good for the brain.

- **Overall,** this recipe is a good source of vitamins B6, E, and C, as well as complex antioxidants. It is also an excellent source of folate.

> **DID YOU KNOW?** Pepper contains a component called piperine, which helps in the absorption of fat-based antioxidants.

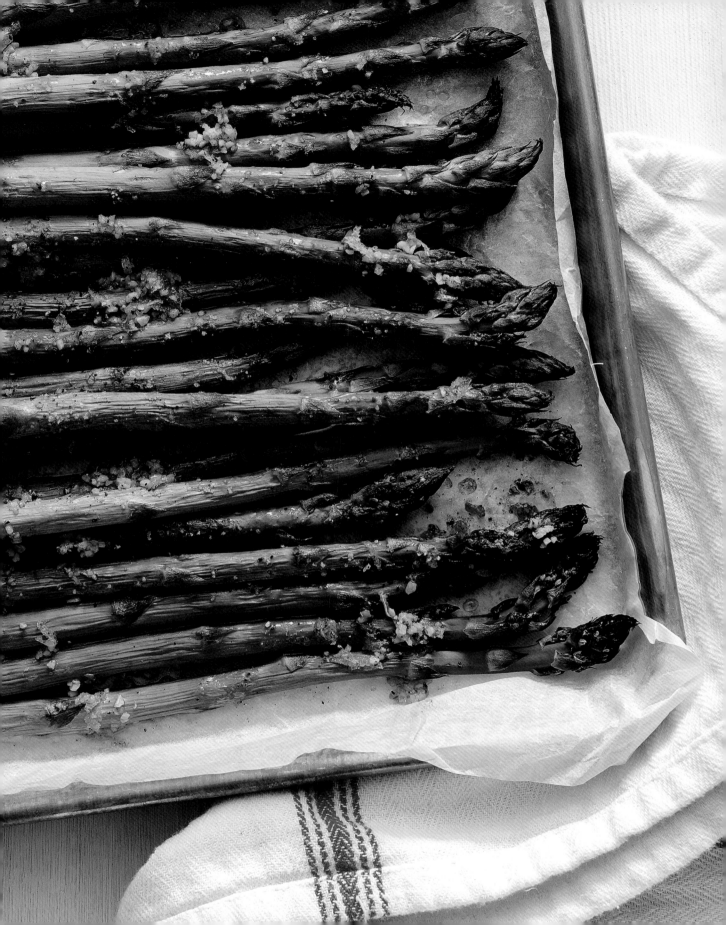

SESAME-ROASTED BROCCOLI

PAREVE | GLUTEN-FREE | PASSOVER OPTION | DO NOT FREEZE |
MAKES 4 SERVINGS

1 large bunch broccoli
(about 1½ lb/750 g)

2 Tbsp (30 mL) olive oil

2 Tbsp (30 mL) lemon juice
(preferably fresh)

2–3 cloves garlic, minced
(about 2 tsp/10 mL)

1 tsp (5 mL) dried basil

¼ tsp (1 mL) dried oregano

¼ tsp (1 mL) dried thyme

Salt and freshly ground
black pepper

¼ cup (60 mL) sesame seeds

Roasting broccoli transforms it, enhancing the flavor. If you prefer using fresh herbs instead of dried, add them during the last few minutes of cooking—dried herbs should be added at the beginning of cooking. Broccoli shrinks in volume during roasting, so consider doubling the recipe. This perfect low-carb snack is addictive!

1. Preheat oven to 400°F (200°C). Line a rimmed baking sheet with parchment paper.

2. Trim and discard woody ends from broccoli. Cut broccoli into spears or large pieces. Soak thoroughly in cold salted water for a few minutes, then drain well.

3. Spread broccoli out on the prepared baking sheet and drizzle with olive oil and lemon juice. Sprinkle with garlic and seasonings. Toss broccoli gently with your hands, coating on all sides. Sprinkle with sesame seeds.

4. Roast, uncovered, in the lower third of the oven for 15–20 minutes, until broccoli is tender-crisp and lightly browned. Use tongs to turn the broccoli once or twice during roasting. Serve hot or at room temperature.

168 calories per serving, 13 g carbohydrates, 6 g fiber, 3 g sugar, 7 g protein, 12 g fat (2 g saturated fat), 52 mg sodium, 671 mg potassium

NORENE'S NOTES:

- **Mix it up!** Strips of red or yellow bell pepper can be roasted together with the broccoli.

- **Sesame-roasted asparagus:** Substitute asparagus for broccoli. Cooking time will be slightly less, depending on the thickness of the asparagus. For a dairy option, sprinkle with Parmesan cheese before roasting

- **Passover option:** Omit sesame seeds. If desired, sprinkle roasted broccoli with toasted slivered almonds as a garnish.

- **Broccoli** is a very good source of the brain antioxidants lutein and zeaxanthin. It is also very high in vitamin C and has a high ratio of fiber to total carbs (39% of solids).

- **Sesame seeds,** which are very nutrient-dense, add a wallop of extra nutrients to the recipe.

- **Overall,** the recipe is extremely high in vitamin C at 178 mg per serving, and is an excellent source of the brain-important B vitamins B6 and folate, as well as the minerals magnesium and zinc.

DID YOU KNOW? Broccoli, a member of the cruciferous group of vegetables, contains glucosinolates that convert to potent cancer-fighting compounds during food processing.

STEAMED BROCCOLI WITH OLIVE OIL, GARLIC, AND HERBS

PAREVE | GLUTEN-FREE | PASSOVER | DO NOT FREEZE | MAKES 4 SERVINGS

1 large bunch broccoli (about 1½ lb/750 g)

4 tsp (20 mL) extra virgin olive oil

2–3 cloves garlic (about 2 tsp/10 mL minced)

½ tsp (2 mL) dried basil

¼ tsp (1 mL) dried thyme

Salt and freshly ground black pepper

Steaming retains maximum nutrients because very little water is used. Full steam ahead!

1. Trim and discard woody ends from broccoli. Cut broccoli into spears or large pieces. Soak thoroughly in cold salted water for a few minutes, then drain well. Place in a steamer basket.

2. Bring 1 inch (2.5 cm) water to a boil in a large saucepan. Place steamer basket in the saucepan. Cover saucepan and simmer broccoli for 5–6 minutes, until tender-crisp and bright green. Don't overcook!

3. Transfer broccoli to a serving bowl. Add oil, garlic, and seasonings. Toss gently to combine. Serve immediately.

95 calories per serving, 10 g carbohydrates, 4 g fiber, 3 g sugar, 6 g protein, 5 g fat (<1 g saturated fat), 51 mg sodium, 618 mg potassium

NORENE'S NOTES:

- **Less-than-seven rule:** Always cook broccoli less than 7 minutes to preserve its bright green color, and to prevent it from forming an unpleasant, sulphur-like odor. For even cooking, cut florets no larger than 1½ inches (4 cm) and cut stems into ½-inch (1 cm) slices.

- **Quick broccoli for one:** Rinse 1 cup (250 mL) broccoli florets and drain well. Place in a 2-cup (500 mL) glass measure. Microwave on high, covered, for 1–2 minutes, until tender-crisp. Drizzle with either lemon juice or low-calorie salad dressing and garnish with sesame seeds (but not during Passover).

- **Fresh or frozen?** Frozen broccoli contains more beta carotene than fresh. However, it contains twice as much sodium and less iron, thiamine, riboflavin, calcium, and vitamin C.

- **This recipe** provides similar levels of brain nutrition as Sesame-Roasted Broccoli (p. 444) and Oven-Roasted Asparagus (p. 441), though at slightly lower concentrations.

- **Overall,** this recipe is a good source of vitamin E, magnesium, and zinc, without being an excellent source. However, it still retains "excellent" status for the folate and vitamin B6, as well as for being an outstanding source of vitamin C at 175 mg per serving.

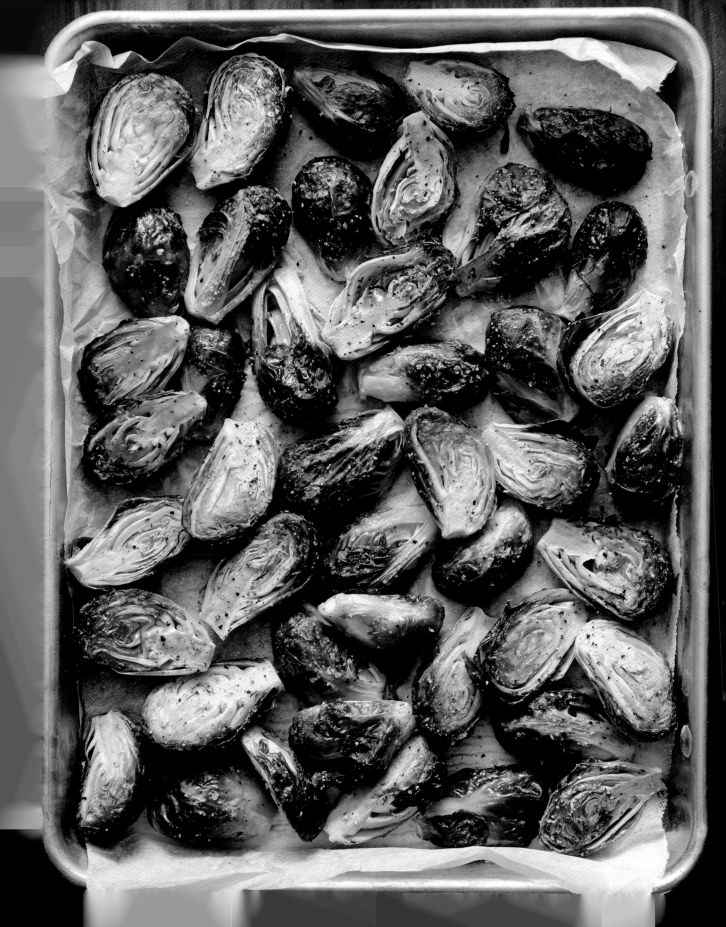

ROASTED BRUSSELS SPROUTS

PAREVE | GLUTEN-FREE | PASSOVER | DO NOT FREEZE | MAKES 4–6 SERVINGS

The fresher the sprouts, the finer the flavor. This addictive recipe was shared with me by Risa Golding. It multiplies easily and makes a fabulous snack. When you roast them, everyone will shout for more sprouts!

1½ lb (750 g) Brussels sprouts (about 30–36)

2–3 Tbsp (45 mL) olive oil

Salt and freshly ground black pepper

1. Preheat oven to 425°F (220°C). Line a large, rimmed baking sheet with parchment paper.

2. Trim ends from Brussels sprouts and remove any yellow leaves. Cut sprouts in half and soak in salted cold water for 10 minutes to rid them of any hidden insects. Drain well.

3. Transfer to a bowl and toss with olive oil, salt, and pepper. Spread out the sprouts in a single layer on the prepared baking sheet.

4. Roast, uncovered in the lower third of the oven, for 20–30 minutes, until crispy and well browned. Halfway through cooking, turn sprouts over for more even browning. Serve hot or at room temperature.

140 calories per serving, 17 g carbohydrates, 7 g fiber, 4 g sugar, 6 g protein, 7 g fat (1 g saturated fat), 47 mg sodium, 729 mg potassium

NORENE'S NOTES:

- **Shaved brussels sprouts:** Follow Steps 1–2. In a food processor fitted with the slicer, slice Brussels sprouts in batches, using very light pressure. Transfer to a bowl and continue as directed in Step 3. Roasting time will be 15–18 minutes.

- **Variations:** Brussels sprouts are also fabulous drizzled with freshly squeezed lemon juice or sprinkled with finely minced lemon or lime zest. Experiment with various seasonings such as minced garlic or thyme.

- **What's in store?** Brussels sprouts resemble mini cabbages. Smaller sprouts are more tender than larger ones, which tend to be bitter and woody in the center. Choose small dark green sprouts that are tightly closed, about 1–1½ inches (2.5–4 cm) in diameter. There are about 2 dozen (3 cups/750 mL) sprouts in 1 lb (500 g).

RECIPE CONTINUED . . .

DR. ED SAYS:

· **Brussels sprouts** have many of the nutrient characteristics of cruciferous vegetables, but perhaps not in as large a quantity as others. Nevertheless, they are good sources of vitamins B6 and folate, as well as the important antioxidants lutein and zeaxanthin. Typical of the cruciferous group, they are also very high in vitamin C.

· **Overall,** this recipe is excellent in folate and vitamin C, and is a good source of B6, vitamin E, and the complex antioxidants lutein and zeaxanthin.

DID YOU KNOW? An excess of cruciferous vegetables can cause hypothyroidism, which can be mitigated by cooking—so if you are taking thyroid medication and consume large amounts of cruciferous vegetables, talk to your doctor, and cook your cruciferous vegetables.

ROASTED RAINBOW CARROTS

PAREVE | GLUTEN-FREE | PASSOVER | DO NOT FREEZE | MAKES
6 SERVINGS

These multihued roasted carrots are a show-stopper at any meal! Heir-loom carrots range in color from orange to yellow to red, and even purple. If you can't find them, feel free to use the standard orange ones. For maximum flavor, choose fresh bunched carrots.

3 bunches heirloom carrots (about 18)

2 Tbsp (30 mL) olive oil

2 Tbsp (30 mL) honey or maple syrup

2 tsp (10 mL) dried thyme or rosemary

Salt and freshly ground black pepper

1. Preheat oven to 425°F (220°C). Line a large, rimmed baking sheet with parchment paper.

2. Trim tops and ends of carrots, leaving some green. Scrub, rinse well, then pat dry with paper towels. Cut carrots lengthwise in halves or quarters, depending on their size.

3. Spread carrots in a single layer on the prepared baking sheet. Drizzle with olive oil and honey. Sprinkle with thyme, salt, and pepper; toss with your hands to coat.

4. Roast, uncovered, for 40–45 minutes, or until carrots are tender and caramelized, stirring occasionally. Serve hot or at room temperature.

96 calories per serving, 14 g carbohydrates, 3 g fiber, 9 g sugar, 1 g protein, 5 g fat (1 g saturated fat), 58 mg sodium, 273 mg potassium

NORENE'S NOTES:

- **Garlic-roasted carrots:** Instead of thyme, add 3-4 tsp (15-20 mL) minced fresh garlic. If desired, add 1 large red onion, halved and sliced.

- **Sweet and tangy carrots:** Add a drizzle of balsamic vinegar or lemon juice. Use dill instead of thyme.

- **Size counts:** Small-to-medium carrots are best. Large carrots have tough, tasteless, woody cores, and are less sweet.

RECIPE CONTINUED . . .

ROASTED RAINBOW CARROTS (continued)

DR. ED SAYS:

- **Carrots,** which are the main ingredient in this recipe, supply reasonable levels of brain-friendly nutrients, but they cannot be considered at the good or excellent level. This is because they contain 40% sugar on a dry weight basis when water is removed (though this translates to only 5% by weight as consumed, due to the high water content in carrots). The distinguishing characteristic of carrots is their very high content of carotenoid antioxidants beta carotene and vitamin A, which is the major benefit of the recipe.

- **Thyme and rosemary** will also add a potent punch of complex antioxidants.

- **Sweet option:** If you want to cut back on the 9 g of sugar per serving, try reducing the amount of honey and maple syrup used.

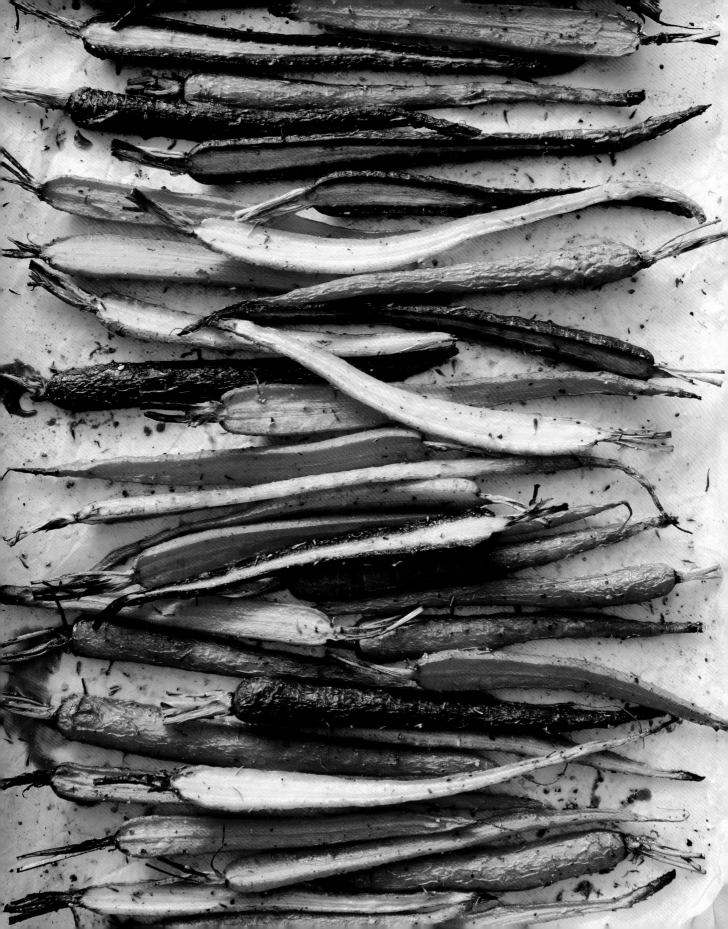

CARROT & SWEET POTATO TZIMMES

PAREVE | GLUTEN-FREE | PASSOVER | REHEATS AND/OR FREEZES
WELL | MAKES 12 SERVINGS

2 large sweet potatoes, peeled and cut into 1-inch (2.5 cm) pieces

1 acorn or butternut squash, peeled, seeded, and cut into 1-inch (2.5 cm) pieces

4 carrots, peeled and cut into ½-inch (1 cm) slices

12–15 prunes, pitted and halved

½ cup (125 mL) orange juice

½ cup (125 mL) water

1 tsp (5 mL) orange zest

Sweetener equivalent to ¼ cup (60 mL) brown sugar

1 tsp (5 mL) ground cinnamon

Salt and freshly ground black pepper

My late friend Bev Gordon shared this holiday family favorite with me. I've modified her recipe to reduce the carbs. Bev told me: "I associate September with Rosh Hashanah, Yom Kippur, and new beginnings. This wonderful holiday dish contains a delicious blend of root vegetables, plentiful at this time of the year."

1. Preheat oven to 375°F (190°C). Spray a 9- × 13-inch (23 × 33 cm) baking dish with nonstick cooking spray.

2. Combine sweet potatoes, squash, carrots, and prunes in a large bowl. Add orange juice, water, zest, sweetener, cinnamon, salt, and pepper. Toss to combine. Transfer to the prepared dish and cover with foil.

3. Bake for 40 minutes. Uncover and bake 20 minutes longer, stirring occasionally. Serve hot.

69 calories per serving, 17 g carbohydrates, 3 g fiber, 5 g sugar, 1 g protein, 0 g fat (0 g saturated fat), 29 mg sodium, 343 mg potassium

NORENE'S NOTES:

- **Time-saver:** You can buy cubed squash and sweet potatoes in many supermarkets. Another way to save on prep time is to use 2 cups (500 mL) bagged baby carrots instead of slicing whole carrots.

DR. ED SAYS:

- **This tasty High Holiday recipe** is on the high side for starch, carbs, and sugar, and only moderate in some of the key brain nutrients. However, what it lacks in this area, it makes up for by being an excellent source of carotenoid antioxidants and a good source of vitamins C and B6, as well as fiber.

DID YOU KNOW? One measure of the concentration of antioxidants in a food is by its color—the deeper the color, the more antioxidant it contains.

CURRIED ROASTED CAULIFLOWER

PAREVE | GLUTEN-FREE | PASSOVER OPTION | DO NOT FREEZE |
MAKES 4–6 SERVINGS

Thanks to Shelley Sefton for introducing this dish to me. Whenever she makes this high-fiber, high-flavor dish for family and friends, they devour it. If making this for a crowd, double or triple the recipe. Shelley says she can eat the whole thing herself—so can I!

1 large cauliflower

1 red bell pepper, cut into long narrow strips

2 Tbsp (30 mL) olive oil

2 tsp (10 mL) curry powder

½ tsp (2 mL) salt (or to taste)

¼ cup (60 mL) minced green onions or chives

1. Preheat oven to 400°F (200°C). Line a large, rimmed baking sheet with parchment paper.

2. Wash cauliflower well and cut into large florets. Place in a large bowl together with red pepper strips. Drizzle with oil and sprinkle with curry powder and salt; toss to combine. Spread in a single layer on the prepared baking sheet. (Can be prepared a few hours in advance and set aside.)

3. Roast, uncovered, for 40–45 minutes, until golden and crispy. Halfway through cooking, stir the vegetables. When done, some of them will be blackened around the edges—that's okay.

4. Remove pan from oven and transfer vegetables to a serving dish; sprinkle with green onions. Serve immediately or at room temperature.

127 calories per serving, 13 g carbohydrates, 6 g fiber, 5 g sugar, 5 g protein, 8 g fat (1 g saturated fat), 356 mg sodium, 720 mg potassium

NORENE'S NOTES:

- **Curry powder** is usually a mixture of turmeric, chili powder, ground coriander, ground cumin, ground ginger, and pepper. It can be bought in mild, medium, or hot strengths.

- **Roasted cauliflower medley:** Add 1–2 cups (250–500 mL) each of sliced mushrooms and unpeeled Japanese eggplant. Sliced zucchini and Spanish onions are also delicious. If you add more vegetables, use 3–4 Tbsp (45–60 mL) olive oil and 1 Tbsp (15 mL) curry powder.

- **Passover option:** Instead of curry powder, use 2 tsp (10 mL) dried rosemary and 2–3 cloves minced garlic.

RECIPE CONTINUED . . .

DR. ED SAYS:

· **Cauliflower, bell pepper, and olive oil** are the main contributing ingredients. They provide an excellent source of vitamin C, vitamin B6, folate, and fiber, and a good source of magnesium, zinc, and choline.

DID YOU KNOW? A major component of curry is turmeric, whose key ingredient is curcumin—an excellent antioxidant and anti-inflammatory. It is one of the supplements we recommend as worth trying for cognitive maintenance.

CHIMICHURRI CAULIFLOWER STEAKS

PAREVE | GLUTEN-FREE | PASSOVER | DO NOT FREEZE | MAKES
6 SERVINGS

Chimichurri is a bold-flavored herb sauce that is as common in Argentina as ketchup is in North America. This scrumptious side also makes a delicious vegetarian main dish when served over tri-colored quinoa or zucchini noodles.

---

1. **CHIMICHURRI SAUCE:** In a food processor fitted with the steel blade, process garlic, green onions, and parsley until minced, about 8–10 seconds. Add olive oil, vinegar, oregano, red pepper flakes, and salt. Process until combined, 5–10 seconds. Transfer sauce to a large glass measure. Cover and refrigerate up to 48 hours. Bring to room temperature before serving.

2. **CAULIFLOWER STEAKS:** Preheat oven to 425°F (220°C). Line a large, rimmed baking sheet with parchment paper. Arrange cauliflower slices in a single layer on the prepared baking sheet and brush both sides with olive oil. Roast, uncovered, about 15 minutes, just until tender, turning slices over half-way through cooking.

3. Remove cauliflower steaks from oven and transfer carefully to a large serving platter. Serve hot, topped with sauce.

286 calories per serving, 13 g carbohydrates, 5 g fiber, 5 g sugar, 5 g protein, 26 g fat (4 g saturated fat), 363 mg sodium, 745 mg potassium

NORENE'S NOTES:

- **Waste not, want not:** Don't throw away the small pieces that crumble after slicing the cauliflower—use them to make Popcorn Cauliflower (p. 459).

- **Pesto cauliflower steaks:** Instead of Chimichurri Sauce, top with Power Pesto (p. 492), using half the recipe.

RECIPE CONTINUED . . .

CHIMICHURRI SAUCE:

3 cloves garlic

4 green onions, trimmed

¾ cup (185 mL) tightly packed fresh flat-leaf parsley (washed and well dried, stems trimmed)

⅓ cup (80 mL) extra virgin olive oil

3 Tbsp (45 mL) white wine vinegar

½ tsp (2 mL) dried oregano

¼–½ tsp (1–2 mL) red pepper flakes (or to taste)

½ tsp (2 mL) salt

CAULIFLOWER STEAKS:

1 large or 2 medium heads cauliflower, trimmed, cored, and cut into ½-inch (1 cm) thick slices (see Norene's Notes)

2 Tbsp (30 mL) olive oil

CHIMICHURRI CAULIFLOWER STEAKS (continued)

DR. ED SAYS:

- **Olive oil and cauliflower** are the main nutritional contributors here, while the spices provide various antioxidants. This recipe is an excellent source of vitamin C, vitamin B6, and folate, and a good source of magnesium.

> DID YOU KNOW? Olive oil, aside from its benefits in lowering harmful LDL cholesterol, also contains unknown factors that make it especially useful in reducing cognitive decline. The best type of olive oil is cold-pressed extra virgin olive oil.

POPCORN CAULIFLOWER

PAREVE | GLUTEN-FREE | PASSOVER | DO NOT FREEZE | MAKES
4–6 SERVINGS

Cauliflower shrinks a lot when roasted, so be sure to make a lot! This makes a fabulous snack or side dish and is delicious at any temperature with just about anything.

1 large cauliflower

2 Tbsp (30 mL) olive oil

3–4 cloves garlic (about 1 Tbsp/ 15 mL minced)

Salt and freshly ground black pepper

1 tsp (5 mL) dried basil

1 tsp (5 mL) dried oregano

1. Preheat oven to 425°F (220°C). Line a large, rimmed baking sheet with parchment paper.

2. Wash cauliflower well and break into very small florets. Place in a large bowl and drizzle with oil. Add garlic, salt, pepper, basil, and oregano; toss to combine. Spread out in a single layer on the prepared baking sheet. Can be prepared a few hours in advance and set aside.

3. Roast, uncovered, in the lower third of the oven for 30–35 minutes, until well browned and tender-crisp. Stir occasionally for even browning. Transfer to a serving bowl. Serve immediately or at room temperature.

117 calories per serving, 11 g carbohydrates, 4 g fiber, 4 g sugar, 4 g protein, 8 g fat (1 g saturated fat), 64 mg sodium, 645 mg potassium

NORENE'S NOTES:

• **Spice it up!** Instead of basil and oregano, use chili flakes, turmeric, and paprika for a spicy kick.

• **What's in store:** White cauliflower is the most popular, but it also comes in various colors, including yellow, green, and purple. Choose cauliflower with compact florets and no brown spots.

• **Size counts:** A medium cauliflower (6–7 inches/15–18 cm in diameter) yields about 8 cups (2 L) florets. Soak florets in cold water for 10 minutes to help remove any hidden insects; drain well.

RECIPE CONTINUED . . .

POPCORN CAULIFLOWER (continued)

DR. ED SAYS:

- **Oregano and basil** provide antioxidants, otherwise this recipe is very similar in nutritional benefits to Chimichurri Cauliflower Steaks (p. 457).

- **Garlic** has been shown to have a strong anti-inflammatory effect that keeps arteries in a healthy state and reduces the risk of cardiovascular diseases.

DID YOU KNOW? Dried oregano has a fiber content of 42 g per 100 g, and is a powerhouse of concentrated nutrients. Unfortunately, we don't get most of that because we use it in such small quantities.

GARLIC MASHED FAUX-TATOES

DAIRY-FREE OPTION | GLUTEN-FREE | PASSOVER | REHEATS WELL
(DO NOT FREEZE) | MAKES 4 SERVINGS

Cauliflower is a sneaky substitute for mashed potatoes. The potato version contains more than triple the carbs and double the calories of this scrumptious, creamy alternative. The dairy-free version goes great with fish!

1 medium head cauliflower, trimmed, cored, and cut into florets

1 Tbsp (15 mL) olive oil

3–4 cloves garlic (about 1 Tbsp/ 15 mL minced)

¼ cup (60 mL) grated Parmesan cheese

3–4 Tbsp (45–60 mL) plain Greek yogurt (skim or 1%)

Salt and freshly ground black pepper

2 green onions, trimmed and finely minced (for garnish)

1. Place a steamer insert into a large saucepan and fill with water to just below the bottom of the steamer. Bring water to a boil. Add cauliflower florets, cover, and steam on low for 12–15 minutes, until very tender.

2. Meanwhile, heat oil in a small nonstick pan over medium heat. Add garlic and sauté until translucent, about 2 minutes. Remove from heat.

3. Transfer cauliflower florets to a food processor fitted with the steel blade. Process for 25–30 seconds, until very smooth, scraping down the sides of the bowl as needed.

4. Add sautéed garlic, Parmesan, yogurt, salt, and pepper. Process for a few seconds longer to combine.

5. Transfer to a serving bowl and garnish with green onions.

92 calories per serving, 9 g carbohydrates, 3 g fiber, 3 g sugar, 5 g protein, 5 g fat (1 g saturated fat), 126 mg sodium, 476 mg potassium

NORENE'S NOTES:

- **No steamer?** Use your microwave. Rinse cauliflower florets, place in a microwave-safe dish, and sprinkle with 2 Tbsp (30 mL) water. Cook, covered, for 7-8 minutes on high. Let stand for 2 minutes longer (cauliflower continues to cook as it stands).

- **Dairy-free option:** Omit Parmesan cheese and Greek yogurt. In Step 4, add ¼-⅓ cup (60-80 mL) almond milk or dairy-free milk. Amount needed will depend on the size of the cauliflower.

- **Smash hit:** Replace half the potatoes with cauliflower when making mashed potatoes. You can use a potato masher or ricer instead of a food processor.

RECIPE CONTINUED . . .

GARLIC MASHED FAUX-TATOES (continued)

DR. ED SAYS:

- **It's a great idea** to substitute potatoes with cauliflower as it replaces such a large amount of starch, which is so easily converted to sugar in the body!

- **Nutritionally,** this is in the same range as the other recipes where cauliflower is the major ingredient.

FAUX FRIED "RICE"

PAREVE | GLUTEN-FREE | PASSOVER OPTION | REHEATS WELL
(DO NOT FREEZE) | MAKES 6–8 SERVINGS

This colorful, versatile dish tastes just like fried rice, but with a fraction of the carbs. Feel free to add your favorite vegetables—bean sprouts, grated broccoli stems or carrots, sliced water chestnuts, bamboo shoots, or bok choy. Always add the longer-cooking vegetables first. Faux-tastic!

1. Grate cauliflower in a food processor fitted with the grater, using medium pressure. Set aside. (The grated cauliflower is the "rice.")

2. Heat oil in a large nonstick wok or skillet on medium-high. Stir-fry garlic, ginger, and green onions for 1 minute. Add celery, mushrooms, and red pepper; stir-fry for 2–3 minutes.

3. Add "rice" and stir-fry 3–4 minutes longer, just until tender-crisp.

4. Add soy sauce and sesame oil and stir-fry 1–2 minutes longer. Stir in peas.

5. Make a well in the center of the mixture. Add beaten eggs and scramble for 1–2 minutes, just until set. Mix eggs into the "rice" and season with pepper. Serve immediately.

100 calories per serving, 10 g carbohydrates, 3 g fiber, 4 g sugar, 6 g protein, 5 g fat (1 g saturated fat), 268 mg sodium, 439 mg potassium

NORENE'S NOTES:

- **Cauliflower rice:** You can buy cauliflower rice in 12- or 16-oz (340 or 454 g) packages, and they come with a 16-day shelf life. What a "grate" time-saver!

- **Be prepared:** Get all your veggies ready in advance and place them on a large platter. Stir-fry them quickly just before mealtime.

- **Meal deal:** To transform this into a main dish, add diced firm tofu, cooked chicken, or turkey for the last 2 minutes of stir-frying.

- **Passover option:** Omit green peas, soy sauce/tamari, and sesame oil. Garnish with ½ cup (125 mL) toasted slivered almonds and ½ cup (125 mL) chopped fresh parsley.

RECIPE CONTINUED . . .

½ large cauliflower, trimmed and cut into large chunks (see Norene's Notes)

1 Tbsp (15 mL) olive or grapeseed oil

4 cloves garlic (about 2 tsp/10 mL minced)

1 tsp (5 mL) minced ginger

6 green onions, sliced

2 stalks celery, diced

2 cups (500 mL) sliced mushrooms

1 red bell pepper, diced

2 Tbsp (30 mL) soy sauce or tamari (preferably low-sodium)

1 tsp (5 mL) toasted sesame oil

½ cup (125 mL) frozen green peas (no need to thaw)

2 large eggs, lightly beaten

Freshly ground black pepper

FAUX FRIED "RICE" (continued)

DR. ED SAYS:

- **Cauliflower:** Now you can enjoy "rice" without guilt, as cauliflower rice has very low available carbohydrates and good levels of dietary fiber. In addition to providing protein and antioxidants, cauliflower also has anti-cancer properties.

- **Bell peppers, as well as the spices,** provide excellent antioxidants in this recipe.

- **Mushrooms** provide antioxidants and an additional bonus of protein. When possible, choose shiitake, oyster, or other wild mushrooms, as they contain compounds that enhance immune functions.

- **Overall,** this delicious vegetable dish is an excellent source of vitamin C and a good source of vitamin B6 and folate.

DID YOU KNOW? Mushrooms contain the highest food concentration of the unique biological antioxidants ergothioneine and glutathione, which the body uses to protect its cells. People who have low levels of these antioxidants are more prone to AD/dementia and other neurodegenerative diseases.

CORNBREAD STUFFING MOUNDS

PAREVE | REHEATS AND/OR FREEZES WELL | MAKES ABOUT 18 MOUNDS

Instead of stuffing a turkey or chicken, shape this vegetable-packed cornbread mixture into mounds. It "a-mounds" to a superb side dish! Use your food processor to speed up preparation.

Fiesta Corn Muffins (p. 139)

2 Tbsp (30 mL) olive oil

2 medium onions, chopped

2 stalks celery, chopped

1 red bell pepper, chopped

3 cups (750 mL) zucchini, chopped (about 1 large zucchini, unpeeled)

2 cloves garlic (about 1 tsp/5 mL minced)

2 large eggs, slightly beaten

½–1 tsp (1–2 mL) salt

¼ tsp (1 mL) black pepper

½ tsp (2 mL) dried thyme

½ cup (125 mL) chopped fresh parsley (or 2 Tbsp/30 mL dried)

1. Bake muffins as directed. Once cooled, cut into ½-inch (1 cm) cubes and place in a large mixing bowl.

2. Heat oil in a large nonstick skillet on medium-high. Sauté onions, celery, red pepper, zucchini, and garlic for 6–8 minutes, until softened. Remove from heat and cool slightly before adding to the cornbread; mix well.

3. Add eggs, salt, pepper, thyme, and parsley; mix well. (Can be made up to a day or two in advance and refrigerated.)

4. Preheat oven to 375°F (190°C). Line a large, rimmed baking sheet with parchment paper.

5. With an ice cream scoop or a ⅓-cup (80 mL) dry measure, scoop the stuffing mixture into mounds on the prepared baking sheet, leaving about 2 inches (5 cm) between each mound.

6. Bake, uncovered, for 25–30 minutes, or until golden and crusty.

33 calories per mound, 3 g carbohydrates, 1 g sugar, 1 g fiber, 1 g protein, 2 g fat (trace saturated), 70 mg sodium, 104 mg potassium

NORENE'S NOTES:

· **Multigrain stuffing mounds:** Instead of corn muffins, substitute 6 cups (1.5 L) multigrain, whole wheat, or rye bread, cut into cubes.

DR. ED SAYS:

· **Zucchini** is a very good source of the important carotenoid antioxidants lutein and zeaxanthin.

· **Corn bread** is an excellent source of folate and a good source of fiber.

RECIPE CONTINUED . . .

CORNBREAD STUFFING MOUNDS (continued)

- **Overall,** this recipe is low-carb, low-sugar, and low-sodium, and is notable primarily for its fiber and vitamin C, as well as the antioxidants contributed by the zucchini and bell pepper.

DID YOU KNOW? High-maize corn starch has a high content of resistant starch, which means that instead of being converted to sugar, the starch acts like a dietary fiber.

CURRIED EGGPLANT & CHICKPEAS

PAREVE | GLUTEN-FREE | REHEATS AND/OR FREEZES WELL |
MAKES 6 CUPS (1.5 L)

My friend the late Maurice Borts called this dish the "Seven-Time Winner," because he served it seven times and on each occasion his guests asked for the recipe. This makes a big batch, but leftovers freeze well. Vegetarians love it!

1. Cut eggplant into ½-inch (1 cm) chunks (see Norene's Notes)—you'll have about 8 cups (2 L). Place in a colander and lightly sprinkle with salt. Let stand for 20–30 minutes. Rinse well and squeeze gently to remove any excess liquid and bitter juices from the eggplant.

2. Steam eggplant in a vegetable steamer until tender, about 10–12 minutes (or microwave, covered, in a large microwaveable bowl for 10 minutes). Don't overcook.

3. Heat oil in a large pot on medium-high. Add onion and sauté until tender-crisp, about 6–8 minutes.

4. Add steamed eggplant and drained chickpeas to the pot and mix well. Add curry powder, cumin, water, lemon juice, honey, and ketchup. Stir to combine and bring to a boil. Reduce heat to low and simmer, uncovered, for 8–10 minutes, stirring occasionally. Season with salt and pepper to taste and serve.

106 calories per ½-cup (125 mL) serving, 19 g carbohydrates, 5 g fiber, 8 g sugar, 4 g protein, 2 g fat (0 g saturated fat), 47 mg sodium, 313 mg potassium

2 medium eggplants

Salt

1 Tbsp (15 mL) olive oil

1 large red onion (about 2 cups/ 500 mL chopped)

1 can (19 oz/540 g) chickpeas, drained and rinsed

3–4 tsp (15–20 mL) curry powder

½ tsp (2 mL) ground cumin

½ cup (125 mL) cold water

6 Tbsp (90 mL) lemon juice (preferably fresh)

2 Tbsp (30 mL) honey (or to taste)

2 Tbsp (30 mL) ketchup

Salt and freshly ground black pepper

NORENE'S NOTES:

• **What's in store:** Eggplants come in all shapes, sizes, colors, and varieties. Choose shiny, smooth, firm eggplants with no soft spots.

• **Size counts:** Large eggplants tend to be bitter and are often full of seeds. Small, slender eggplants have smaller seeds and are usually more tender.

RECIPE CONTINUED . . .

- **To peel or not to peel?** That is the question! Peel eggplants when making an eggplant spread, or if the skin is tough. Otherwise, the choice is yours (I usually don't bother).

- **Sponge-blob eggplant:** Eggplant acts like a sponge, soaking up as much oil as you give it. Salting eggplant before cooking draws out the bitter juices and excess moisture, so it needs less oil and you won't turn into a blob! Smaller varieties usually don't need to be salted before cooking.

DR. ED SAYS:

- **Eggplant** is notable primarily for its contributions of antioxidants and fiber, although it is somewhat high in carbs.

- **Chickpeas** are an excellent source of fiber, high in protein at 7%, and have good levels of magnesium and folate.

- **Overall,** this recipe is a good source of fiber, protein, folate, and magnesium, although it is somewhat high in sugars and carbs. If you are sensitive to sugar and carbs, try reducing the honey and ketchup, or use sugar-free syrup and ketchup.

> DID YOU KNOW? Soluble fiber can combine with cholesterol and thus reduce the risk of cardiovascular disease, which in turn can reduce the risk of AD/dementia.

SESAME GREEN BEANS

PAREVE | GLUTEN-FREE | PASSOVER OPTION | DO NOT FREEZE | MAKES 4 SERVINGS

For a colorful presentation, use a combination of green and yellow beans. Cut the bell peppers into strips about the same size as the beans. Prepare all the ingredients in advance and cook just before serving. This recipe will be ready to eat in minutes.

---

1. In a small bowl, combine the water, soy sauce, and honey; set aside.

2. Heat olive oil in a wok or a large nonstick skillet over medium-high. Add green onions, garlic, and ginger, and stir-fry for 1 minute. Add green beans and bell pepper strips; mix well. Cook for 1 minute longer.

3. Add reserved soy sauce mixture and bring to a boil. Cover, reduce heat to low, and simmer for 4–5 minutes, or until tender-crisp. Season with pepper to taste and toss with sesame oil.

4. Transfer cooked beans to a platter. Sprinkle with sesame seeds and serve immediately.

143 calories per serving, 15 g carbohydrates, 5 g fiber, 7 g sugar, 4 g protein, 9 g fat (1 g saturated fat), 299 mg sodium, 390 mg potassium

NORENE'S NOTES:

- **No strings attached:** Today's green beans are stringless and less work to prepare. Either snap off the tough ends by hand or snip them off with scissors.

- **It's a snap!** To test for freshness when buying beans, snap one in half and taste for sweetness. They should snap, not bend. Thinner beans are sweeter and more tender.

- **Passover-friendly asparagus almondine:** Substitute asparagus for green beans. Instead of 2 Tbsp (30 mL) soy sauce, use 1 Tbsp (15 mL) balsamic vinegar. Instead of sesame seeds, sprinkle with ¼ cup (60 mL) toasted sliced almonds.

RECIPE CONTINUED . . .

¼ cup (60 mL) water or vegetable broth

2 Tbsp (30 mL) low-sodium soy sauce or tamari

1 tsp (5 mL) honey

1 Tbsp (15 mL) olive oil

2 green onions, trimmed and chopped

3–4 cloves garlic (about 1 Tbsp/15 mL minced)

2 tsp (10 mL) minced fresh ginger

1 lb (500 g) green beans, trimmed

1 red or orange bell pepper, cut into long, narrow strips

Freshly ground black pepper

2 tsp (10 mL) toasted sesame oil

2 Tbsp (30 mL) sesame seeds

SESAME GREEN BEANS (continued)

DR. ED SAYS:

- **Green beans** have good quantities of folate, fiber, and vitamin C. They also have some antioxidants, but these are undefined.

- **Sesame seeds,** a powerhouse of dense nutrition, are high in fiber, high in protein, and low in carbs. In addition, they are very high in magnesium, potassium, zinc, folate, and vitamin B6. The fat content is mostly of the type that is good for you, so don't spare the sesame seeds.

- **Overall,** this recipe is a good source of vitamin E, magnesium, zinc, and folate, and is an excellent source of vitamins B12, B6, and C.

> DID YOU KNOW? Sesame seeds, one of the oldest oilseed crops known to man, were first cultivated about 3000 years ago.

ROASTED PORTOBELLO MUSHROOMS

PAREVE | GLUTEN-FREE | PASSOVER | DO NOT FREEZE | MAKES
6–8 SERVINGS

These large, meaty mushrooms are delicious with chicken, fish, or beef. They also make an excellent vegetarian alternative to burgers. Add roasted portobello mushrooms to salads and wraps or use them as part of a mixed vegetable platter.

6–8 large portobello mushrooms

2 Tbsp (30 mL) olive oil

2 tsp (10 mL) balsamic vinegar

2–3 cloves garlic (about 2 tsp/10 mL minced)

½ tsp (2 mL) dried thyme (or 1 tsp/5 mL fresh)

Salt and freshly ground black pepper

2 Tbsp (30 mL) chopped fresh parsley (for garnish)

1. Preheat oven to 400°F (200°C). Line a large baking sheet with parchment paper.

2. Rinse mushrooms quickly and dry well. Trim stems and cut mushrooms into ½-inch (1 cm) slices. Spread out in a single layer on the prepared baking sheet.

3. Drizzle with oil and vinegar and sprinkle with garlic, thyme, salt, and pepper. Using your hands, toss slices to coat all sides with oil and seasonings.

4. Roast, uncovered and stirring occasionally, for 20–25 minutes, or until nicely browned.

5. Transfer to a platter, garnish with parsley, and serve.

62 calories per serving, 4 g carbohydrates, 1 g fiber, 2 g sugar, 2 g protein, 5 g fat (1 g saturated fat), 9 mg sodium, 320 mg potassium

NORENE'S NOTES:

- **Grilled portobello mushrooms:** Preheat grill or BBQ. Leave mushrooms whole and place them in a medium bowl; season as directed. Grill over medium-high heat until tender, about 5 minutes per side.

- **Be a mushroom maven:** There are three types of button mushrooms—white, cremini/coffee-colored, and portobello (grown-up cremini mushrooms). Shiitake mushrooms have a smoky flavor and meaty texture, but are more expensive. Oyster mushrooms are cheaper than shiitakes. Store mushrooms in a loosely closed paper bag in the refrigerator up to 1 week.

RECIPE CONTINUED . . .

- **Raw or cooked?** Many people love to eat raw mushrooms, but it's best to cook them thoroughly as most types are carcinogenic if eaten raw. Heat destroys many toxins, makes mushrooms more digestible, and improves their taste and texture—so cook them, for goodness sake!

- **Wash or not?** Fresh mushrooms are 90% water and, surprisingly, don't absorb much water when rinsed. Rinse quickly before cooking, then wrap in a towel to absorb moisture. Any excess moisture will evaporate during cooking. You can also clean mushrooms by wiping them with a damp paper towel or using a mushroom brush.

DR. ED SAYS:

- **Mushrooms** are a major source of two unique antioxidants, ergothioneine and glutathione, which have been shown to be associated with a lower risk of AD/dementia. So, it's always good to include a mushroom dish every so often. The great thing about these compounds is that they are not destroyed when the mushrooms are cooked.

STIR-FRY SPINACH WITH MANDARINS

PAREVE | GLUTEN-FREE | PASSOVER | DO NOT FREEZE | MAKES
6 SERVINGS

This quick, garlicky stir-fry tastes terrific and is so healthy. Spinach shrinks a lot when cooked—eat spinach more often and hopefully your waistline will also shrink!

1. Wash spinach, dry well, and set aside.

2. Heat a nonstick wok or a large skillet over medium heat. Add nuts and toast for 2–3 minutes, or until golden, stirring often. Remove from the wok and set aside.

3. Add oil to the wok and increase heat to medium-high. Add onion, bell pepper, and garlic; stir-fry for 2 minutes. Add spinach in batches and stir-fry for 2–3 minutes, or until spinach has wilted and all liquid has evaporated.

4. Add lemon juice, salt, and pepper. Stir in orange segments and transfer to a serving dish. Garnish with almonds and serve immediately.

128 calories per serving, 13 g carbohydrates, 4 g fiber, 5 g sugar, 4 g protein, 8 g fat (1 g saturated fat), 64 mg sodium, 159 mg potassium

1 lb (500 g) baby spinach
(about 10 cups/2.5 L raw)

⅓ cup (80 mL) slivered almonds

2 Tbsp (30 mL) grapeseed oil

1 medium onion, sliced

1 red or yellow bell pepper, sliced

3–4 cloves garlic (about
1 Tbsp/15 mL minced)

1 Tbsp (15 mL) lemon juice
(preferably fresh)

Salt and freshly ground
black pepper

1 can (11 oz/312 g) mandarin
orange segments, drained and
well rinsed

NORENE'S NOTES:

- **I be-leaf:** Baby spinach is the ultimate fast food. Its flat, tender, dark green leaves require just a quick rinse, and there's no need to remove the stems. An easy way to dry spinach is in a salad spinner.

- **Cook it right:** There's no need to dry spinach well if boiling, steaming, or microwaving it. However, if sautéing or stir-frying spinach in oil, dry it well to avoid splattering during cooking. The shorter the cooking time, the higher the nutrient content.

- **Weighing in:** A cello bag of spinach usually contains 10 oz (300 g, or about 7 cups/1.65 L raw) and yields about 1–1½ cups (250–375 mL) cooked. One bunch of fresh spinach weighs 12 oz (340 g, or about 10 cups/2.5 L raw) and yields about 1½ cups (375 mL) cooked. A 1-lb (454 g) tub contains about 10 cups (2.5 L) raw spinach. Greens shrink a lot during cooking: 3 cups (750 mL) raw yields about 1 cup (250 mL) cooked.

RECIPE CONTINUED . . .

- **It's in the bag:** Store spinach in the refrigerator for 4–5 days. Place a few paper towels inside the bag to absorb any moisture.

- **Frozen assets:** Frozen spinach defrosts quickly in the microwave. Microwave on high power for 3 minutes. Once cooled, squeeze dry. Spinach will reduce to about one-third of its original volume.

- **Green cuisine:** Swiss chard or bok choy can be substituted for spinach in most recipes; cooking time is about the same.

- **Swiss chard with garlic:** Instead of spinach, use Swiss chard. Cut leaves into 1-inch (2.5 cm) pieces and the tender part of the stems into ½-inch (1 cm) pieces. Sauté 2 cups (500 mL) sliced mushrooms along with the onion, bell pepper, and garlic.

- **How sweet it is:** Choose water-packed canned mandarins. Look for a brand that is sugar-free. Alternatively, use fresh mandarins, peeled and segmented.

DR. ED SAYS:

- **Spinach,** the main component of this recipe, has been the most associated with a reduced risk of AD/dementia among leafy greens. This is probably due to the very high content of antioxidants lutein and zeaxanthin, as well as other carotenoids. It is also rich in vitamin C, magnesium, and manganese, as well as the important B vitamins.

- **Almonds** add a good wallop of much needed natural vitamin E, which has been shown to reduce cognitive decline.

- **Overall,** this recipe is an excellent source of vitamin E, vitamin C, and folate, and a good source of vitamin B6 and magnesium. The sugar content tends to be somewhat high, so choose no-sugar-added mandarins, as described above.

> DID YOU KNOW? The beneficial effect of the B vitamins contained in leafy vegetables is greatly enhanced if combined with a fish meal containing Omega-3 fats.

SPINACH & BROCCOLI KUGEL

DAIRY OPTION | PAREVE | GLUTEN-FREE OPTION | PASSOVER |
REHEATS AND/OR FREEZES WELL | MAKES 12 SERVINGS

This colorful kugel, packed with healthy leafy greens and vegetables, is lower in carbs than most traditional kugels. You can also make miniature kugels instead of a big one. If you don't feel like turning on the oven, use the vegetables as a scrumptious stir-fry (see Norene's Notes).

1 pkg (10 oz/300 g) fresh baby spinach (about 7 cups/1.75 mL)

1–2 Tbsp (15–30 mL) olive oil

2 medium onions, chopped

1 red bell pepper, chopped

2 cloves garlic, minced

1 cup (250 mL) grated carrots (or 2 medium carrots, grated)

1 pkg (10 oz/284 g) broccoli slaw (or 2 cups/500 mL grated broccoli stems)

¾ tsp (4 mL) salt (or to taste)

¼ tsp (1 mL) freshly ground black pepper

½ tsp (2 mL) dried basil

4 eggs (or 2 eggs + 4 egg whites)

1 cup (250 mL) matzo meal (whole wheat or gluten-free)

1. Preheat oven to 350°F (175°C). Spray a 7- × 11-inch (18 × 28 cm) glass baking dish with nonstick cooking spray.

2. Rinse spinach thoroughly but do not dry. Cook in a covered saucepan, with just the water that is already clinging to the leaves, for 3 minutes (or microwave on high for 3 minutes). Do not add any water. The water clinging to the leaves provides enough steam to cook them. Once cooled, squeeze dry.

3. Heat oil in a large nonstick wok or skillet. Sauté onions, red pepper, and garlic over medium-high heat until golden, about 5 minutes. Add carrots and broccoli slaw and stir-fry 2 minutes longer. Stir in cooked spinach and seasonings. Let cool.

4. In a large mixing bowl, lightly beat eggs. Add sautéed vegetables and matzo meal; mix well. Spread mixture evenly in the prepared pan.

5. Bake, uncovered, for 45–50 minutes, until firm. Cut into squares to serve.

84 calories per serving, 12 g carbohydrates, 2 g fiber, 3 g sugar, 4 g protein, 3 g fat (1 g saturated fat), 199 mg sodium, 88 mg potassium

NORENE'S NOTES:

- **Dairy option:** Sprinkle ½ cup (125 mL) grated low-fat cheese (e.g., Parmesan, cheddar, Swiss) on top before baking.

- **Switch your greens:** Use Swiss chard, regular spinach, or baby kale (or a mix) instead of baby spinach. Wash thoroughly and spin dry in a lettuce spinner. Trim, discarding any tough stems.

RECIPE CONTINUED . . .

SPINACH & BROCCOLI KUGEL (continued)

- **Mini kugels:** Spray compartments of a muffin pan with nonstick spray. In Step 4, spoon mixture into the sprayed compartments. Bake at 350°F (175°C) for 35–40 minutes, until nicely browned.

- **Spinach and broccoli stir-fry:** Prepare veggies up to the end of Step 3 but do not cool. Add a drizzle of light soy sauce and sesame oil and serve immediately. Makes 4 servings.

DR. ED SAYS:

- **Spinach** is the one green leafy vegetable that has been specifically shown to reduce the risk of AD/dementia (see Kale Chips, p. 193, for more information.) This recipe is a great combination of two of the most important vegetables for brain health—spinach and broccoli.

- **Broccoli,** a member of the cruciferous family, provides good quantities of vitamin C, lutein, zeaxanthin, B vitamins, and fiber.

- **Onions, garlic, olive oil, and bell peppers** are staples of the Mediterranean diet, which has consistently been shown to reduce the risk of AD/dementia (see Rosemary Chicken & Vegetables, p. 310.)

- **Basil** rounds out the nutritional contribution with antioxidants as well as flavor.

- **Carrots** are also a source of vitamins C and B6, fiber, and potassium. They may have a small beneficial effect on memory because of their carotenoid antioxidant content.

- **Omega-3 eggs,** as opposed to regular eggs, will provide some Omega-3 fat to the diet, but you will get substantially more from fish, algae, or certain plant oils such as flax, chia, and hemp. Omega-3 eggs are a way for lacto-ovo vegetarians and non-fish eaters to get some Omega-3 in their diet.

- **Overall,** this versatile recipe has excellent vitamin C levels and good amounts of folate, antioxidants, and plant Omega-3 fats.

SPINACH STUFFING

PAREVE | GLUTEN-FREE | PASSOVER | REHEATS AND/OR FREEZES
WELL | MAKES ABOUT 2 CUPS (500 ML)

This versatile stuffing is packed with phytonutrients, vitamins, and flavor. It makes a super low-carb stuffing for turkey, chicken, or salmon.

1 Tbsp (15 mL) olive oil

2 medium onions, chopped

1 red bell pepper, chopped

2 cloves garlic (about 2 tsp/10 mL minced)

1 pkg (10 oz/300 g) frozen chopped spinach, thawed and squeezed dry

½ cup (125 mL) chopped fresh parsley

½ cup (125 mL) chopped dried apricots

1 tsp (5 mL) dried basil

Salt and freshly ground black pepper

1. In a large nonstick skillet, heat oil on medium. Add onions, bell pepper, and garlic and sauté about 6–8 minutes, or until tender. If the mixture begins to stick, add a little water.

2. Stir in spinach and cook 2–3 minutes longer, until most of the moisture disappears.

3. Remove pan from heat and stir in parsley, apricots, basil, salt, and pepper. Let cool before using. Stuffing can be prepared up to a day in advance and refrigerated.

63 calories per ¼-cup (60 mL) serving, 11 g carbohydrates, 3 g fiber, 6 g sugar, 2 g protein, 2 g fat (trace saturated fat), 31 mg sodium, 315 mg potassium

NORENE'S NOTES:

- **Get stuffed!** Instead of red bell pepper, substitute 1 cup (250 mL) chopped sun-dried tomatoes. Instead of frozen spinach, substitute 2 cups (500 mL) packed chopped fresh spinach. A medley of your favorite leftover roasted vegetables combined with 1 cup (250 mL) cooked quinoa (or any cooked grain) also makes a scrumptious stuffing.

DR. ED SAYS:

- **Spinach,** once again, is the main component, and presents a similar nutritional profile to the other spinach recipes in this book.

- **Dried apricots** give a boost of carotenoid antioxidants, which they have in high concentration, but they also boost the sugar content per serving since they contain over 50% sugar. Compensating for this, they are very high in fiber and potassium, low in sodium, and high in natural vitamin E. They are also a good source of B vitamins and vitamin C.

DID YOU KNOW? The orange and yellow color of the apricots is due to their carotenoid content.

SPAGHETTI SQUASH NOODLES

PAREVE | GLUTEN-FREE | PASSOVER | REHEATS WELL (DO NOT FREEZE) | MAKES 3–4 SERVINGS

1 large spaghetti squash (about 3–4 lb/1.5–1.8 kg)

Desired toppings (see Norene's Notes)

When spaghetti squash is cooked, the pale golden flesh turns into long thin strands that resemble pasta, with a fraction of the carbs. For short strands, see Norene's Notes. This also makes an excellent meatless main dish.

1. Preheat oven to 400°F (200°C). Line a baking dish with parchment paper.

2. Pierce squash in several places with the point of a sharp knife. Microwave, uncovered, on high for 5 minutes—this makes it easier to cut in half. Cool slightly.

3. Cut squash in half crosswise around its waist (not lengthwise). Using a spoon or melon baller, scrape out and discard seeds and stringy fibers.

4. Place squash halves, cut side down, in a prepared baking dish. Bake, uncovered, for 40–45 minutes, until tender. Cool slightly.

5. Run a fork around the inside perimeter of the squash, releasing long, spaghetti-like strands.

104 calories per serving (squash only), 25 g carbohydrates, 5 g fiber, 10 g sugar, 3 g protein, 1 g fat (trace saturated fat), 69 mg sodium, 451 mg potassium

NORENE'S NOTES:

- **Short strand version:** In Step 3, cut the squash in half lengthwise, not crosswise. Discard seeds and stringy fibers. Continue as directed in Step 4. Use a fork to scrape squash flesh into short strands.

- **Use your (squash) noodle:** Spaghetti squash will fill you up without filling you out! It has just 42 calories per 1 cup (250 mL) and is very low in fat, with less than 0.5 g fat/cup. A 4-lb (1.8 kg) squash yields about 5 cups (1.25 L) when cooked.

- **Top it up:** Serve with a drizzle of extra virgin olive oil and salt and pepper, or top with Oven-Roasted Vegetable Medley (p. 488) or Oven-Roasted Tomato Sauce (p. 490).

- **Spaghetti squash:** The serving size is quite high at almost 1 lb (500 g), but it shrinks substantially during cooking. Since most of it is water (about 92%), the caloric intake is quite low for this serving size (especially compared to traditional pasta). Another advantage of such a large serving size is that it magnifies the nutritional content of an otherwise non-remarkable food, resulting in a good intake of vitamin C, vitamin B6, folate, magnesium, and zinc, as well as providing excellent fiber consumption. The disadvantage of the serving size is that consumption of digestible carbs and sugars is high.

> **DID YOU KNOW?** Squash is considered a fruit because it contains the seeds of the plant. Eggplant, string beans, avocado, and bell peppers are also considered fruits.

ROASTED BUTTERNUT SQUASH

PAREVE | GLUTEN-FREE | PASSOVER | DO NOT FREEZE | MAKES 4–6 SERVINGS

1 medium butternut squash, peeled, seeded, and cubed (about 4 cups/1 L cubed)

2 Tbsp (30 mL) olive oil

2 cloves garlic, minced

1 tsp (5 mL) minced fresh thyme or rosemary leaves

Salt and freshly ground black pepper

Roasting butternut squash enhances its natural sweetness. Short on time? You can buy precut squash cubes at many grocery stores and supermarkets. Don't be tempted to use frozen squash cubes in this recipe as they won't turn glazed and golden.

1. Preheat oven to 400°F (200°C). Line a rimmed baking sheet with parchment paper.

2. Place squash cubes on the prepared baking sheet and drizzle with oil. Sprinkle with garlics, thyme, salt, and pepper; toss to coat well. Spread out in a single layer.

3. Roast, uncovered, for 30–35 minutes, until tender and golden, stirring once or twice.

125 calories per serving, 17 g carbohydrates, 3 g fiber, 3 g sugar, 2 g protein, 7 g fat (1 g saturated fat), 6 mg sodium, 500 mg potassium

NORENE'S NOTES:

- **How a-peeling!** Here's an easy way to peel tough-skinned squash. Wash, then poke holes all over with a fork or the point of a sharp knife. Microwave squash on high power for 3–4 minutes. Once cooled, place squash on its side and slice off both ends. Using a vegetable peeler, remove and discard the skin.

- **How to cube squash, part 1:** Cut squash in two at its neck. Cut the narrow neck into 1-inch (2.5 cm) rounds. Slice rounds into long rectangles and then into cubes.

- **How to cube squash, part 2:** Cut bottom part of the squash in half. Use a spoon to scoop out and discard seeds and pulp. Slice each squash half into strips and cut each strip into cubes.

- **Buying info:** A 3-lb (1.4 kg) butternut squash yields about 4 cups (1 L) raw 1-inch (2.5 cm) cubes.

- **Spice it up!** Omit thyme and pepper. Sprinkle squash cubes lightly with salt, ground cinnamon, and a drizzle of honey or maple syrup (requires certification for Passover).

- **The serving size** for the butternut squash in this recipe is smaller than for the spaghetti squash, and the sugar and carb contents are also less, thus reducing the intake of these components to more-manageable levels. At the same time, butternut squash has very high carotenoid levels, natural vitamin E, and vitamin C, and provides good amounts of fiber, vitamin B6, folate, and magnesium.

- **Thyme and rosemary** round out the contribution of a variety of antioxidants.

- **Overall,** this recipe reflects the nutritional contribution of butternut squash.

SMASHED POTATO "LATKES"

PAREVE | DAIRY OPTION | GLUTEN-FREE | PASSOVER | DO NOT
FREEZE | MAKES 12 LATKES

12 baby red-skinned potatoes
(2 inches/5 cm in diameter)

Lightly salted water

1–2 Tbsp (15–30 mL) olive oil

Salt and freshly ground
black pepper

Additional seasonings (to taste):
dried basil, rosemary, thyme,
garlic powder, onion powder,
paprika

A no-grate alternative to potato latkes, these are a wonderful way to get rid of your frustration—just smash away! This recipe multiplies easily for a crowd.

1. Boil potatoes in enough lightly salted water to cover them for 15–20 minutes, until fork-tender. Drain well. (If desired, potatoes can be prepared in advance up to this point and refrigerated for a day or two.)

2. Preheat oven to 400°F (200°C). Line a large, rimmed baking sheet with parchment paper or sprayed foil.

3. Place potatoes in a single layer, about 3 inches (8 cm) apart, on the prepared baking sheet. Cover them with a piece of parchment paper. Smash each potato once or twice with the flat part of your palm, making a flat disc. Round off any ragged edges by pushing them together with your fingers.

4. Brush tops lightly with olive oil and sprinkle with seasonings.

5. Bake, uncovered, for 20–25 minutes, until golden and crispy. If desired, turn potatoes over halfway through baking.

54 calories per latke, 10 g carbohydrates, 1 g fiber, trace sugar, 1 g protein, 1 g fat (trace saturated fat), 3 mg sodium, 204 mg potassium

NORENE'S NOTES:

- **Easy hack:** In Step 1, instead of boiling potatoes, roast on a rimmed baking sheet for about 1 hour at 350°F (175°C), until fork tender. Continue as directed in Steps 2–5.

- **Whack away!** In Step 3, use the flat side of a meat tenderizer instead of the palm of your hand to smash the potatoes. (Alternatively, flatten with a potato masher.)

- **Dairy option:** During the last 5 minutes of baking, sprinkle each potato with 2 Tbsp (30 mL) grated low-fat Swiss, cheddar, or mozzarella cheese, finely chopped red bell pepper, and minced parsley. Almost like pizza!

- **Potatoes** contain high levels of fiber and vitamin C, reasonably good levels of brain-benefitting minerals, and B vitamins. Baby potatoes require minimal preparation, but their main disadvantage, as with all potatoes, is the high starch content (1 baby potato contains 9 g of starch), which converts easily into sugar.

- **Overall,** this dish is recommended as an occasional treat—save it for a special occasion.

DID YOU KNOW? Green potatoes and potato sprouts contain toxins that are poisonous, taste bitter, and can cause an upset stomach. Although you can peel and discard the green part, it's best not to use them at all.

WINTER VEGETABLE LATKES

PAREVE | GLUTEN-FREE | PASSOVER OPTION | REHEATS AND/OR
FREEZES WELL | MAKES 24 LATKES

1 medium sweet potato

1 large carrot or 6–8 baby carrots

1 large parsnip

1 large Idaho potato

¼ Vidalia or sweet onion,
cut into chunks

2–3 green onions, trimmed

2 Tbsp (30 mL) fresh dill

3 large eggs

½ cup (125 mL) whole wheat
flour or matzo meal

¾ tsp (4 mL) salt (or to taste)

¼ tsp (1 mL) freshly ground
black pepper

2 Tbsp (30 mL) grapeseed or
canola oil (add more as needed)

Everyone loves latkes! This luscious recipe from Beverley Corber of Vancouver, BC, doubles easily if you're cooking for a crowd. Grapeseed oil has a high smoke point, so you can cook latkes at a higher temperature without burning them.

1. Peel sweet potato, carrot, parsnip, and Idaho potato and cut them into large pieces.

2. In a food processor fitted with the grater, grate the cut-up vegetables using medium pressure. Transfer to a large bowl and set aside.

3. Remove grater and insert the steel blade. Process Vidalia onion, green onions, and dill until finely minced, about 8–10 seconds. Add eggs and process 5 seconds longer. Transfer mixture to the grated vegetables along with flour, salt, and pepper. Mix well.

4. Spray a large nonstick skillet with nonstick cooking spray. Add 2 Tbsp (30 mL) oil and heat over medium high. Using a large spoon, drop mixture into the hot oil and flatten slightly. Brown well on both sides, about 2–3 minutes per side.

5. Remove browned latkes from the skillet and drain well on paper towels. Add additional oil to the skillet as needed, stirring the batter before cooking each new batch.

54 calories per latke, 8 g carbohydrates, 1 g fiber, 1 g sugar, 2 g protein, 2 g fat (trace saturated fat), 88 mg sodium, 149 mg potassium

NORENE'S NOTES:

- **Eggs-actly!** Instead of 3 eggs, substitute 2 eggs and 2 egg whites.

- **Grate tip:** Beverley rinses the grated potatoes and then squeezes out the excess moisture, but I don't bother.

- **Gluten-free/passover option:** Use matzo meal (whole wheat or gluten-free) instead of flour.

- **Warm it up:** To keep cooked latkes warm, arrange in a single layer on a large baking sheet and place in a 250°F (120°C) oven. Do not cover.

- **Frozen assets:** To save space when freezing or reheating latkes, stand them upright in loaf pans. Reheat, uncovered, in a preheated 400°F (200°C) oven for about 10 minutes, or until crispy. There's no need to defrost them first.

DR. ED SAYS:

- **A single serving** of these vegetable latkes has relatively moderate levels of brain-healthy nutrients and reasonable starch levels—but who can eat just one? When you consume three, the nutrient contribution becomes significant, but the starch level, which is converted to sugar, increases dramatically, so that a serving of three latkes contains 21 g of starch.

- **Eggs, onions, and carrots** mitigate this problem somewhat by contributing protein, choline, vitamin B12, and antioxidants, but the same recommendation holds here as for Smashed Potato "Latkes" (p. 482) —consider them an occasional treat.

SWEET POTATO "FRIES"

PAREVE | GLUTEN-FREE | PASSOVER | REHEATS AND/OR FREEZES
WELL | MAKES 4 SERVINGS

3 medium sweet potatoes, well
scrubbed (do not peel)

2 Tbsp (30 mL) olive oil

Salt and freshly ground
black pepper

1 tsp (5 mL) sweet paprika

1 tsp (5 mL) garlic powder

Sweet potato fries are a delicious and healthier alternative to traditional French fries made from regular potatoes. Yam good!

1. Preheat oven to 425°F (220°C). Line a large, rimmed baking sheet with foil. Place the baking sheet in the lower third of the oven to heat up.

2. Meanwhile, cut sweet potatoes into ¼-inch (0.5 cm) strips or wedges and place in a large bowl. Add oil, salt, pepper, paprika, and garlic powder. Using your hands, toss together to coat sweet potatoes on all sides.

3. When the oven is fully heated, spread out sweet potatoes in a single layer on the hot baking sheet.

4. Bake in the lower third of the oven for 20 minutes. Turn sweet potato pieces over with a spatula and continue baking until brown and crispy, about 20–25 minutes longer. Serve immediately.

162 calories per serving, 24 g carbohydrates, 4 g fiber, 5 g sugar, 2 g protein, 7 g fat (1 g saturated fat), 63 mg sodium, 404 mg potassium

NORENE'S NOTES:

- **Lighter fare:** Instead of olive oil, use 1 egg white to coat the fries.

- **Spice it up!** Season with salt and pepper and omit the paprika and garlic powder. Sprinkle with ground cinnamon and nutmeg, or sprinkle with seasoning salt, chili flakes, Cajun spices, basil, curry powder, rosemary, or any spices you like. (Not all spices are certified for Passover.)

- **Frozen assets:** Cooked sweet potatoes freeze well, unlike white potatoes. There's no need to thaw them when reheating—just spread the frozen "fries" on a foil-lined baking sheet and bake, uncovered, at 400°F (200°C), for 10–12 minutes.

- **What's the difference?** Sweet potatoes are not yams, although they are often marketed that way. Sweet potatoes usually have orange flesh, but can also have yellow, white, or even purple flesh. The darker the flesh, the moister and sweeter they are. Sweet potatoes with dark orange flesh have more vitamin A than those with lighter-colored flesh. The skin can be different colors, including red-orange, brown, and purple. Yams are bigger, usually have white flesh, have a thick, dark-brown skin, and tend to be bland, floury, and starchy—they are never sweet.

DR. ED SAYS:

- **Sweet potatoes** are still potatoes and contain high carb and sugar levels, even higher than regular potatoes. However, they have more nutrition than regular potatoes, especially in carotenoid antioxidants as well as vitamin A and fiber. Interestingly enough, reports have been published concluding that sweet potatoes can stabilize sugar levels in diabetics. So, there may be something in the sweet potato that counteracts its high carb and sugar levels.

OVEN-ROASTED VEGETABLE MEDLEY

PAREVE | GLUTEN-FREE | PASSOVER | REHEATS WELL (DO NOT FREEZE) | MAKES 6 SERVINGS

2 medium onions, halved and sliced

2 red bell peppers, cut into strips

2 cups (500 mL) sliced mushrooms

1 lb (500 g) asparagus (tough ends trimmed), cut diagonally into 2-inch (5 cm) pieces

1 large zucchini or yellow squash, cut into strips (no need to peel)

3–4 cloves garlic (about 1 Tbsp/ 15 mL minced)

3 Tbsp (45 mL) olive oil

3 Tbsp (45 mL) lemon juice (preferably fresh) or rice vinegar

2 tsp (10 mL) sea salt or kosher salt

Freshly ground black pepper

2 Tbsp (30 mL) minced fresh dill + extra for garnish

1 Tbsp (15 mL) minced fresh thyme (or 1 tsp/5 mL dried)

½ cup (125 mL) sesame seeds

This versatile vegetable medley, or any of its variations, makes for a colorful side dish. Leftovers make a scrumptious snack straight from the refrigerator, or can be chopped and added to cooked whole grains. To transform this medley into a meatless main dish, see "Spaghetti" with Oven-Roasted Vegetables (p. 367).

1. Place prepared vegetables in a large bowl. Add minced garlic, oil, lemon juice, salt, pepper, dill, and thyme; mix well. (If desired, vegetables can be prepared in advance up to this point, covered, and refrigerated for several hours or overnight.)

2. Preheat oven to 425°F (220°C). Line a large, rimmed baking sheet with parchment paper.

3. Spread vegetables in a single layer on the prepared baking sheet and sprinkle with sesame seeds. Roast, uncovered, for 18–20 minutes, or until golden brown and tender-crisp, stirring once or twice.

4. Transfer to a serving platter and garnish with additional dill. Serve hot or at room temperature. (To reheat, bake uncovered at 375°F/190°C for 10–12 minutes.)

191 calories per serving, 16 g carbohydrates, 5 g fiber, 7 g sugar, 6 g protein, 13 g fat (2 g saturated fat), 206 mg sodium, 626 mg potassium

NORENE'S NOTES:

- **Variation:** Substitute trimmed green beans for asparagus (but not during Passover). For a spicy kick, add 1 tsp (5 mL) red pepper flakes or paprika to the seasoning mixture in Step 1. Turmeric makes a great addition.

- **Mixed vegetable medley:** Use your favorite vegetable combo (e.g., onions, colored bell peppers, cauliflower florets, thinly sliced beets or carrots, diced butternut squash). Drizzle with 3 Tbsp (45 mL) each olive oil and balsamic vinegar. Sprinkle with salt, pepper, and dried basil; toss to combine. Spread out in a single layer on the prepared baking sheet. Roast, uncovered, at 425°F (220°C), for about 20 minutes, until tender-crisp, stirring once or twice. (If using beets, carrots, or squash, increase roasting time by 10–15 minutes.)

DR. ED SAYS:

- **Bell peppers, asparagus, zucchini, and squash** provide a varied mixture of flavonoid and carotenoid antioxidants, including lutein and zeaxanthin.

- **Mushrooms** provide the unique and powerful biological antioxidants ergothioneine and glutathione.

- **Onions** contain quercetin, which helps in the absorption of certain antioxidants. All of this will maximize the beneficial impact on the brain. The contribution of other important nutrients per serving is also worth noting, and the only drawback is that the sugar is somewhat on the high side.

- **Sesame seeds,** which are nutrient-dense, also contribute significantly to the nutritional benefits of this recipe. One serving has excellent levels of vitamin E, vitamin C, folate, zinc, magnesium, and fiber, and even has a respectable level of plant-based Omega-3 fats.

- **Overall,** this powerhouse recipe is one of my favorites because it combines several vegetables to get a wide spectrum of antioxidants, which is important for optimum brain function.

OVEN-ROASTED TOMATO SAUCE

PAREVE | GLUTEN-FREE | PASSOVER | REHEATS AND/OR FREEZES
WELL | MAKES 3 CUPS (750 ML)

12–14 ripe plum (Roma) tomatoes
(about 4 lb/2 kg)

2 medium onions, chopped

6–8 cloves garlic (about
2 Tbsp/30 mL minced)

½ tsp (2 mL) kosher salt

Freshly ground black pepper

2 Tbsp (30 mL) olive oil

¼ cup (60 mL) coarsely chopped
fresh basil

This garden-fresh sauce is superb in the summertime when tomatoes are sweet, plentiful, and inexpensive. Although you can roast any kind of tomatoes any time of the year, plum tomatoes work best because of their thicker skins. Best of all, you can control the sodium content. This scrumptious sauce is perfect on pasta, spiralized vegetables, chicken, or fish. Sauce it up!

1. Preheat oven to 375°F (190°C). Spray a 9- × 13-inch (23 × 33 cm) baking dish with nonstick cooking spray.

2. Core tomatoes; if they are large, cut into halves or quarters. Place tomatoes in the baking dish together with onions and garlic. Sprinkle with salt and pepper and drizzle with oil. Mix well.

3. Roast, uncovered, for about 1½ hours or until tender, stirring occasionally. When done, tomatoes will collapse and reduce in volume by half—their skins will be slightly brown and cracked.

4. Remove baking dish from oven and coarsely mash the tomato mixture together with the pan juices—the resulting texture should be chunky. Stir in basil.

5. Either serve hot or transfer the cooled mixture to a container. Seal tightly and refrigerate or freeze until needed.

114 calories per ½-cup (125 mL) serving, 16 g carbohydrates, 4 g fiber, 10 g sugar, 3 g protein, 5 g fat (1 g saturated fat), 177 mg sodium, 788 mg potassium

NORENE'S NOTES:

- **Roast and boast!** Roast other vegetables along with the tomatoes (e.g., zucchini, mushrooms, bell peppers, and/or eggplant). Italian seasoning and/or red pepper flakes make for tasty additions. Always delicious, always different!

- **We like lycopene:** Tomatoes are rich in lycopene, a powerful antioxidant. Cooked tomatoes contain more lycopene than raw ones. Fat is necessary for proper absorption of lycopene, so adding a little olive oil makes tomatoes tastier and healthier.

DR. ED SAYS:

- **Tomatoes** are the name of the game. As Norene has pointed out, they contain high levels of the powerful carotenoid antioxidant lycopene, which has been shown to help prevent a multiplicity of diseases including cancer. Also, cooked tomatoes release more lycopene than raw ones. This is because cooking and macerating breaks down the tomato cell walls so the lycopene can be released.

- **Overall,** this recipe provides excellent levels of fiber, vitamin E, vitamin C, vitamin B6, folate, and magnesium.

> **DID YOU KNOW?** Eighty percent of the lycopene ingested in America comes from tomatoes; guava and watermelon also have high concentrations of lycopene.

POWER PESTO

DAIRY OPTION | PAREVE | MEAT OPTION | GLUTEN-FREE |
PASSOVER | FREEZES WELL | MAKES ABOUT 2 CUPS (500 ML)

4 large cloves garlic, peeled

½ cup (125 mL) unsalted almonds

1 cup (250 mL) fresh basil leaves,
stems discarded

1 cup (250 mL) baby spinach
leaves

½ cup (125 mL) flat-leaf parsley

1 cup (250 mL) extra virgin
olive oil

½ tsp (2 mL) salt

⅛ tsp (0.5 mL) freshly ground
black pepper

Pesto is ready "presto" with the help of your food processor! Leafy greens such as baby spinach and parsley are not only used for salads, they can also be used in this terrific pesto as another way to incorporate brain-boosting ingredients into your meals. Use it on its own with whole grain pasta or spiralized vegetables as a meatless meal, or add a little pesto to salad dressings, marinades, or pasta sauces. So versatile!

1. In a food processor fitted with the steel blade, drop garlic through the feed tube while the machine is running. Process until minced. Add almonds, basil, spinach, and parsley. Process until fine, about 15–20 seconds.

2. Slowly drizzle in oil through the feed tube while the machine is running and process until well blended. Texture should be fairly creamy. If too thick, add a little water. Add salt and pepper.

3. Store in a tightly closed glass jar in the refrigerator.

72 calories per 1 Tbsp (15 mL), 1 g carbohydrates, trace sugar, <1 g fiber, 1 g protein, 8 g fat (1 g saturated), 38 mg sodium, 29 mg potassium

NORENE'S NOTES:

- **Store it right:** Pesto keeps for 2–3 weeks in the refrigerator if covered with a thin layer of olive oil. It also freezes well.

- **Go nuts!** Instead of almonds, substitute walnuts or pine nuts.

- **Nut-free option:** Use pumpkin or sunflower seeds as a nut-free alternative.

- **Dairy option:** Blend in ½ cup (125 mL) grated Parmesan at the end of Step 2, or add a spoonful or two of Parmesan cheese to whole grain pasta dishes along with the pesto.

- **Low-carb dinner:** Add a spoonful or two of pesto to lightly steamed zucchini noodles or Spaghetti Squash Noodles (p. 478). Stir in a little grated Parmesan cheese and light table cream (5% cream).

- **Meat option:** Pesto is perfect on grilled chicken and scrumptious on salmon. For a vegetarian twist, see Pesto Cauliflower Steaks (p. 457).

- **Spinach** is the most documented ingredient in this recipe for brain health, but parsley and basil follow closely. This pesto is a power-house for the brain with its three nutrient-rich leafy greens.

- **Parsley** is high in fiber, vitamin C, and folate, and is a good source of magnesium while being low in sugars and digestible carbs. Although it is high in carotenoid antioxidants, including lutein and zeaxanthin (which are good for the brain), its main claim to fame is probably the large quantity of the bioflavonoid apigenin, which has been shown to be a powerful anti-inflammatory, antioxidant, and anti-cancer agent.

- **Basil** is high in vitamin C, folate, and magnesium. It is also very high in carotenoid antioxidants, including lutein and zeaxanthin. However, because the leaves are so light (1 cup/250 mL only weighs 6 g), we probably don't get the full impact of all its brain nutrients.

- **Olive oil and almonds** round out the brain-nutrition profile. Olive oil is a key staple of the Mediterranean diet, and almonds provide wide-spectrum vitamin E.

- **Overall,** this healthful recipe stands out for its excellent mix of antioxidants.

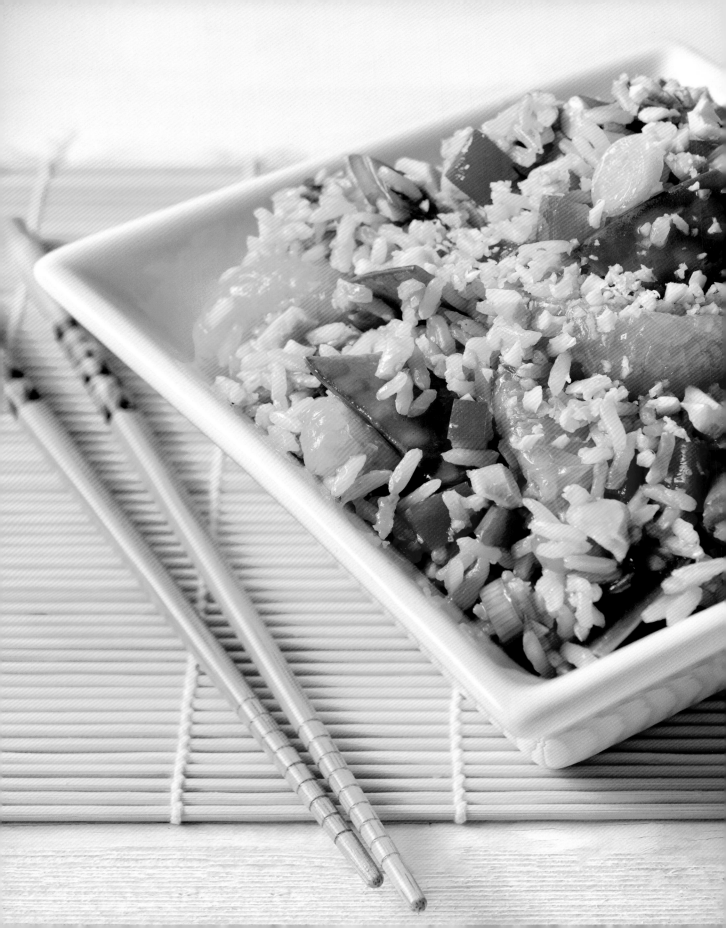

BRAINY GRAINS

THE GRAIN TRAIN: Our dietician, Sharona Abramovitch, recommends that you hop on board and include more whole grains in your diet. Experiment with barley, bulgur, whole wheat couscous, farro, freekeh, kasha/buckwheat groats, quinoa, black/brown rice, and wheat berries. Some of the best whole grains, as mentioned in the first part of this book, are flax, oats, and quinoa. To sneak more whole grains into your diet, add them to soups, salads, side dishes, and casseroles.

GLUTEN ALERT! Some people are gluten intolerant and/or suffer from celiac disease. Grains that contain gluten are wheat, rye, oats, barley, and spelt. Gluten-free grains include corn, quinoa, kasha, and rice.

THE WHOLE TRUTH: Whole grains tend to be darker, chewier, and more flavorful because all three layers of the kernel are included, which makes them nutritionally superior to refined grains. Whole grains provide protein, antioxidants, fatty acids, fiber, and many phytochemicals.

A SALUTE TO THE KERNEL: Most of the fiber in kernels is found in the bran, which is the outer layer of the kernel. The germ is in the center, where many of the vitamins, minerals, and fatty acids are found. The endosperm is in the core and contains most of the starch and the least amount of vitamins and minerals. When grains are refined, the germ and the bran are discarded, resulting in starchy and fluffy white foods with little fiber or nutritional value.

WHAT'S IN STORE: Look for the words "whole" or "100% whole" before the name of the grain when buying grains, pastas, cereals, breads, and crackers. Another option is to look at the ingredient list and look for whole grain or whole wheat flour as the first ingredient.

HEALTH GAINS FROM GRAINS: Whole grains offer protection against diabetes, heart disease, cancer, and many digestive problems because of their fiber content—food with more fiber takes longer to digest, which is a good thing. On the other hand, refined grains are quickly digested, resulting in higher levels of blood sugar, insulin, and triglycerides, and higher levels of LDL. A note of caution: Although whole grains do have a place in a brain-healthy diet, they are also a group of foods that has one of the highest carb levels, and therefore should be used in moderation, as described in the first part of this book.

FIBER FACT: Soluble fiber helps lower your body's glycemic response to a food. Grains that are digested slowly and have a lower GI value include barley, bulgur, buckwheat groats (kasha), farro, freekeh, oats, rice (wild and black), and wheat berries.

NO-BRAIN GRAINS: Grains are very simple to cook and very versatile. If you can boil water, you'll have no problem cooking grains. Bulgur doesn't require cooking—soaking is sufficient.

COOK IT RIGHT: Place grains in a strainer, rinse, and drain well. Transfer to a saucepan and add water as directed, along with a pinch of salt. You can also cook grains in vegetable or chicken broth. A clove of garlic in the cooking liquid won't hurt either (but not for breakfast)! Bring to a boil; reduce heat to low and simmer, covered tightly, until all the water is absorbed. No peeking allowed! If any water remains, just drain it off.

READY OR NOT? If grains aren't cooked to your liking, add a little more water, cover, and cook for a few minutes longer. Fluff with a fork before serving. However, the longer a grain is cooked, and the higher the temperature, the higher its GI will be.

BE PREPARED: Since grains are so easy to prepare, why not cook extra? Grains can be cooked in advance, cooled, and stored in a covered container in the refrigerator up to 4–5 days. Cook once, eat twice!

FROZEN ASSETS: Most grains freeze well but sometimes there's a change in texture. Pack cooked grains in small airtight containers or resealable bags for quick convenience. Either thaw overnight in the refrigerator or transfer to a microwaveable container. Microwave for 2 minutes per 1 cup (250 mL) on high power to defrost and heat. To heat defrosted grains, microwave on high for 1 minute per 1 cup (250 mL).

PUMP UP THE VOLUME: Add raw or cooked veggies such as onions, bell peppers, celery, carrots, tomatoes, or zucchini to whole grains. Vegetables will increase the volume and help lower the GI.

PROTEIN POWER: To turn grains into a main dish, add some protein such as chicken, turkey, fish, tofu, cheese, or cooked/canned beans or chickpeas.

BOOST THE FLAVOR: Add a drizzle of extra virgin olive oil and some lemon, orange, or lime juice—fresh is best. Balsamic, red wine, or rice vinegar can be used instead of citrus juices. Vinegars and citrus foods can also help lower the GI. For an additional flavor boost, add some minced garlic, dill, basil, thyme, parsley, rosemary, or other herbs. Toasted (Asian) sesame oil and soy/tamari sauce work well in Asian-inspired dishes. Use your imagination.

HIDDEN TREASURES: Cooked grains are ideal as a stuffing for poultry or meat and can be used to stuff vegetables like cabbage rolls, peppers, squash, or zucchini.

BREAKFAST BONANZA: Cooked whole grains make an excellent breakfast. Choose from barley, bulgur, whole wheat couscous, farro, freekeh, kasha/buckwheat, rolled oats, or quinoa. Combine with yogurt, berries, seeds, and/or nuts for a nutritional boost.

"POP" CULTURE: Amaranth, barley, wild rice, wheat berries, and millet will pop like popcorn, or at least puff.

RICE AROUND THE WORLD: Rice is a staple food for over half the world's population. Soup, salad, or a stir-fry based around whole-grain rice, plus lean proteins such as chicken, turkey, lean meat, fish, or tofu, and lots of colorful vegetables will provide a healthy balance of carbs, fat, and protein, plus some fiber, vitamins, and minerals.

BEST BETS: Make the switch from white rice to brown, which has a wonderful, nutty flavor. Brown rice is nutritious and contains several B vitamins, minerals, dietary fiber, and protein. White rice has had its husk, bran, and germ removed, so it's less nutritious than brown rice. Black rice is an excellent choice.

TO RINSE OR NOT TO RINSE: Rice is a leading dietary source of inorganic arsenic, both because of how commonly it's eaten and because the plant and grain tend to absorb arsenic more readily than other food crops as it grows. Always rinse rice thoroughly under cold running water before cooking. As an added bonus, the cooked rice will be far less likely to clump together.

BROWN RICE IN HALF THE TIME: For each 1 cup (250 mL) brown rice, add 2 cups (500 mL) water and a pinch of salt. Place in a saucepan and soak at room temperature for several hours or overnight. When ready to cook, rinse rice, refill the pot with fresh water, and bring to a boil over high heat. Reduce heat and simmer, tightly covered, for 22 minutes. Turn off the heat and let stand, covered, for 10 minutes. Fluff with a fork before serving.

PASTA-BILITIES: Like people, pasta comes in different shapes, sizes, and colors. Below are some helpful guidelines on "healthy weighs" to enjoy pasta.

WHAT'S IN STORE: Whole-grain pasta, made from durum whole wheat semolina, is higher in fiber and chewier than traditional pasta.

PORTION DISTORTION: Did you know that a serving of cooked pasta is only ½ cup (125 mL) and contains about 100 calories? Most people can easily eat 2–3 cups (500–750 mL) of pasta at a meal, which is the equivalent of 4–6 slices of bread.

CUT THE CARBS: Replace half the pasta with steamed spiralized vegetables like zucchini, beet, squash, or carrot noodles. Now that's using your noodle!

COOK IT RIGHT: Cook pasta until al dente (firm to the bite)—don't overcook it or you will boost the GI value. Start testing for doneness about 2 minutes before the cooking time indicated on the package directions.

EXPAND WITHOUT EXPANDING: By adding vegetables to pasta, you'll consume fewer calories and will still be able to enjoy a full plate. Add asparagus, broccoli, carrots, cauliflower, eggplant, spinach, or zucchini. Sauté vegetables in olive oil and add garlic, onions, and herbs for flavor. Toss in some lean protein such as chicken, fish, tofu cubes, or grated reduced-fat cheese. Avoid creamy, calorie-packed sauces.

FIBER UP: Add 1 cup (250 mL) puréed kidney beans or lentils to any pasta sauce to thicken it and increase the fiber content. They'll never know!

SAUCY SECRETS: Bottled and canned sauces are convenient when you're rushed for time. Always check nutrition labels for fat, calories, sodium, and serving size—you may be surprised! It's always better to make your own.

BARLEY MUSHROOM RISOTTO WITH SUN-DRIED TOMATOES

DAIRY-FREE OPTION | REHEATS AND/OR FREEZES WELL | MAKES
4 CUPS (1 L)

1 Tbsp (15 mL) olive oil

1 medium onion, chopped

1½–2 cups (375–500 mL) chopped
portobello mushrooms

2 cloves garlic (about 2 tsp/10 mL
minced)

1 cup (250 mL) hulled, pot,
or pearl barley (see
Norene's Notes)

3 cups (750 mL) hot vegetable
broth (preferably low-sodium or
no-salt-added)

4–5 sun-dried tomatoes

2–3 Tbsp (30–45 mL) grated
Parmesan cheese

2 Tbsp (30 mL) minced fresh basil
(or 1 tsp/5 mL dried)

½ tsp (2 mL) dried thyme

Salt and freshly ground
black pepper

Portobello mushrooms and sun-dried tomatoes add a rich elegance to this humble grain. Although it's not as creamy as traditional risotto, there will barely be any barley left once people taste it!

1. Heat oil in a large saucepan over medium-high heat. Add onion, mushrooms, and garlic; sauté for 5 minutes, or until tender. Stir in barley and cook for 3–4 minutes, or until lightly toasted.

2. Reduce heat to medium-low and slowly stir in ½ cup (125 mL) hot broth. Cook and stir for about 2 minutes, or until broth evaporates. Add another ½ cup (125 mL) broth and continue stirring until almost no liquid remains. Repeat once more, adding another ½ cup (125 mL) broth. Continue stirring until most of the liquid has evaporated.

3. Pour in the remaining broth. Reduce heat and simmer, covered and stirring occasionally, for about 45–55 minutes, until barley is tender.

4. While barley is cooking, soak sun-dried tomatoes in enough boiling water to cover for 10 minutes. Drain, then cut into bite-sized pieces with scissors.

5. Add sun-dried tomatoes, cheese, basil, thyme, salt, and pepper to barley; mix well. Remove from heat, cover, and let stand for 5 minutes longer.

118 calories per ½-cup (125 mL) serving, 21 g carbohydrates, 5 g fiber, 2 g sugar, 4 g protein, 3 g fat (<1 g saturated fat), 78 mg sodium, 224 mg potassium

NORENE'S NOTES:

• **Hulled barley,** which is also referred to as whole grain hull-less barley, is interchangeable with pearl and pot barley in most recipes, so use what you have on hand, adjusting the cooking time accordingly. Refer to Barley Basics in Barley Vegetable Salad (p. 406) for more information.

- **Variations:** Substitute ½ cup (125 mL) dry white wine for part of the broth. Instead of mushrooms, use 1 bunch asparagus with the ends trimmed. Cut diagonally into 1-inch (2.5 cm) slices and lightly steam for 3–4 minutes. Add to barley at the beginning of Step 5. Frozen peas also make a great "green" option.

- **Dairy-free option:** Instead of Parmesan cheese, either use nutritional yeast or omit the cheese.

DR. ED SAYS:

- **Barley** is high in carbs but also one of the lowest glycemic-index grains at about 28 (which helps control blood sugar), primarily because of its soluble fiber content. This, in combination with its relatively high amounts of magnesium, potassium, zinc, and vitamin B6, makes it one of the high-tier preferred grains.

- **Portobello mushrooms,** which have been previously discussed, are a good source of protein, as well as the usual nutrients found in vegetables. In addition, mushrooms are the only fruit or vegetable source of vitamin D.

- **Antioxidants** in this recipe are provided by the barley, tomatoes, and spices, especially basil with its high concentrations of lutein and zeaxanthin.

- **Sun-dried tomatoes** have had their nutrients concentrated sixfold due to dehydration. This means they are an excellent source of magnesium, potassium, zinc, vitamin C, B vitamins, and choline. They are especially high in the proven antioxidant lycopene, at 46 mg per 100 g. Their main drawback is their sugar content, at 38% by weight.

> DID YOU KNOW? When you see "multigrain" on a grain-containing food, this does not mean that the grains are whole grains. Always look for 100% whole grains.

BRING ON THE BULGUR

PAREVE | MEAT OPTION | GLUTEN-FREE OPTION | PASSOVER
OPTION | DO NOT FREEZE | MAKES 6 CUPS (1.5 L)

1 cup (250 mL) medium bulgur

1 cup (250 mL) boiling water
or vegetable broth (preferably
low-sodium or no-salt-added)

½ cup (125 mL) slivered almonds

¼ cup (60 mL) raw
sunflower seeds

4 green onions, thinly sliced

1 red bell pepper, seeded
and chopped

1 yellow bell pepper, chopped

2 stalks celery, chopped

¾ cup (185 mL) dried cranberries

¾ cup (185 mL) slivered
dried apricots

DRESSING:

¼ cup (60 mL) extra virgin
olive oil

1–2 Tbsp (15–30 mL) honey
(to taste)

2 Tbsp (30 mL) lemon or orange
juice (preferably fresh)

1 tsp (5 mL) salt (or to taste)

Freshly ground black pepper

½ tsp (2 mL) ground cumin

½ tsp (2 mL) ground cinnamon

So versatile! This fiber-packed, grain-based salad is excellent for a buffet and does double duty as a side dish. Leftovers are a perfect lunch-box addition. Experiment with other grains (see Norene's Notes).

1. Place bulgur in a large bowl and add boiling water. Cover and let stand for 20–30 minutes, until water is absorbed. Fluff with a fork and set aside. (You should have about 2 cups/500 mL.)

2. Meanwhile, combine almonds and sunflower seeds in an ovenproof dish. Toast in a 350°F (175°C) oven for 5–10 minutes, watching carefully to prevent burning. Add to the bulgur, along with green onions, bell peppers, celery, cranberries, and apricots.

3. **DRESSING:** In a glass measure, combine oil, honey, juice, and seasonings. Add to the bulgur and mix well. Cover and refrigerate up to 24 hours. Serve chilled or at room temperature.

188 calories per ½-cup (125 mL) serving, 28 g carbohydrates, 4 g fiber, 14 g sugar, 4 g protein, 9 g fat (1 g saturated fat), 205 mg sodium, 269 mg potassium

NORENE'S NOTES:

- **Go with the grain(s):** Instead of bulgur, soak 1 cup (250 mL) whole wheat couscous in 1½ cups (375 mL) boiling water for 10 minutes. Alternatively, cook 1 cup (250 mL) brown basmati rice in 2 cups (500 mL) boiling water for 40–45 minutes. Experiment with other cooked whole grains (e.g., farro, freekeh, black rice, quinoa, or wheat berries), following cooking instructions on the package.

- **How sweet it isn't!** Omit the dried cranberries and apricots. Alternatively, check online sources for unsweetened dried fruits.

- **Protein power:** Add sliced cooked chicken or turkey, flaked salmon or tuna, or extra-firm tofu cubes.

- **Gluten-free/passover option:** Instead of bulgur, use 1 cup (250 mL) quinoa. Rinse well, then cook in 2 cups (500 mL) boiling water for 15 minutes. Let stand, covered, for 15 minutes, then fluff with a fork and let cool. Replace sunflower seeds with pecans, pistachios, or walnuts. Omit the cumin.

DR. ED SAYS:

- **Moderation is key:** This recipe is somewhat high in carbs (to be expected with grains) and sugar, so enjoy it in moderation. The relatively high fiber content mitigates the blood glucose spiking caused by the carbs to a reasonable extent. The high sugar is primarily contributed by apricots and cranberries, so if you use unsweetened dried fruits, or reduce the amount, it will help.

- **Almonds and sunflower seeds,** which are nutrient-dense powerhouses, are the main source of natural vitamin E in this recipe.

- **Overall,** although high in sugar, this recipe is a good source of natural vitamin E and vitamin C, and provides good amounts of antioxidants from different sources.

> **DID YOU KNOW?** Fruits are the major source of total sugars (both added and natural) in a North American diet.

BULGUR WITH ALMONDS & RAISINS

PAREVE | REHEATS AND/OR FREEZES WELL | MAKES 4 CUPS (1 L)

1½ cups (375 mL) medium bulgur

1½ cups (375 mL) boiling water or vegetable broth (preferably low-sodium or no-salt-added)

½ cup (125 mL) slivered almonds

2 Tbsp (30 mL) extra virgin olive oil

3 Tbsp (45 mL) lemon or orange juice (preferably fresh)

¼ cup (60 mL) chopped fresh basil (or 1 tsp/5 mL dried)

½ cup (125 mL) raisins

Salt and freshly ground black pepper

Bulgur is actually precooked cracked wheat, so it doesn't require cooking, just soaking. While the bulgur soaks in water, take a soak in your bathtub and you'll both be ready at the same time!

1. Place bulgur in a heat-resistant bowl and add boiling water (or broth). Cover the bowl with a large plate and let stand about 20–30 minutes, until liquid is absorbed and bulgur is tender. Fluff with a fork and set aside (you should have about 3 cups/750 mL).

2. Meanwhile, toast almonds in a skillet over medium heat, stirring frequently, about 5 minutes, until golden and fragrant. Let cool.

3. Stir oil, juice, basil, and raisins into the bulgur. Season with salt and pepper and top with toasted almonds. Serve hot or at room temperature. (If freezing, top with almonds at serving time.)

255 calories per ¾-cup (175 mL) serving, 40 g carbohydrates, 6 g fiber, 9 g sugar, 7 g protein, 10 g fat (1 g saturated fat), 10 mg sodium, 325 mg potassium

NORENE'S NOTES:

- **Variations:** Instead of raisins, add dried cranberries or diced dried apricots (preferably unsweetened). For a lower-sugar version, use pomegranate seeds. Instead of almonds, substitute toasted walnuts, pecans, or pine nuts.

- **Grain power:** Instead of bulgur, substitute 3 cups (750 mL) cooked farro, freekeh, quinoa, or kasha, following cooking instructions on the package.

- **Love me tender:** Bulgur has a tender, chewy texture, and makes a nice alternative to rice. Although this dish is best made with medium bulgur, you can use fine bulgur as well. If you use coarse bulgur, you will have to cook it first.

- **Bulgur** is one of the moderate GI grains, which means it will help control blood sugar spiking due to the breakdown of carbs and sugar. Although high in carbs, it is also high in fiber, B vitamins, and important minerals, as well as being a source of antioxidants.

- **Basil** provides the important brain antioxidants lutein and zeaxanthin.

- **Almonds, extra virgin olive oil, raisins, and lemon juice** round out the contribution of antioxidants in this recipe, each contributing different types of the important nutrients.

- **Overall,** we have a good and varied supply of plant antioxidants, with a similar profile to the previous recipe. As well, this recipe is a very good or excellent source of vitamin E, magnesium, and vitamin B6. It's still on the high side with sugar, but less than the previous recipe.

DID YOU KNOW? Although bulgur is also a wheat, it has a much lower glycemic index than wheat flour because it is still a partially intact grain, and the carbs in the grain are more difficult to break down into glucose.

COUSCOUS, MEDITERRANEAN-STYLE

PAREVE | REHEATS AND/OR FREEZES WELL | MAKES 8 SERVINGS

2 Tbsp (30 mL) olive oil

2 medium onions, chopped

1 red bell pepper, chopped

1 yellow bell pepper, chopped

2 cloves garlic (about 2 tsp/10 mL minced)

1½ cups (375 mL) whole wheat pearl couscous

1 tsp (5 mL) ground cumin

2¼ cups (560 mL) hot vegetable broth (preferably low-sodium or no-salt-added)

½ cup (125 mL) finely chopped dried apricots or dates

Salt and freshly ground black pepper to taste

½ cup (125 mL) chopped fresh parsley or mint

½ cup (125 mL) toasted slivered almonds or pine nuts

Experience the fabulous flavors of the Mediterranean with this colorful, versatile dish. Whole wheat pearl couscous is higher in fiber than other varieties of couscous. Or, as an alternative to couscous, get on the "grain train" (see Norene's Notes).

1. Heat oil in a large, deep skillet over medium heat. Add onions, bell peppers, and garlic; sauté for 6–7 minutes, or until golden.

2. Stir in couscous and cumin. Slowly add hot broth and bring to a boil. Reduce heat and simmer, covered, for 12–15 minutes, until couscous is tender.

3. Stir in apricots and season with salt and pepper. Transfer to a large serving bowl, or 8 individual bowls; sprinkle with parsley and almonds. Serve hot.

231 calories per serving, 37 g carbohydrates, 5 g fiber, 7 g sugar, 6 g protein, 8 g fat (1 g saturated fat), 45 mg sodium, 289 mg potassium

NORENE'S NOTES:

- **The ancient grain train:** Instead of couscous, use hulled barley, buckwheat groats, bulgur, farro, freekeh, or quinoa, following cooking instructions on the package.

- **Israeli couscous with sun-dried tomatoes:** Omit cumin, dried fruit, and nuts. In Step 3, stir in 1 tsp (5 mL) Italian seasoning and ½ cup (125 mL) chopped sun-dried tomatoes, rinsed and drained. If desired, add ½ cup (125 mL) sliced pitted black olives.

- **Israeli couscous with mushrooms and chickpeas:** Sauté 2 cups (500 mL) sliced mushrooms with onions, bell peppers, and garlic. Instead of cumin, add 1 tsp (5 mL) dried basil or thyme. If you replace the dried fruit and nuts with 1½ cups (375 mL) canned chickpeas (rinsed and drained), you'll reduce the sugars.

RECIPE CONTINUED . . .

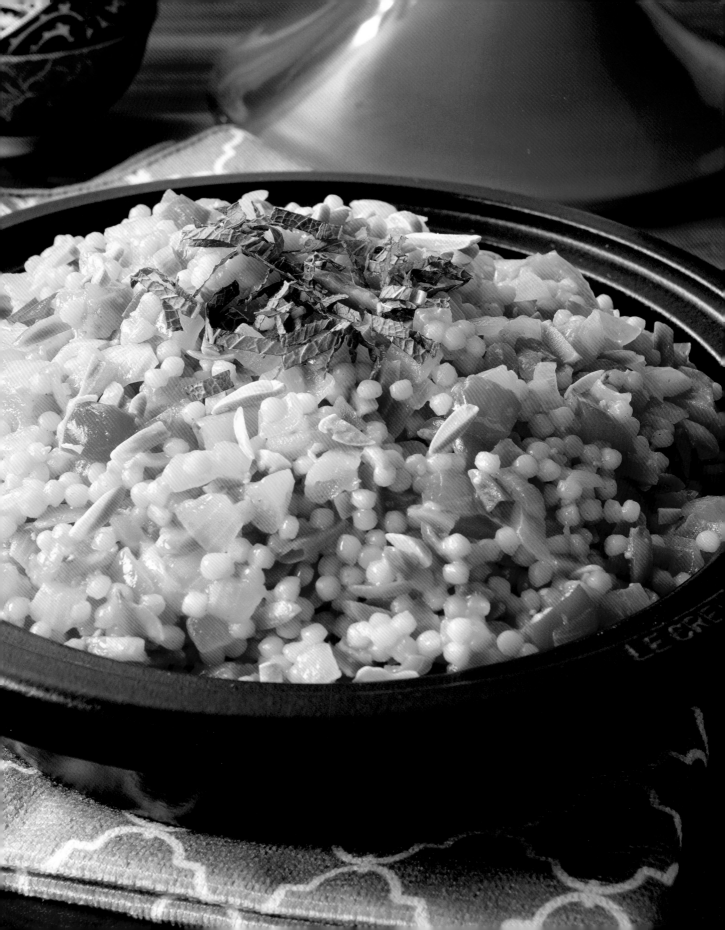

COUSCOUS, MEDITERRANEAN-STYLE (continued)

DR. ED SAYS:

- **Moderation is key:** This is another recipe to enjoy in moderation because of its high carb and sugar content (dried fruits are always a major source of sugar).

- **Couscous** is not a star in the nutrient content field except for its excellent level of the antioxidant selenium (1 cup/250 mL contains about 60% of the recommended daily intake). The non-remarkable nutritional quality of couscous is because, unlike bulgur, it is made from semolina wheat flour and will therefore have a much higher GI than bulgur, which is a cracked whole grain. Therefore, couscous will not control blood sugar as well as bulgur or barley.

- **Apricots, dates, almonds, parsley, and mint** do offer a range of beneficial brain nutrients and antioxidants. Dried apricots, in particular, are high in fiber and rich in carotenoid antioxidants.

- **Overall,** this recipe is an excellent source of vitamins E and C, and a good source of magnesium and vitamin B6. Also, it provides ample and varied plant antioxidants.

> DID YOU KNOW? Couscous is not really a natural whole grain. It is more like a pasta because it is formed into spheres from flour.

COUSCOUS, MOROCCAN-STYLE

PAREVE | REHEATS AND/OR FREEZES WELL | MAKES 4 SERVINGS

This delicious one-pot dish, with its blend of exotic Moroccan flavors, is an updated version of Shayla Goldstein's recipe. It's great for busy families, especially since it doubles or triples easily.

1½ cups (375 mL) vegetable broth (preferably low-sodium or no-salt-added)

⅛ tsp (0.5 mL) ground cumin

⅛ tsp (0.5 mL) ground coriander

⅛ tsp (0.5 mL) ground ginger

1 cup (250 mL) whole wheat couscous

2 green onions, finely chopped

⅓ cup (80 mL) dried cranberries or chopped dried apricots

¼ cup (60 mL) shelled pistachios or pine nuts (for garnish)

1. In a small saucepan over high heat, bring broth, cumin, coriander and ginger to a boil. Stir in couscous.

2. Remove pan from heat and stir in green onions and cranberries. Let stand, covered, for 5–10 minutes. Fluff with a fork, transfer to 4 individual bowls, garnish with pistachios, and serve.

238 calories per serving, 45 g carbohydrates, 5 g fiber, 9 g sugar, 7 g protein, 4 g fat (trace saturated fat), 54 mg sodium, 105 mg potassium

NORENE'S NOTES:

- **The ancient grain train:** Instead of couscous, stir in barley, buckwheat groats, bulgur, farro, or quinoa at the end of Step 1. Follow cooking times directed on the package. Continue as directed in Step 2.

DR. ED SAYS:

- **This recipe** is similar to Couscous Mediterranean-Style, with its choice of couscous and dried fruits, nuts, and spices—similar comments apply.

DID YOU KNOW? Foods made from whole wheat flour have a higher GI than foods made with whole wheat kernels or groats. That's because their starches are more easily broken down into sugars. However, you can control this to some extent since higher temperatures and a longer cooking time tend to increase the GI of the grain starch. So, boiling instead of baking, and baking for shorter times, will reduce the GI.

FREEKEH PILAF

PAREVE | REHEATS AND/OR FREEZES WELL | MAKES 5 SERVINGS

1½ Tbsp (22 mL) olive or grapeseed oil

1 medium onion, chopped

2 stalks celery, chopped,

1 orange bell pepper, chopped

1 cup (250 mL) coarsely chopped mushrooms

2 cloves garlic, minced

1 cup (250 mL) cracked roasted freekeh

1 cup (250 mL) vegetable broth (preferably low-sodium or no-salt-added)

½ cup (125 mL) dried cranberries, rinsed and drained (optional)

¼ cup (60 mL) minced fresh parsley

¼ cup (60 mL) minced fresh dill

¼ tsp (1 mL) ground cinnamon

Salt and freshly ground black pepper

¼ cup (60 mL) toasted almonds, coarsely chopped

Freekeh, a fiber-packed grain that comes from wheat, is harvested when the wheat is green. It's then roasted and rubbed, resulting in a coarsely textured grain with a smoky, somewhat earthy flavor that goes well with sweet spices such as cinnamon. Freekeh is usually sold cracked and is delicious in pilafs and salads.

1. Heat oil in a large skillet or saucepan on medium. Sauté onion, celery, and bell pepper for 3–4 minutes, until softened. Add mushrooms and garlic and sauté for 3–4 minutes longer.

2. While vegetables are sautéing, soak freekeh in cold water for 5 minutes. Drain in a sieve and rinse well under cold running water.

3. Add freekeh to the skillet and stir well. Add broth and cranberries

4. Reduce heat and simmer, covered, for 15 minutes. Remove pan from heat and let stand, covered, for 5 minutes.

5. Add parsley, dill, cinnamon, salt, and pepper; mix well. Transfer to a serving bowl or divide into 5 portions, sprinkle with almonds, and serve hot.

200 calories per serving, 30 g carbohydrates, 6 g fiber, 3 g sugar, 7 g protein, 8 g fat (1 g saturated fat), 46 mg sodium, 422 mg potassium

NORENE'S NOTES:

- **Grain power:** Combine freekeh with other cooked grains in salads and pilafs. Use barley, bulgur, whole wheat couscous, farro, buckwheat groats, millet, quinoa, rice, or wheat berries. Follow cooking instructions on the package.

- **Nuts and seeds:** Instead of almonds, garnish with toasted chopped pecans, walnuts, pine nuts, or pistachios. Instead of nuts, use toasted sunflower or pumpkin seeds.

DR. ED SAYS:

- **Freekeh** is a young, green, whole wheat grain that has been roasted. It is very high in fiber and protein and compares favorably with quinoa. It has a moderate GI of 43, which is relatively good for grains and therefore makes it useful in controlling blood sugar spikes. This recipe is also much lower in sugar than the couscous recipes, while being high in brain-friendly nutrients and a variety of good antioxidants.

- **Mushrooms** also contribute their own unique antioxidants, while helping reduce the carbohydrate load.

- **Overall,** this recipe is an excellent source of vitamin E, vitamin C, vitamin B6, folate, magnesium, and zinc—all important for brain health. As a bonus, it is also high in natural antioxidants and has high levels of fiber and protein.

KASHA & BOW TIES

PAREVE | GLUTEN-FREE OPTION | REHEATS AND/OR FREEZES WELL |
MAKES 6 SERVINGS

2 Tbsp (30 mL) olive oil

2 medium onions, halved
and sliced

2 cups (500 mL) sliced
mushrooms

1 cup (250 mL) mini bow tie pasta
(whole grain or gluten-free)

1 cup (250 mL) coarse or medium
kasha (buckwheat groats)

1 egg white

2 cups (500 mL) hot vegetable
broth (preferably low-sodium or
no-salt-added)

¼ cup (60 mL) chopped fresh dill

Salt and freshly ground
black pepper

Comfort food that's actually good for you! Kasha, also known as buck-wheat groats, is excellent hot as a breakfast cereal or super as a side dish. Use kasha instead of rice or other grains in casseroles, salads, and pilafs. Kasha has a toasty, nutty flavor, and triples in volume when cooked. Try it instead of rice or noodles in chicken soup.

1. Heat oil in a large nonstick skillet or pot over medium heat. Add onions and mushrooms; sauté for 8–10 minutes, until golden. Transfer to a bowl.

2. Meanwhile, cook pasta according to the package directions.

3. In the same skillet, combine kasha with egg white. Cook over medium heat, stirring constantly, until dry and toasted.

4. Reduce heat and gradually add hot broth—be careful, it splatters! Simmer, covered, for 15–18 minutes, until most of the liquid has been absorbed and holes appear on the surface. (Medium kasha takes a few minutes less than coarse grain.)

5. Combine kasha with bow ties and the onion/mushroom mixture. Stir in dill and season with salt and pepper. Serve hot.

185 calories per serving, 31 g carbohydrates, 4 g fiber, 3 g sugar, 6 g protein, 6 g fat (1 g saturated fat), 62 mg sodium, 272 mg potassium

NORENE'S NOTES:

- **Use your noodle:** As a general guideline, 2 oz (60 g) uncooked mini bow ties, shells, spirals, ziti, and so on are roughly equal to ½ cup (125 mL) dry or 1 cup (250 mL) cooked. Larger, bulkier shapes may yield more, while smaller shapes may yield less.

- **No yolk-ing!** Toasting kasha with an egg white before adding the liquid keeps the grains separate and prevents them from becoming sticky.

- **Double without trouble:** If you want to double the recipe, use the whole egg instead of just the egg white.

- **Kasha (buckwheat groats)** falls into the category of whole or partially whole grains as opposed to flours, so it tends to have a lower glycemic index than wheat and therefore is useful in controlling blood sugar from the carbs.

- **Wheat,** in the form of pasta in this recipe, also tends to have a lower GI than wheat flour, especially if the pasta is cooked al dente.

- **Mushrooms,** as in previous recipes, offer one of the only plant sources of vitamin D, as well as unique antioxidants and protein.

- **Dill** is a good source of the brain-helpful antioxidant kaempferol, and is a source of B vitamins and magnesium.

- **Overall,** this recipe is a good source of vitamin B6, folate, magnesium, and zinc, and has reasonable plant antioxidants.

> DID YOU KNOW? Although the word "wheat" is part of the word buckwheat, it is actually wheat-free, and therefore gluten-free!

KASHA & SQUASH CASSEROLE

PAREVE | GLUTEN-FREE OPTION | REHEATS AND/OR FREEZES WELL |
MAKES 12 SERVINGS

Don't be deterred by the length of this recipe—it's a winner! Although it takes a little time to prepare, it's well worth it. This makes a wonderful side dish, especially for a crowd, but vegetarians can enjoy it as a main dish.

ONION MIXTURE:

1 Tbsp (15 mL) olive oil

3 medium onions, chopped

KASHA MIXTURE:

1 cup (250 mL) medium or coarse kasha (buckwheat groats)

1 large egg, separated + extra 1 large egg

2 cups (500 mL) hot vegetable broth (preferably low-sodium or no-salt-added)

½ tsp (2 mL) salt (or to taste)

¼ tsp (1 mL) freshly ground black pepper

SQUASH MIXTURE:

2 pkg (14 oz/398 mL) butternut squash cubes (about 4 cups/1 L)

2 large eggs

2 Tbsp (30 mL) olive oil

¼ cup (60 mL) crushed whole grain crackers (preferably low-sodium)

1 Tbsp (15 mL) brown sugar or granulated Splenda

½ tsp (2 mL) salt

¼ tsp (1 mL) freshly ground black pepper

1. **ONION MIXTURE:** Heat oil in a large nonstick skillet over medium heat. Add onions and sauté for 8–10 minutes, until golden. If the mixture begins to stick, just add a little water. Remove onions from the skillet; reserve half for the kasha mixture and half for the squash mixture.

2. **KASHA MIXTURE:** In the same skillet, combine kasha with egg white; reserve yolk. Cook kasha over medium heat, stirring constantly until dry and toasted, about 5 minutes. Reduce heat and gradually add hot broth—be careful, it splatters! Simmer, covered, for 12–15 minutes, until most of the liquid is absorbed and holes appear on the surface. (Coarse kasha takes a few minutes longer than medium grain.) Remove from heat and let stand, covered, for 5 minutes. Fluff with a fork and cool slightly.

3. Combine kasha with half the onions. Add salt, pepper, reserved yolk, and additional egg; mix well. Spread evenly in a sprayed 9- × 13-inch (23 × 33 cm) glass baking dish, pressing down lightly to form a base.

4. **SQUASH MIXTURE:** In a medium saucepan, combine squash with enough boiling water to cover. Bring to a boil, reduce heat, and simmer, covered, for 20 minutes, until tender. Drain well and return to the saucepan. Cool slightly, then mash. Add the remaining onions, eggs, oil, crackers, brown sugar, salt, and pepper; mix well. Spread evenly over the kasha layer.

5. **TOPPING:** Combine nuts, sugar, and cinnamon in a medium bowl; mix well. Sprinkle evenly over the squash layer. (Can be assembled up to this point, covered, and refrigerated overnight.)

6. Bake, uncovered, in a preheated 350°F (175°C) oven for 45 minutes, or until golden. Cool slightly before cutting into squares.

191 calories per serving, 25 g carbohydrates, 4 g fiber, 5 g sugar, 6 g protein, 9 g fat (2 g saturated fat), 250 mg sodium, 372 mg potassium

NORENE'S NOTES:

- **Gluten-free option:** Use gluten-free crackers or quinoa flakes.

DR. ED SAYS:

- **Kasha,** as mentioned in previous recipes, is a preferred grain because of its moderate GI, which helps to control blood glucose. It is also very high in fiber and protein and is an excellent source of vitamin B6, zinc, and potassium, while also providing a good source of folate.

- **Butternut squash** is a great source of fiber and carotenoid antioxidants.

- **Eggs** are excellent sources of choline and high-quality protein, as well as good sources of zinc, B6, folate, and vitamins D and E. They are also very low in carbs and sugar.

- **Overall,** this recipe provides a good source of vitamin E, vitamin C, vitamin B6, folate, magnesium, zinc, and carotenoid plant antioxidants.

> **DID YOU KNOW?** Choline is a precursor to the neurotransmitter acetylcholine and is important in a brain-healthy diet.

> **DID YOU KNOW?** Kasha, also known as buckwheat groats, is actually not a wheat and is gluten-free, which makes it ideal for people with celiac disease.

TOPPING:

½ cup (125 mL) crushed walnuts or pecans

1 Tbsp (15 mL) brown sugar or granulated Splenda

½ tsp (2 mL) ground cinnamon

POLENTA WITH REFRIED BLACK BEANS

PAREVE | GLUTEN-FREE | POLENTA REHEATS AND/OR FREEZES
WELL (DO NOT FREEZE REFRIED BLACK BEANS) | MAKES 6 SERVINGS

POLENTA:

4 cups (1 L) lightly salted water

1 cup (250 mL) cornmeal (preferably stone-ground whole grain)

1 Tbsp (15 mL) olive oil

REFRIED BLACK BEANS:

2 tsp (10 mL) olive oil

1 medium onion, chopped

1 can (19 oz/540 g) black beans,
drained (do not rinse)

2 cloves garlic (about 1 tsp/5 mL
minced)

¼ tsp (1 mL) ground cumin
(or to taste)

½ tsp (2 mL) chili powder
(or to taste)

Salt and freshly ground
black pepper

1 medium tomato, chopped

¼ cup (60 mL) minced fresh
cilantro or flat-leaf parsley

4–6 drops hot sauce (optional)

There are "plenta" of wonderful ways to eat polenta. Enjoy for breakfast as a gluten-free cereal, top with refried black beans as a fiber-packed side dish, or use as a pizza base (see Norene's Notes). The recipe for refried black beans comes from my friend Kathy Guttman. It makes a zesty side dish with grilled chicken or salmon and is great in burritos.

---

1. **POLENTA:** Bring water to a boil in a large, heavy-bottomed saucepan. Gradually add cornmeal, whisking constantly. Reduce heat and simmer for 20 minutes, stirring every few minutes with a wooden spoon or silicone spatula. Polenta will become thick and pull away from the sides of the pan.

2. Remove from heat and stir in oil. Cover and keep warm. If polenta becomes too firm, just whisk in a little water. You'll have about 4 cups (1 L).

3. **REFRIED BLACK BEANS:** Heat oil in a large nonstick skillet over medium heat. Add onion and sauté for 3–4 minutes, or until softened. Stir in black beans, garlic, cumin, chili powder, salt, and pepper. Continue sautéing for 3–4 minutes to blend flavors. Stir in tomato, cilantro, and hot sauce, if using.

4. Remove pan from heat. Using a potato masher or immersion blender, mash until the mixture is somewhat creamy, but with some beans still whole or partially mashed. You'll have about 2 cups (500 mL) in total.

5. **ASSEMBLY:** Use an ice cream scoop to scoop out polenta onto 6 serving plates; top each serving with ⅓ cup (80 mL) of the bean mixture.

204 calories per serving, 34 g carbohydrates, 9 g fiber, 2 g sugar, 8 g protein, 5 g fat (1 g saturated fat), 197 mg sodium, 428 mg potassium

NORENE'S NOTES:

• **Mamaliga:** Cook polenta as directed in Step 1. Stir in ½ cup (125 mL) milk (skim or 1%) and 1 Tbsp (15 mL) olive oil. Use an ice cream scoop to scoop out polenta onto 6 serving plates. Top each serving with ½ cup (125 mL) low-fat (1%) cottage cheese and ¼ cup (60 mL) plain (skim or 1%) yogurt. So dairy good!

- **Polenta pizza:** Evenly spread hot polenta in a sprayed 10-inch (25 cm) pie plate and top with ¾ cup (185 mL) tomato sauce (preferably low-sodium or no-salt-added). Add any of the following: sliced tomatoes, mushrooms, bell peppers, roasted peppers, sun-dried tomatoes, onions, marinated artichoke hearts, basil, or other herbs. Drizzle lightly with olive oil and sprinkle with salt and pepper. Top with ¾– 1 cup (185–250 mL) grated low-fat mozzarella, Monterey Jack, or Swiss cheese. Bake, uncovered at 375°F (190°C), for 15 minutes, until cheese is melted and golden. Cut into 6 wedges and serve.

- **The new black!** Black beans are easier to digest than most beans. They're packed with antioxidants and fiber, are high in protein, and have a fairly low GI. Look for low-sodium or no-salt-added brands.

DR. ED SAYS:

- **Black beans** are one of the main ingredients in this recipe. They are rich in fiber and protein and contain significant amounts of antioxidants, while also being a good source of B vitamins and minerals for the brain. They are low in sugar and have a low GI, making them suitable for controlling blood sugar.

- **Cornmeal** is very high in starch, which can cause a high GI (about 68) and spikes in blood sugar. The way to reduce the impact of this starch is to choose a coarse-grind cornmeal and a high-amylose maize (corn starch).

- **Overall,** this recipe is a good source of vitamin E, vitamin C, vitamin B6, folate, magnesium, and zinc, and provides some plant antioxidants. It's also extremely high in fiber.

> **DID YOU KNOW?** There are two types of starches—amylose and amylopectin. The former has a low GI because it is hard to digest, while the latter has a high GI because it is easier to digest. Beans and corn tend to have higher amylose than other grains, but you should always look for high-amylose maize cornmeal as some corn varieties can be low in amylose.

CRIMSON QUINOA WITH ROASTED BEETS

DAIRY OPTION | PAREVE | MEAT OPTION | GLUTEN-FREE |
PASSOVER | DO NOT FREEZE | MAKES 6 SERVINGS

ROASTED BEETS:

1 bunch small red or rainbow beets (about 4), scrubbed and trimmed (see Norene's Notes)

QUINOA:

2 cups (500 mL) water or vegetable broth (preferably low-sodium or no-salt-added)

1 cup (250 mL) quinoa

½ cup (125 mL) diced red onion (or 4 green onions, sliced)

3 Tbsp (45 mL) extra virgin olive oil

3 Tbsp (45 mL) balsamic vinegar

2 Tbsp (30 mL) minced fresh basil or dill

Salt and freshly ground black pepper

Keen on quinoa? Although there are several steps, this comes together quickly, resulting in a show-stopping dish that can't be "beet!"

1. **ROASTED BEETS:** Preheat oven to 350°F (175°C). Spray a large piece of heavy-duty aluminum foil with nonstick cooking spray. Center beets on the foil and wrap tightly, pinching the edges together. Bake for 1 hour, or until tender. Carefully open up the foil packet and let beets stand until cool enough to handle.

2. Use paper towels to rub off beet skins and discard. Slice beets into rounds, then dice them. Place in a large bowl.

3. **QUINOA:** Meanwhile, place water in a medium saucepan and bring to a boil over high heat. Place quinoa in a fine-mesh strainer and rinse under cold running water for 1–2 minutes; drain well. (Rinsing removes the bitter coating.) Add quinoa to the boiling liquid. Reduce heat to low and simmer, covered, for 15 minutes. Remove from heat and let stand, covered, for 5 minutes. Fluff with a fork and let cool.

4. **ASSEMBLY:** Combine beets with quinoa, onion, oil, vinegar, basil, salt, and pepper; mix gently. Serve chilled or at room temperature.

200 calories per serving, 26 g carbohydrates, 4 g fiber, 6 g sugar, 5 g protein, 9 g fat (1 g saturated fat), 50 mg sodium, 368 mg potassium

NORENE'S NOTES:

- **Can't "beet" this!** To save time, use 1 package (about 1 lb/454 g) vacuum-packed whole, peeled, cooked beets—no roasting required!

- **Dairy option:** At serving time, top with 1 cup (250 mL) crumbled goat or feta cheese and/or a handful of coarsely chopped toasted nuts of your choice. For a fruity option, add 1 cup (250 mL) mandarin or grapefruit segments.

- **Meat option:** Add leftover cooked diced chicken or turkey for an easy meal.

- **Beets,** one of the two primary ingredients in this recipe, are mainly known for their high content of betaine, which helps control heart disease. Two other major sources of this beneficial chemical are wheat bran and spinach.

- **Quinoa** is one of the top three whole grains I most recommend (see Part 1 of this book). Quinoa is very high in protein and fiber, and its protein, unlike most plant proteins, is very nutritious. It also has a moderate GI at about 53 and, like beets, is a good source of betaine. The key reason it is recommended is because it contains a chemical called hydroxyecdysone, which increases lifespan and reduces inflammatory markers, glycation products, and blood sugar that can accelerate cognitive decline.

- **Overall,** this recipe is an excellent source of folate and magnesium, and is a good source of vitamin B6 and zinc. However, its key features are the unique contribution of betaine and hydroxyecdysone.

> **DID YOU KNOW?** Betaine, a natural chemical, controls a harmful chemical called homocysteine, which is implicated in heart disease. It also helps in proper functioning of the liver. Vitamins B6 and B12 and folate also lower homocysteine levels—some researchers believe this attribute is what makes these compounds beneficial to the brain.

RAINBOW QUINOA, TWO WAYS

PAREVE | GLUTEN-FREE | PASSOVER | DO NOT FREEZE SALAD
(PILAF FREEZES WELL) | MAKES 6 CUPS (1.5 L)

3 cups (750 mL) vegetable broth
(preferably low-sodium or
no-salt-added)

1½ cups (375 mL) quinoa

2 cloves garlic

½ cup (125 mL) fresh parsley
(or 1 Tbsp/15 mL dried)

¼ cup (60 mL) fresh basil or dill
(or 2 tsp/10 mL dried)

4 green onions, cut into thirds

1 red bell pepper, cut into chunks

1 orange bell pepper,
cut into chunks

1 cup (250 mL) mandarin
orange segments

½ cup (125 mL) dried cranberries

¼ cup (60 mL) extra virgin
olive oil

¼ cup (60 mL) orange juice
(preferably fresh)

Salt and freshly ground black
pepper to taste

Serve quinoa cold as a colorful salad or hot as a pilaf (see Norene's Notes). A food processor helps speed up preparation. For a low-carb option, use cauliflower "rice" instead of cooked quinoa (see Norene's Notes).

---

1. Place broth in a medium saucepan and bring to a boil over high heat. Place quinoa in a fine-mesh strainer and rinse under cold running water for 1–2 minutes; drain well. (Rinsing removes the bitter coating.) Add quinoa to the boiling liquid. Reduce heat to low and simmer, covered, for 15 minutes. Remove from heat and let stand, covered, for 5 minutes. Fluff with a fork.

2. In a food processor fitted with the steel blade, process garlic, parsley, and basil until minced, about 10 seconds. Combine with cooled quinoa in a large bowl.

3. Process green onions and bell peppers with several quick on/off pulses until coarsely chopped. Add to quinoa along with mandarins and dried cranberries.

4. Add oil, orange juice, salt, and pepper. Mix gently to combine. Cover and refrigerate up to 1 day in advance. Adjust seasonings to taste before serving.

246 calories per 3/4-cup (185 mL) serving, 37 g carbohydrates, 5 g fiber, 13 g sugar, 6 g protein, 9 g fat (1 g saturated fat), 60 mg sodium, 370 mg potassium

NORENE'S NOTES:

- **Quinoa pilaf:** Cook quinoa as directed in Step 1. Reduce olive oil to 2 Tbsp (30 mL) and heat in a large, deep skillet. Add chopped green onions and bell peppers. Sauté over medium heat for 5–7 minutes, until tender-crisp. Add quinoa to the skillet along with orange juice, minced garlic, parsley, basil, salt, and pepper (don't add any more oil). Mix gently, cover, and cook for 5–10 minutes, until heated through. Stir in orange segments and cranberries.

- **Cauliflower rice:** Instead of quinoa, use cauliflower rice. Defrost one 32-oz (907 g) package of frozen cauliflower florets and pat dry with paper towels. In a food processor fitted with the steel blade, process florets in batches, using quick on/off pulses. Transfer to a large bowl and continue as directed in Steps 2–4. (Alternatively, riced cauliflower can be found in many supermarkets' fresh and frozen aisles.)

DR. ED SAYS:

- **Quinoa** has multiple sources of a variety of plant antioxidants, as well as other benefits discussed in Crimson Quinoa with Roasted Beets (p. 518).

- **Spices, bell peppers, and mandarin oranges** are the main contributors of brain-healthy nutrients to this recipe. Basil is very high in carotenoid antioxidants, especially lutein and zeaxanthin, and dill provides kaempferol, also thought to benefit the brain. Cranberries and mandarin oranges contain among the highest concentrations of antioxidants found in fruits.

- **Overall,** this recipe is an excellent source of vitamin C, vitamin B6, folate, and magnesium, as well as a good source of zinc and vitamin E. Its main drawback is the high concentration of sugar, but this can be reduced by using unsweetened cranberries or less orange juice.

> **DID YOU KNOW?** Quinoa is not actually a grain. It is a seed, but is commonly grouped into the grain family.

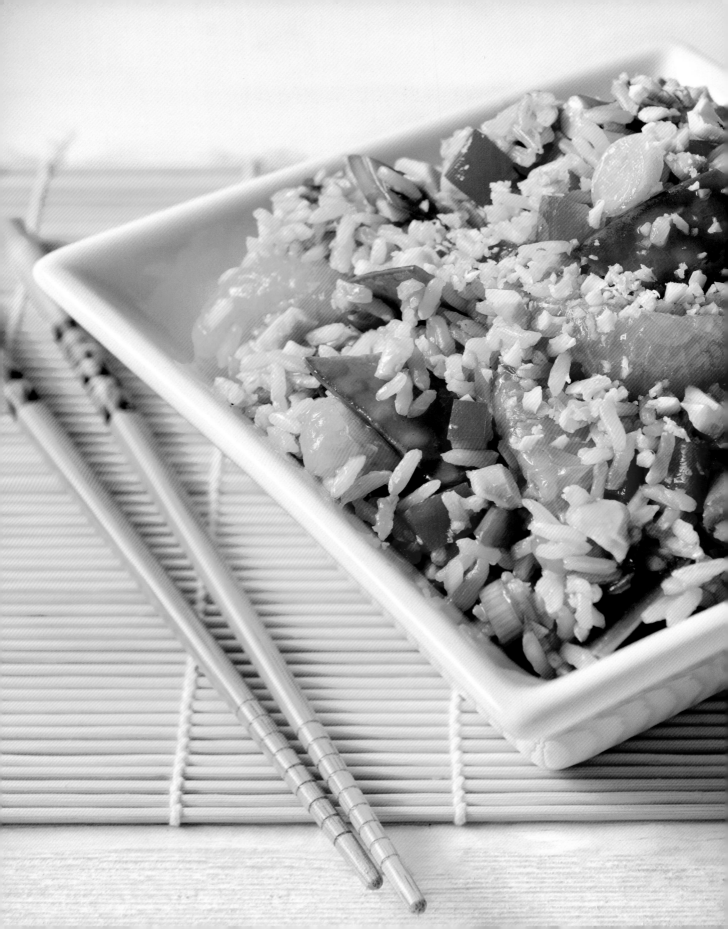

ASIAN RICE WITH SNOW PEAS & CASHEWS

PAREVE | GLUTEN-FREE | DO NOT FREEZE | MAKES ABOUT 8 CUPS (2 L)

This elegant dish was inspired by a recipe from food writer Felisa Billet. Cooked rice, snow peas, mandarin segments, and cashews are combined with an Asian-style dressing, resulting in a colorful presentation.

---

1. **DRESSING:** Combine all ingredients in a jar, cover tightly, and shake well. Refrigerate.

2. **RICE:** In a medium saucepan or a rice cooker, cook rice according to the package instructions. You will have about 4 cups (1 L). Transfer to a large bowl and cool slightly.

3. Add snow peas, green onions, bell pepper, and orange segments. Add dressing and toss to combine. Season with salt and pepper. Cover and refrigerate for at least 1 hour, or preferably overnight, to allow flavors to blend.

4. Serve chilled, garnishing with cashews at serving time.

156 calories per ½-cup (125 mL) serving, 19 g carbohydrates, 2 g fiber, 4 g sugar, 3 g protein, 8 g fat (1 g saturated fat), 255 mg sodium, 160 mg potassium

NORENE'S NOTES:

- **Switch it up!** Experiment with different types of rice (e.g., brown basmati or wild rice, or your favorite rice blend). Black rice (also known as forbidden rice) makes for a spectacular presentation. Follow cooking instructions on the package.

- **Grain power!** Try this with cooked buckwheat groats or quinoa for a gluten-free version. If gluten is not a concern, use wheat berries, freekeh, farro, or whole wheat pearl couscous.

- **Go nuts!** Instead of cashews, use chopped almonds, pecans, or pistachios.

- **Go for green:** Serve on a bed of dark leafy greens garnished with toasted pumpkin seeds or chopped pistachios. For a protein boost, add grilled salmon.

- **Variation:** If snow peas are not available, use snap peas or edamame.

RECIPE CONTINUED . . .

DRESSING:

¼ cup (60 mL) tamari (preferably low-sodium)

3 Tbsp (45 mL) canola oil

1 Tbsp (15 mL) toasted sesame oil

2 Tbsp (30 mL) rice vinegar

2 Tbsp (30 mL) orange juice (preferably fresh)

1–2 Tbsp (15–30 mL) honey (or to taste)

2 cloves garlic (about 2 tsp/ 10 mL minced)

1 tsp (5 mL) minced ginger

RICE:

1⅓ cups (310 mL) uncooked brown rice, rinsed and drained

1 cup (250 mL) snow peas, cut diagonally into 1-inch (2.5 cm) pieces

5–6 green onions, sliced

1 red bell pepper, finely diced

1 cup (250 mL) mandarin orange segments

Salt and freshly ground black pepper

1 cup (250 mL) chopped dry-roasted cashews (for garnish)

DR. ED SAYS:

- **Snow peas** have good levels of vitamin B6, fiber, and folate. They also contain significant amounts of carotenoid antioxidants, including lutein and zeaxanthin, and very high levels of vitamin A.

- **Cashews,** like most nuts, are very nutrient-dense, so you don't have to eat a lot to get a lot of nutrition. Cashews have excellent levels of magnesium, potassium, zinc, and selenium, and good levels of fiber, vitamin B6, folate, and vitamin E. They also contain reasonable levels of phytosterols to control cholesterol. Like most nuts, cashews have high fat content, but this is mostly unsaturated fat, which is good.

DID YOU KNOW? Phytosterols are natural plant components that help decrease cholesterol in the body. Some food products, such as certain brands of margarine, add extracted phytosterols.

WHEAT BERRY SALAD

PAREVE | GLUTEN-FREE OPTION | DO NOT FREEZE SALAD (WHEAT BERRIES FREEZE WELL) | MAKES 6 CUPS (1.5 L)

I call this "My Dentist's Favorite Wheat Berry Salad!" Dr. Howard Rosen loves this versatile, grain-based salad, which was inspired by a recipe from Lee Ann Gallant, a Toronto pediatrician. She uses organic foods whenever possible to optimize good nutritional health. The original version of Lee Ann Gallant's versatile, grain-based salad used dried cranberries, but pomegranate seeds make a lower-sugar alternative.

1. Combine wheat berries with lightly salted water in a medium saucepan and bring to a boil. Reduce heat to low, cover, and simmer for 1–1½ hours, or until tender. Drain if necessary and let cool. (Can be prepared in advance and refrigerated.)

2. In a large bowl, combine wheat berries with red and orange peppers, green onions, parsley, apple, celery, and pomegranate seeds. Add vinaigrette, salt, and pepper; mix well. Refrigerate for at least 1 hour to blend flavors.

142 calories per ½-cup (125 mL) serving, 20 g carbohydrates, 4 g fiber, 6 g sugar, 3 g protein, 7 g fat (1 g saturated fat), 45 mg sodium, 147 mg potassium

NORENE'S NOTES:

- **Shop talk!** Wheat berries come in soft and hard varieties, but this doesn't refer to tenderness. Soft wheat berries are low in gluten, while hard wheat berries are high in gluten. They will triple in volume when cooked. Soaking overnight helps reduce the cooking time.

- **Chews right!** Wheat berries have a chewy texture, so be prepared to chew! Use in salads or as a substitute for rice, pasta, or other grains—even as a breakfast cereal.

- **Will they freeze?** Cooked wheat berries will keep up to a week in the refrigerator or can be frozen for 3–4 months, so cook up a big batch and use them throughout the week in different recipes. Now that's using your grain!

RECIPE CONTINUED . . .

1 cup (250 mL) wheat berries (white or red), rinsed and drained

3 cups (750 mL) lightly salted water

1 red bell pepper, finely chopped

1 orange bell pepper, finely chopped

4 green onions, thinly sliced

½ cup (125 mL) chopped fresh parsley

1 green apple, unpeeled, cored, and diced

2 stalks celery, thinly sliced

¾ cup (185 mL) pomegranate seeds

⅔ cup (160 mL) Raspberry Vinaigrette (p. 431) or your favorite dressing

Salt and freshly ground black pepper

- **Herb magic:** Instead of parsley, experiment with other herbs such as cilantro, basil, oregano, thyme, or rosemary.

- **How to seed a pomegranate:** Roll pomegranate to loosen the seeds. Score around the middle without cutting through. Twist, separating it in half. Working with one-half at a time, invert over a bowl, seeds facing down. Tap top firmly with a wooden spoon, squeezing gently to release the seeds into the bowl. Discard the white pith. Seeds will keep 2–3 days in the refrigerator.

- **Tutti-fruiti:** No pomegranate seeds? Use dried cranberries, raisins, dried or fresh cherries or blueberries, or dried apricots. Instead of apples, use firm plums, peaches, nectarines, Asian pears, or mandarin oranges.

- **Mix it up!** Instead of celery, use fennel, jicama, water chestnuts, or hearts of palm.

- **Gluten-free option:** Instead of wheat berries, use whole buckwheat groats, black rice, or quinoa. Cook according to package directions.

DR. ED SAYS:

- **Wheat berries** are the grain contribution to this recipe, and they are a good choice as far as grains go. Wheat products (including whole wheat products) made from wheat flour have a high GI and contribute to spikes in blood sugar. However, by eating the wheat in its granular whole grain form called groats (found in wheat berries, bulgur wheat, and freekeh), we have a much-reduced GI and glycemic effect. This is because the starch in the groats is more difficult to break down into glucose.

- **Bell peppers** are very high in vitamin C, antioxidants, magnesium, and zinc, and are a good contributor of brain-benefitting nutrients.

- **Parsley,** used generously in this recipe, has low sugar and carbs, very high vitamin C and folate, and good magnesium and potassium. It is also high in antioxidants, especially the carotenoid family, including lutein and zeaxanthin.

- **Pomegranate** does have good levels of vitamin C and fiber, but is not exceptional in brain-healthy nutrients. Its main claim to fame is its concentration of a variety of polyphenol antioxidants—in fact, the USDA has placed it among the top plant foods for antioxidants. Its disadvantage is its high sugar and carb levels.

> **DID YOU KNOW?** Parsley contains a flavonoid antioxidant called apigenin that possesses anti-inflammatory, antioxidant, and anti-cancer properties.

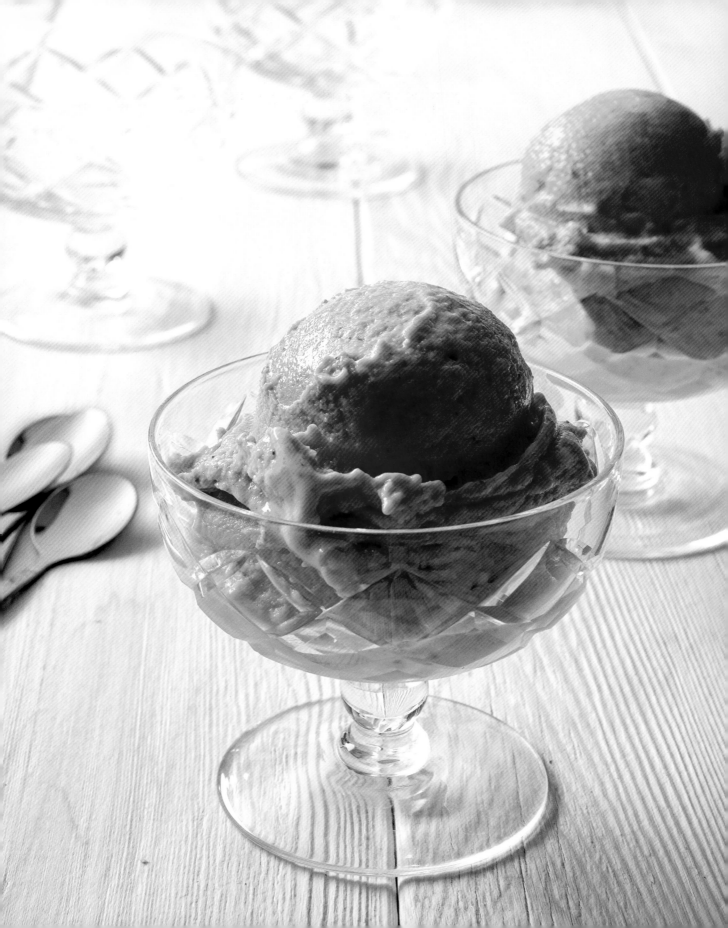

A TOUCH OF SWEET

SWEET OPTIONS: Desserts, by nature, tend to be sweet, and that means significant amounts of sugar, which is increasingly being considered harmful to health. Sweeteners in any form should be consumed in moderation—the World Health Organization recommends that women limit sugar to no more than 40–50 g per day (equivalent to a single can of cola). Below are some sugar alternative options.

HIGH-INTENSITY SWEETENERS: Sucralose (Splenda), stevia, cyclamate, saccharin, aspartame, and so on are in the first category of high-intensity sweeteners, of which you may consider sucralose and stevia. The main problem with this category of sweeteners is that because of the small amounts used, we are missing the bulking contribution of sugar. This can be adjusted for in two ways: (1) commercially, by buying a sweetener with a bulking agent included (usually dextrose or erythritol); or (2) by adding your own bulking agent, such as inulin or polydextrose, both of which are fibers and therefore better than dextrose, which is a sugar. These bulking agents can often be found at health food stores or online.

SUGAR ALCOHOLS: These are in the second category, and are favored commercially because they are used in larger portions to approximate the bulking effects of sugar. These include sorbitol, maltitol, and erythritol. One note of caution is that excessive use of sugar alcohols can result in a laxative effect— erythritol has the least effect as a laxative.

SWEET SUGGESTIONS: If a sweetener is needed, consider using stevia or Splenda, along with a fiber-bulking agent such as inulin or polydextrose. Some experimentation may be required. All sweeteners are plant-derived or synthetic and would qualify as kosher, but aspartame, which is fermented, may not be acceptable for Passover.

DID YOU KNOW? Maple syrup is a natural source of essential minerals, including calcium, zinc, magnesium, and potassium. Just 2 Tbsp (30 mL) provides half of your recommended daily intake of manganese, which is important for brain function, as well as bone health and metabolism. However, the nutrients it provides can be obtained from many other foods which are not full of sugar.

GI GO! To reduce the glycemic index of a dish, add foods with a low GI (e.g., berries, rolled oats, wheat germ, nuts, Greek yogurt, lemon juice). Keep in mind, however, that the GI is not the be all and end all for choice of carbohydrate-containing foods. Glycemic load (GL), which measures total carbohydrate consumption, is considered more important.

PORTION DISTORTION: The main problem with sweets is their sugar and digestible carb contents. Therefore, we recommend that the recipes in this chapter be eaten in moderation. The other problem with most sweets is that they taste so good, you can't stop at just one serving, and sugar has been found to be addictive. If you share dessert, you'll also share the calories, carbs, sugars, and fat. One plate—two forks!

THE LIGHT SWITCH: Instead of pie, switch to fruit crisp. See Berry-Apple Crisp and its multiple variations (p. 537). Fruit crisps, especially berry-based ones with their juicy fruit fillings and crunchy toppings of rolled oats and nuts, are lower in fat and calories than traditional pie. No rolling of dough is required—and you'll have fewer rolls around your middle!

CLEAN CUISINE: To remove pesticides and other harmful chemicals, peel fruit or wash it thoroughly in a solution of water mixed with 2 or 3 drops of liquid dish detergent, vinegar, or a little baking soda. Always wash melons such as cantaloupe, honeydew, or watermelon before cutting.

BERRIES ARE BEST: Fruits contain an abundance of vitamins, minerals, phytochemicals, antioxidants, and fiber that help reduce the risks of disease. They'll satisfy your sweet tooth and also provide nutritional benefits. Enjoy them fresh, frozen, roasted, grilled, or poached. Keep in mind, however, that fruits are the number one source of sugars in the diet—so even though they are a better alternative than baked goods and sweets, they should still be used in moderation (see the Brain Boosting Diet menu plan in the first part of this book.)

BERRY VERSATILE: Try berries in fruit crisps, smoothies, muffins, quick breads, pancakes, and fruit salad. Use berries as a topping for your breakfast cereal or as a satisfying snack. Berry good!

GET CULTIVATED! Fresh blueberries are cultivated and are larger and sweeter than wild ones.

GO WILD! Wild blueberries may be tiny, but they're mighty good for you. Wild blueberries are packed with more phytonutrients (potent antioxidants found in plants that strengthen the immune system) than cultivated ones.

PLATTER POWER: Arrange fresh fruit (e.g., cut-up watermelon, pineapple, kiwi, nectarines, plums, strawberries, blueberries, blackberries, raspberries) on a large serving platter. Garnish with slices of star fruit for a simply stellar dessert.

FRUIT KABOBS: Place colorful cubes of fruit on wooden skewers and arrange on a serving platter for a pretty presentation. If you plan to grill the fruit, first soak the skewers in cold water for 20–30 minutes.

LEMON AID: Sprinkle fresh fruit with lemon juice to prevent it from discoloring.

NEAT TRICK: To save on cleanup, line a baking sheet (or sheets) with parchment paper. If you wipe the baking sheet first with a damp cloth, the parchment won't roll up!

POSITION IS EVERYTHING: Bake cookies, cakes, and muffins on the middle rack of your oven. If baking two pans at once that won't both fit on the same rack, place racks so that they divide the oven space evenly into thirds. For even browning, switch (from top to bottom) and rotate the pans (from back to front) for the last few minutes of baking.

AQUAFABA: The drained liquid from canned or cooked chickpeas (aquafaba) can either be used as an egg substitute in baking or whipped into semisoft peaks to make egg-free meringue. Excellent for those with egg allergies!

EGG-FREE MERINGUE: Shake the unopened can vigorously, then drain chickpeas through a fine-mesh strainer over a bowl; save chickpeas for future use. Whisk the drained liquid, then measure. Beat 1 cup (250 mL) chickpea liquid with ½ tsp (2 mL) cream of tartar in a stand mixer on high speed until stiff peaks form, about 5 minutes. Voila—vegan meringue!

STORE IT RIGHT: Either store drained chickpea liquid in the refrigerator up to a week or freeze it in ice cube trays. When frozen solid, transfer aquafaba cubes to an airtight container for future use.

TIME FOR A DIP! For a delicious dip for fresh fruit, melt dark chocolate in a small microwaveable bowl. Place the dip in the center of a platter, surrounded by a colorful array of fruit. Dip a-weigh!

CHOCOLATE DIPPED APRICOTS: Dip the tips of dried apricots in melted chocolate, then coat with chopped pistachios, almonds, or walnuts. Place on parchment paper and refrigerate until set.

CHOCOLATE-STUFFED RASPBERRIES: Stuff hollowed-out raspberries with semisweet or dark chocolate chips—so berry good!

CALLING ALL CHOCOHOLICS! The darker the chocolate, the higher the antioxidant content. Dark chocolate can provide as much as 3 g of fiber in a 1-oz (30 g) serving. The "dark side" is that chocolate is high in calories, so watch your portions!

CHOCOLATE MELTDOWN: Microwave 1–2 oz (30–60 g) chocolate (or 1 cup/250 mL chocolate chips) uncovered on medium for 2–3 minutes, stirring once every minute. Your bowl must be dry and the chocolate shouldn't be covered or it will "seize" (become lumpy and grainy).

FANCY THAT! For an elegant presentation, arrange alternate layers of colorful fruit in wine or parfait glasses. Top with a swirl of Coconut "Whipped Cream" (see below) and chocolate shavings.

COCONUT "WHIPPED CREAM" is dairy-free! Chill 1 can (14 oz/398 mL) organic unsweetened full-fat coconut milk overnight. Open the can and pour off liquid (save it for smoothies). Whip thickened coconut cream in a chilled bowl for 3–5 minutes, until soft peaks form. Blend in 1–2 Tbsp (15–30 mL) icing sugar or desired sweetener and 1 tsp (5 mL) vanilla extract. Use immediately or refrigerate up to a week. Makes 1½ cups (375 mL).

MOCK-SICKLES! For an easy treat, freeze individual containers of sugar-free yogurt. Insert a wooden stick before freezing and wrap well. Enjoy!

FROZEN GRAPES: Place washed grapes on top of a clean towel and pat dry. Transfer to a rimmed baking sheet or baking dish. Freeze until grapes are solid, about 2 hours. Transfer to a large resealable freezer bag and store in the freezer.

SMART SNACKS: For more ideas, see Better Breakfasts (p. 119) and Splendid Spreads & Starters (p. 161).

ALMOND CRUST

PAREVE | PASSOVER | IF FROZEN, CRUST MAY BECOME SOGGY |
MAKES 1 CRUST

1½ cups (375 mL) finely ground almonds (almond flour)

2 Tbsp (30 mL) sugar or sweetener

1 tsp (5 mL) ground cinnamon

1 Tbsp (15 mL) vegetable oil

1 egg white

This low-carb crust is perfect for those who are watching their carb intake. Even though it's fairly high in fat, this almond crust contains mainly heart-healthy unsaturated fat.

1. Preheat oven to 350°F (175°C). Spray a 9-inch (23 cm) glass pie plate with nonstick cooking spray.

2. In a mixing bowl, combine almonds, sugar, and cinnamon. Add oil and egg white and mix well. Pat mixture evenly into the bottom and partway up the sides of the prepared pan.

3. Bake for 10–12 minutes, until lightly browned. Fill as desired.

133 calories per 1/8 crust, 7 g carbohydrates, 4 g sugar, 2 g fiber, 4 g protein, 11 g fat (1 g saturated), 7 mg sodium, 139 mg potassium

NORENE'S NOTES:

- **Go nuts:** Replace half the ground almonds with other nuts (e.g., ground walnuts, pecans, or hazelnuts).

- **Chocolate almond crust:** Add 2 Tbsp (30 mL) unsweetened cocoa powder to the nut mixture.

- **Pan-tastic!** You can also bake this crust in a 9- or 10-inch (23 or 25 cm) springform pan and use it for your favorite cheesecake. If you line the pan with parchment paper first, it will be easier to remove the finished crust from the pan.

DR. ED SAYS:

- **Almonds** account for this recipe's substantial fiber and protein content, as well as its high vitamin E and other nutrients.

- **Overall,** this is a great substitute for a wheat-based crust because of its low digestible carb level, high fiber, and vitamin E content, as well as other nutrients present in the almonds.

APPLE-LICIOUS CAKE

PAREVE | FREEZES WELL (SEE NORENE'S NOTES) | MAKES 1 CAKE
(12 SLICES)

An apple a day will keep the doctor a-weigh! This is a higher-fiber, lower-carb version of my fabulous apple cake from *Second Helpings, Please!* Serve it for the Jewish High Holidays or as an occasional treat.

1. Preheat oven to 350°F (175°C). Spray a 7- × 11-inch (18 × 28 cm) glass baking dish with nonstick cooking spray.

2. **FILLING:** In a large bowl, combine apples with sweetener and cinnamon; mix well and set aside.

3. **BATTER:** In a food processor fitted with the steel blade, process almonds until finely ground, about 25–30 seconds. Transfer to a bowl and set aside.

4. Add eggs, sugar, vanilla extract, oil, and applesauce to the food processor. Process for 2 minutes, or until smooth and creamy. Don't insert the pusher into the feed tube while processing. Add the ground almonds along with flour, baking powder, cinnamon, and salt; process just until combined.

5. **ASSEMBLY:** Using a rubber spatula, spread about half the batter in the prepared pan. Spread apple filling evenly over the batter. Top with the remaining batter and spread evenly. Some of the apples will peek through, but that's okay!

6. Bake for 50–60 minutes, until golden brown.

236 calories per slice, 38 g carbohydrates, 24 g sugar, 4 g fiber, 4 g protein, 9 g fat (1 g saturated), 14 mg sodium, 289 mg potassium

NORENE'S NOTES:

- **Berry good variation:** Replace half the apples with your favorite berries, for a total of 4–5 cups (1–1.25 L) fruit.

- **Nut allergies?** Replace almonds with either ½ cup (125 mL) wheat germ or whole wheat pastry flour.

RECIPE CONTINUED . . .

FILLING:

6 large apples, peeled, cored, and thinly sliced (Cortland, Spartan, or Honeycrisp)

Sweetener equivalent to ¼ cup (60 mL) brown sugar, lightly packed

2 tsp (10 mL) ground cinnamon

BATTER:

½ cup (125 mL) whole blanched almonds (or ½ cup/125 mL almond meal)

2 large eggs

⅔ cup (160 mL) sugar

1 tsp (5 mL) pure vanilla extract

¼ cup (60 mL) canola oil

½ cup (125 mL) unsweetened applesauce

1¼ cups (310 mL) whole wheat flour

2 tsp (10 mL) baking powder

½ tsp (2 mL) ground cinnamon

Pinch of salt

- **Fiber up:** Apples and almonds help boost this cake's fiber content. Replacing part of the flour with ground almonds helps to lower the carbs.

- **Deep-dish apple cake:** In Step 5, spread apples evenly in the prepared pan. Spoon batter over the apples and bake as directed.

- **Freezer alert:** If frozen, the cake will become very moist. Just reheat it uncovered in a preheated 350°F (175°C) oven for 10 minutes and it will taste just baked!

DR. ED SAYS:

- **Apples** are not overly rich in brain nutrients, but do have good fiber and antioxidant content, especially the important polyphenol catechin antioxidants. Although about 70% of the dry weight of an apple is made up of sugars, more than half is from fructose. The fructose and the fiber help to give apples reasonably low GIs and GLs.

- **Cinnamon** is in a group of spices that contains the highest antioxidant levels of any foods.

- **Overall,** this recipe is quite high in sugar due to the apples, but more than half is due to fructose, which does not contribute much to blood glucose response. It also contains good amounts of vitamin E and reasonable amounts of vitamins C, B6, and B12 and folate, as well as magnesium and zinc.

> **DID YOU KNOW?** A Canadian study in 2005 found that the highest antioxidant content in apples was found in Red Delicious, Northern Spy, and Ida Red apples.

BERRY-APPLE CRISP

DAIRY OPTION | PAREVE | GLUTEN-FREE OPTION | REHEATS AND/
OR FREEZES WELL | MAKES 10 SERVINGS

Berry delicious! I've modified my favorite recipe for Jumbleberry Crisp, transforming it into a brain-boosting, heart-healthy dessert by using almond flour (finely ground almonds) instead of regular flour in the topping. I often use a sugar substitute, but you can use sugar if you prefer.

1. **FILLING:** Preheat oven to 375°F (190°C). Combine ingredients for filling in a large bowl and toss together. (If using frozen berries, there's no need to thaw them first.) Transfer to a sprayed 10-inch (25 cm) ceramic quiche dish or 7- × 11-inch (18 × 28 cm) glass baking dish and spread evenly.

2. **TOPPING:** Using the same large bowl (no washing required), combine topping ingredients and mix until crumbly. Sprinkle topping evenly over the filling.

3. Bake, uncovered, for 40–45 minutes, until topping is golden and juices are bubbly. To test for doneness, insert a knife into the center of the dish. It should be hot to the touch. Serve warm or at room temperature.

263 calories per serving, 37 g carbohydrates, 7 g fiber, 26 g sugar, 6 g protein, 12 g fat (1 g saturated) 2 mg sodium, 56 mg potassium

NORENE'S NOTES:

- **Any kind of fruit crisp:** Use a total of 6-7 cups (1.5-1.75 L) fruit (e.g., sliced apples, peaches, plums, pears, rhubarb). I like to use 4 cups (1 L) blueberries and/or strawberries and 3-4 cups (750-1000 mL) sliced fruit.

- **Individual fruit crisps:** Spray 8-10 ramekins with nonstick cooking spray. Place on a parchment-lined rimmed baking sheet. Bake for 35-40 minutes, until golden.

- **Frozen assets:** If you freeze the crisp, thaw it before serving. Reheat for a few minutes to crisp up the topping.

- **Dairy option:** Serve with a dollop of plain Greek yogurt (skim or 1%) for a protein boost.

RECIPE CONTINUED . . .

FILLING:

4 cups (1 L) fresh or frozen mixed berries (wild blueberries, strawberries, raspberries, cranberries, and/or blackberries)

2 large apples, peeled, cored, and sliced

⅓ cup (80 mL) whole wheat flour or gluten-free flour

Sweetener equivalent to ½ cup (125 mL) sugar

1 tsp (5 mL) ground cinnamon

TOPPING:

1⅓ cups (310 mL) rolled oats (preferably large flake)

⅓ cup (80 mL) Splenda Brown Sugar Blend or brown sugar, lightly packed

⅓ cup (80 mL) almond flour (finely ground almonds)

⅓ cup (80 mL) canola oil

1 tsp (5 mL) ground cinnamon

BERRY-APPLE CRISP (continued)

- **Do-ahead:** Make a batch of topping and store it in the freezer in a resealable bag. When needed, make a batch of your favorite fruit filling and sprinkle with the frozen crumb mixture. Bake as directed.

DR. ED SAYS:

- **Berries:** The magic in berries is in their antioxidant levels. They have some of the highest antioxidant concentrations of all foods and have been shown repeatedly to reduce the risk of AD/dementia. Raspberries and blackberries are preferable because they have the least sugar. Wild blueberries have twice the antioxidant power of regular blueberries.

- **Sweeteners:** Since too much sugar is not good for cognition, using Splenda instead of sugar is a good choice.

- **Almond flour:** Almonds are one of the best foods for cognition. They are excellent sources of magnesium, zinc, and fiber, and are good sources of vitamins B6 and folate. More importantly, almonds contain one of the highest concentrations of natural vitamin E of any food. Vitamin E has been repeatedly shown to benefit cognitive health and reduce the risk of AD/dementia.

- **Cinnamon, apples, and whole wheat** round out the recipe with additional antioxidants, fiber, and vitamin C.

- **Overall,** this fabulous fiber-packed dessert is packed with brain-boosting nutrients. The high berry antioxidant content, as well as the almond flour (with its high natural vitamin E) all contribute to brain health.

> **DID YOU KNOW?** In addition to having high antioxidant levels, most common berries are also among the fruits with the least amounts of sugar. This means that they have a low GI and GL, and are very good for controlling blood sugar response.

PLUM CRAZY CAKE

PAREVE | DO NOT FREEZE | MAKES 1 CAKE (15 SLICES)

You'll go plum crazy over this delectable, reduced-carbohydrate cake. It's hard to believe it's made with only 1 cup (250 mL) flour and very little sugar. Serve it for breakfast, or enjoy it with guests. Little Jack Horner would say "Stick in your thumb and pull out a plum—yum!"

---

1. Preheat oven to 350°F (175°C). Spray a 9- × 13-inch (23 × 33 cm) glass baking pan with nonstick cooking spray.

2. **FRUIT:** Spread plums in a single layer in the prepared pan. In a small bowl, mix together Splenda and cinnamon; sprinkle over the plums.

3. **BATTER:** In a food processor fitted with the steel blade, combine oil, applesauce, sugar, Splenda, vanilla extract, and eggs. Process for 1 minute or until smooth and creamy. Don't insert the pusher into the feed tube while processing. Add flour, baking powder, and salt; process with 3 or 4 quick on/off pulses, just until blended. Pour batter evenly over the plums.

4. Bake for 45–55 minutes, until golden.

147 calories per slice, 17 g carbohydrates, 10 g sugar, 2 g fiber, 2 g protein, 9 g fat (1 g saturated), 30 mg sodium, 162 mg potassium

NORENE'S NOTES:

- **Variation:** Instead of plums, use 3 lb (1.4 kg) nectarines, peaches, apricots, pears, or apples.

DR. ED SAYS:

- **Plums:** This recipe is all about the plums, which contain good amounts of vitamin C and a variety of antioxidants. Their sugar content is high at greater than 75% of their dry weight, but two-thirds of this sugar is fructose, which has a very low GI. This, combined with the plums' fiber content and the recipe's fat content, helps reduce the GI and GL to low levels. Nevertheless, even though the GI and GL are low, and we are using Splenda, the digestible carb and sugar contents are high. Therefore, this recipe should be eaten in moderation.

RECIPE CONTINUED . . .

FRUIT:

12 firm, ripe plums, pitted and sliced (do not peel)

Granulated Splenda equivalent to 2 Tbsp (30 mL) sugar

1 tsp (5 mL) ground cinnamon

BATTER:

½ cup (125 mL) canola oil

½ cup (125 mL) unsweetened applesauce

¼ cup (60 mL) sugar

¼ cup (60 mL) granulated Splenda or sugar

1 tsp (5 mL) pure vanilla extract

2 large eggs

1 cup (250 mL) whole wheat flour

1 tsp (5 mL) baking powder

⅛ tsp (0.5 mL) salt

PLUM CRAZY CAKE (continued)

- **Overall,** this recipe provides good amounts of vitamin C, vitamin E, vitamin B6, and plant Omega-3 fat, as well as reasonable amounts of vitamin B12, magnesium, and zinc. However, it is on the high side for digestible carbs and sugars.

> DID YOU KNOW? The riper a fruit, the more sugar it will contain. There is a category of foods called resistant starch—a type of fiber that occurs in some fruits such as bananas—that converts to sugar as the fruit ripens.

MINI CHEESECAKES

DAIRY-FREE OPTION | GLUTEN-FREE | PASSOVER | FREEZES WELL |
MAKES 12 MINI CAKES

These muffin-sized cheesecakes are a terrific "weigh" to exercise portion control—as long as you stop at one! Try the variations below and expand your repertoire without expanding your hips!

⅓ cup (80 mL) finely chopped almonds or pecans

2 cups (500 mL) light cream cheese (1 lb/500 g)

Sweetener equivalent to ⅔ cup (160 mL) sugar

2 large eggs

1 Tbsp (15 mL) lemon juice (preferably fresh)

12 large whole strawberries, hulled

1. Preheat oven to 350°F (175°C). Line each compartment of a muffin pan with a paper liner and sprinkle some chopped nuts in the bottom of each.

2. In a food processor fitted with the steel blade, process cheese with sweetener until blended, about 15 seconds. Add eggs and lemon juice; process for 20–30 seconds, until smooth and creamy. Spoon batter into the prepared muffin pan compartments.

3. Bake for 10–12 minutes, until set.

4. Once cooled, top each cheesecake with a whole strawberry and refrigerate for 3–4 hours, or overnight. Serve chilled.

119 calories per mini cake, 7 g carbohydrates, 3 g sugar, 1 g fiber, 5 g protein, 8 g fat (4 g saturated), 156 mg sodium, 158 mg potassium

NORENE'S NOTES:

- **Variation:** Replace half the cream cheese with pressed cottage cheese; increase processing time to 1 minute, until very smooth.

- **Praline mini cheesecakes:** Replace sweetener with brown sugar sweetener. Instead of strawberries, top each cheesecake with a pecan half.

- **Marbled mini cheesecakes:** Place ⅓ cup (80 mL) chocolate chips in a 2-cup (500 mL) glass measure. Microwave on medium for 1 minute, or until melted. Stir ¾ cup (185 mL) cheesecake batter into the melted chocolate. Spoon the remaining batter into the muffin pan compartments. Drizzle chocolate mixture over the white mixture. Cut through the batter with a knife to marble it. Bake as directed. Garnish each mini cheesecake with a strawberry.

RECIPE CONTINUED . . .

MINI CHEESECAKES (continued)

- **Dairy-free option:** Use imitation cream cheese (e.g., Tofutti) instead of cream cheese (but not during Passover).

DR. ED SAYS:

- **Almonds** provide one of the highest concentrations of natural vitamin E of any food, which is important for brain health. Due to their low moisture, they are rich sources of other important brain nutrients such as antioxidants, magnesium, zinc, fiber, and protein, and they also supply good levels of vitamin B6, folate, and choline. At the same time, they are low in digestible carbs and sugars and have a low GI. Almonds are always good for you!

- **Cream cheese** is very low in digestible carbs and sugars and provides a protein punch while also contributing good levels of vitamin B12, which is usually found in animal-source foods. The light version keeps saturated fats at about half the level of regular cream cheese.

- **Strawberrie**s are one of the main berries found to be beneficial for reducing AD/dementia risk, primarily due to their antioxidants, fiber, and relatively low sugar.

- **Overall,** we have a nice contribution of important brain nutrients thanks to the ingredients chosen, and these include vitamin E, vitamin C, vitamin B12, folate, magnesium, and zinc. At the same time, digestible sugars and carbs are kept low.

> **DID YOU KNOW?** Almonds that were originally found in nature were small and poisonous, and only when our ancestors selectively started cultivating them did they become the nutritious food we have today.

ALMOND COCONUT CRUNCHIES

PAREVE | GLUTEN-FREE | PASSOVER | FREEZES WELL | MAKES
ABOUT 30 COOKIES

There's no need to beat the egg whites for these crunchy chocolate cookies—and you can't beat that! Although coconut is high in saturated fat, it's okay to enjoy it in moderation.

2 egg whites

½ cup (125 mL) sugar

1 tsp (5 mL) pure vanilla extract

2 Tbsp (30 mL) unsweetened cocoa powder

½ tsp (2 mL) ground cinnamon

2 cups (500 mL) sliced almonds

1 cup (250 mL) shredded unsweetened coconut

1. Preheat oven to 350°F (175°C). Place rack in the middle of the oven. Line a large, rimmed baking sheet with parchment paper.

2. In a large mixing bowl, combine egg whites, sugar, and vanilla; mix well with a wooden spoon. Add cocoa, cinnamon, almonds, and coconut; stir to combine.

3. Drop mixture from a tablespoon onto the prepared baking sheet, making small mounds.

4. Bake for 15 minutes, until firm.

5. Cool for 15 minutes before removing from pan.

67 calories per cookie, 6 g carbohydrates, 4 g sugar, 1 g fiber, 2 g protein, 5 g fat (1 g saturated), 4 mg sodium, 72 mg potassium

NORENE'S NOTES:

- **How sweet it is:** Although coconut provides texture and taste, choose unsweetened dried shredded coconut or coconut flakes over sweetened dried coconut, which has 2 tsp (10 mL) added sugar per ounce.

DR. ED SAYS:

- **Coconut** is rich in manganese, potassium, and zinc, and also has reasonable quantities of magnesium, but is not noteworthy for other brain nutrients. It has a very high fat content at about 65% of the coconut meat weight, of which about 90% is saturated. Generally speaking, this is a very high level of saturated fats, though some of these saturated fats are considered good fats in the form of medium-chain triglycerides. However, looking at a total profile of all fats, the American Heart Association came out with an advisory that coconut fat is not recommended because of its effect in increasing LDL cholesterol. Use coconut meat in moderation.

RECIPE CONTINUED . . .

DID YOU KNOW? Medium-chain triglyceride fats contained in coconut fat are good for the brain. These fats go straight to the liver, bypassing the normal route for fat absorption, and are used directly for energy. They can be used very efficiently by the brain, as an alternative to sugar, and there are studies that show it to be a more efficient fuel for the aged brain, with the potential for reduced cognitive decline.

BISCOTTI THINS (SKINNY MANDELBROIT)

PAREVE | FREEZES WELL | MAKES ABOUT 48 SLICES

Addictive! The only fat in this recipe is the natural fat contained in the almonds. This is an adaptation of my Melba Mandel Bread from *Healthy Helpings*.

4 large eggs (or 2 eggs + 4 egg whites)

⅔ cup (160 mL) sugar

1 tsp (5 mL) cinnamon

1 tsp (5 mL) pure vanilla or almond extract

1½ cups (375 mL) whole wheat pastry flour or all-purpose flour

½ tsp (2 mL) baking powder

¾–1 cup (185–250 mL) almonds (whole)

1. Preheat oven to 350°F (175°C). Line a 9- × 5-inch (23 × 12 cm) loaf pan with heavy-duty aluminum foil, leaving enough foil extending over the edges so you can wrap the loaf airtight after baking. Spray foil lightly with nonstick cooking spray.

2. In a large bowl, beat eggs until light. Gradually add sugar, cinnamon, and vanilla; beat well. Mix in flour and baking powder. Stir in almonds.

3. Spread mixture evenly in the prepared pan. Bake at 350°F (175°C) for 50–60 minutes, until golden.

4. Cool loaf for 10 minutes, then wrap up tightly in foil. Remove wrapped loaf from pan and refrigerate for 1–2 days, or freeze (see Norene's Notes).

5. Unwrap loaf. Slice as thinly as possible, using an electric or serrated knife.

6. Arrange slices in a single layer on a parchment-lined baking sheet (or sheets).

7. Bake at 300°F (150°C) for 30–40 minutes, until crisp and toasted.

52 calories per slice, 8 g carbohydrates, 3 g sugar, 1 g fiber, 2 g protein, 2 g fat (0 g saturated), 6 mg sodium, 47 mg potassium

NORENE'S NOTES:

- **Sugar rush:** Replace half the sugar with sweetener (e.g., granulated Splenda).

- **Go nuts:** Instead of almonds, use walnuts, pecans, or pistachios.

- **Freeze with ease:** In my catering business, I would make multiple batches, then freeze the baked loaves at the end of Step 4. When needed, I'd thaw a loaf or two, slice it thinly, and bake as directed in Step 7.

RECIPE CONTINUED . . .

DR. ED SAYS:

- **Almonds** are the primary beneficial ingredient in this recipe because of their high vitamin E, fiber, protein, magnesium, potassium, zinc, and manganese content, along with their good B vitamin content and low sugar and digestible carbs. They are also very high in a type of polyphenol antioxidant called proanthocyanidins.

- **Eggs** are excellent sources of high-quality protein, but because they come from animals they are also rich in vitamin B12, vitamin D, and choline.

- **Overall,** per slice, there is not a lot of nutrition other than vitamin E, and there is a significant amount of digestible carbs and sugar. So, enjoy these in moderation.

TRAIL MIX BISCOTTI

PAREVE | FREEZES WELL | MAKES ABOUT 48 SLICES

Everyone will beat a "trail" to your door when you make these skinny, addictive biscotti, which were inspired by Sandra Gitlin's "secret recipe." Happy and healthy trails!

3 large eggs

⅔ cup (160 mL) sugar

2 tsp (10 mL) grated orange rind

1 tsp (5 mL) grated lemon rind

3 Tbsp (45 mL) orange juice (preferably fresh)

¾ cup (185 mL) all-purpose flour

¾ cup (185 mL) whole wheat flour

½ tsp (2 mL) baking powder

½ cup (125 mL) pistachios

½ cup (125 mL) whole almonds

½ cup (125 mL) raisins

½ cup (125 mL) dried cranberries

1. Preheat oven to 350°F (175°C). Spray a 9- × 5-inch (23 × 12 cm) loaf pan with nonstick cooking spray.

2. In a food processor fitted with the steel blade, process eggs with sugar for 2–3 minutes, until well mixed. Add orange and lemon rinds, orange juice, flours, and baking powder; process just until combined.

3. Transfer batter to a large bowl. Stir in nuts, raisins, and dried cranberries.

4. Spread mixture evenly in the prepared pan. Bake for 50–60 minutes, until golden.

5. Remove pan from oven and let stand for 10 minutes before unmolding loaf from pan. (Loaf can be prepared up to this point, wrapped tightly in foil, and refrigerated for 1–2 days. This makes slicing easier.)

6. Slice baked loaf as thinly as possible, using an electric or serrated knife. Arrange slices in a single layer on parchment-lined cookie sheets.

7. Bake in a preheated 300°F (150°F) oven for 30–40 minutes, until crisp and toasted.

56 calories per slice, 9 g carbohydrates, 5 g sugar, 1 g fiber, 2 g protein, 2 g fat (0 g saturated), 5 mg sodium, 58 mg potassium

NORENE'S NOTES:

- **Mix it up:** Instead of raisins and cranberries, add pumpkin and/or sunflower seeds; instead of pistachios, add cashews. You can also try these with an extra ½ cup (125 mL) mini chocolate chips.

- **"Fat-astic" news!** There's no oil added to these biscotti—the only fat in this recipe comes from the nuts.

- **Nuts to you!** Always store nuts and seeds in the refrigerator or freezer so they won't become rancid.

RECIPE CONTINUED . . .

TRAIL MIX BISCOTTI (continued)

- **Store it right!** Store these in cookie tins and hide them in a safe place or they won't last very long! They'll freeze up to 4 months.

DR. ED SAYS:

- **Pistachios** are part of the seeds and nuts family and therefore show a similarly rich profile in B vitamins, minerals, protein, and fiber, while being low in sugars and digestible carbs. Uniquely, they have a very high content of a type of vitamin E called gamma vitamin E, which is thought to play an important role in brain health. They are also rich in the important carotenoid eye and brain antioxidants lutein and zeaxanthin, as well as polyphenol proanthocyanidin antioxidants. Finally, they have significant levels of phytosterols.

- **Raisins and dried cranberries:** Despite their high contents of important antioxidants and other nutrients, both of these ingredients are very high in sugars. Consider using no-sugar-added dried cranberries instead of the raisins and sweetened cranberries.

- **Overall,** I would consider this recipe to be in the same league as Biscotti Thins (p. 545), and recommend they be eaten in moderation because of their sugar content. Also, see my comments above about raisins and dried cranberries.

> **DID YOU KNOW?** Phytosterols are natural plant compounds that have been shown to reduce cholesterol in humans. The data are significant enough that some food manufacturers like Becel incorporate them into their margarine.

PASSOVER NOTHINGS

PAREVE | PASSOVER | FREEZES WELL | MAKES ABOUT 28 COOKIES

These nothings are really something—they look and taste like the kind you make with regular flour! The secret to these cookies is to start them off in a hot oven so they will expand, then, when they've finished baking, leave them in the oven so the insides will dry out and the cookies won't collapse.

3 large eggs

2 Tbsp (30 mL) sugar
+ extra 2 Tbsp (30 mL), for
sprinkling (optional)

⅛ tsp (0.5 mL) salt

½ cup (125 mL) vegetable oil

½ cup (125 mL) Passover
cake meal

1 Tbsp (15 mL) potato starch

1. Preheat oven to 450°F (230°F). Place rack in the middle of the oven. Line a large, rimmed baking sheet with foil and spray with nonstick cooking spray.

2. In a food processor fitted with the steel blade, process eggs, sugar, and salt for 1 minute, until light. While machine is running, pour oil through the feed tube in a steady stream and process for 1 minute longer. Add cake meal and potato starch and process for 2–3 minutes longer—the batter will become thicker as you beat it.

3. Drop batter by scant teaspoonfuls onto the prepared sheet, using a second spoon to push it off. Leave about 2 inches (5 cm) between cookies for expansion. Sprinkle tops of cookies lightly with additional sugar, if using.

4. Quickly place cookies in the oven, then reduce heat to 400°F (200°C). Bake for 7–8 minutes. Reduce heat to 300°F (150°F) and bake for 10–12 minutes longer. No peeking allowed!

5. Turn off the oven, with the cookies inside, for 20–30 minutes longer to dry.

54 calories per cookie, 3 g carbohydrates, 1 g sugar, trace fiber, 1 g protein, 4 g fat (<1 g saturated), 18 mg sodium, 7 mg potassium

NORENE'S NOTES:

- **Hot stuff:** Newer ovens are better insulated, so they hold the heat longer. You may have to reduce the heat and baking time to prevent these cookies from burning. If your oven door has a window, peek and check—don't open the door!

RECIPE CONTINUED . . .

PASSOVER NOTHINGS (continued)

- **Warning light:** If you have an older oven and the temperature light turns on during baking, drop the temperature slightly until the light turns off. Otherwise, your cookies will be too dark.

- **Cute tip:** A cotton swab will remove sticky dough from the hole on the underside of the steel blade.

DR. ED SAYS:

- **Overall,** this recipe is basically fat, starch, and sugar, with not too much of a nutrient contribution except for eggs (which contribute high-quality protein, vitamin B12, some vitamin D, and choline) and vegetable oil (which contributes vitamin E). In addition, each cookie has significant digestible carbs and sugar. The main benefit is the low-calorie content per serving. Enjoy in moderation.

ROGELACH ROLL-UPS

PAREVE | FREEZES WELL | MAKES 24 ROLL-UPS

Versatile, easy, and dairy-free! Instead of forming individual crescents, this simple technique speeds up preparation. That's the way to roll! These can be addictive, so save them as an occasional treat.

1. **PASTRY:** In a food processor using the steel blade, process flour and margarine with several on/off pulses, until mixture resembles coarse oatmeal. Add liquids through the feed tube while the machine is running. Process just until dough begins to gather in a mass around the blades, 8–10 seconds. Do not over-process.

2. Form dough into 2 balls and wrap in plastic wrap. Refrigerate at least 1 hour, or overnight. The colder the dough, the easier it is to roll.

3. **FILLING:** Process filling ingredients until finely ground, 25–30 seconds.

4. Preheat oven to 375°F (190°C). Line a rimmed baking sheet with parchment paper.

5. **ASSEMBLY:** Thinly roll out one ball of chilled dough on parchment paper into a rectangle. (Tip: Wipe the work surface with a damp cloth and the parchment paper won't move!) Sprinkle filling evenly over the dough, leaving a ½-inch (1 cm) border on all sides. Roll up like a jelly roll starting from the long side. Repeat with the remaining dough and filling.

6. Using a serrated knife, slice each roll into 12 pieces. Place on the prepared sheet.

7. Bake for 18–20 minutes, until golden. Once cooled, store in an airtight container.

80 calories per roll-up, 6 g carbohydrates, 1 g sugar, 0 g fiber, 1 g protein, 6 g fat (1 g saturated), 36 mg sodium, 23 mg potassium

NORENE'S NOTES:

- **Be prepared:** Dough may be frozen, baked, or unbaked, and filling can be refrigerated or frozen—so why not make several batches?

RECIPE CONTINUED . . .

PASTRY:

1 cup + 2 Tbsp (280 mL) flour

½ cup (125 mL) frozen tub margarine or Earth Balance, cut into chunks

¼ cup (60 mL) sugar-free ginger ale or soda water

1½ tsp (7 mL) vinegar or lemon juice

FILLING:

3–4 Tbsp (45–60 mL) Splenda Brown Sugar Blend

½ tsp (2 mL) ground cinnamon

⅓ cup (80 mL) chocolate chips (sugar-free chips work well)

⅓ cup (80 mL) walnut pieces or almonds

- **Traditional rogelach:** Roll one piece of dough at a time into a circle instead of a rectangle. Sprinkle with half the filling, then cut with a sharp knife or a pastry wheel into 12 wedges. Roll up each wedge from the outside edge towards the center and place on the prepared sheet. Repeat with the remaining dough and filling. Bake as directed above.

DR. ED SAYS:

- **Ginger ale pastry:** This is the major source of digestible carbs in the recipe, but the fat and acidity will help to control blood sugar concentration.

- **Filling:** This is where most of the nutrition lies. Reducing the sugar by using Splenda Brown Sugar Blend instead of regular sugar, and using sugar-free chocolate chips, results in a very low sugar content of 1 g per cookie, without holding back on brain nutrition. I recommend using an equal combination of almonds and walnuts as each kind has its own special strength. Almonds provide an excellent source of natural vitamin E, whereas walnuts provide an excellent quantity of plant-based Omega-3 fat in the form of alpha-linolenic acid. The nuts also provide high fiber, high protein, magnesium, zinc, manganese, folate, and antioxidants. The cinnamon and chocolate round out the variety of antioxidants supplied.

DID YOU KNOW? Rogelach is a Yiddish term meaning little twists, referring to the shape of the pastry. Rogelach originated from the Jewish population in Eastern Europe. The filling often varies and may include several dried fruits, nuts, poppy seeds, fruit preserves, and so on. It is believed that the croissant, which is similar in shape, was based on this pastry.

SECRET INGREDIENT BROWNIES

PAREVE | GLUTEN-FREE | FREEZES WELL | MAKES 12 BROWNIES

You'll get brownie points for this one! Thanks to my friend Susan Gould for sharing the recipe for these delicious flourless brownies. She got it from her friend Gloria Sheen, who got it from the internet, and we've adapted it to make it brain-friendly. As an added bonus, these brownies are egg-free, and if made with maple syrup they are vegan-friendly too.

1. Preheat oven to 350°F (175°C). Spray an 8-inch (20 cm) square baking pan with nonstick cooking spray.

2. In a food processor fitted with the steel blade, combine beans, cocoa, oats, maple syrup, oil, vanilla, baking powder, and salt. Process until smooth and well blended, scraping down the sides of the bowl several times with a rubber spatula.

3. Stir in chocolate chips and chopped nuts, if using.

4. Pour batter into the prepared pan and spread evenly. Top with walnut or pecan halves, if using, pressing them slightly into the batter.

5. Bake for 18–20 minutes, until set. Remove from oven and let cool for 10 minutes. If they look undercooked, don't worry—refrigerate them overnight and they will firm up.

6. Cut into squares and store in the refrigerator.

162 calories per brownie, 20 g carbohydrates, 6 g sugar, 3 g fiber, 3 g protein, 8 g fat (3 g saturated), 5 mg sodium, 147 mg potassium

NORENE'S NOTES:

- **Secret ingredient brownie bites:** In Step 1, spray 24 compartments of a mini muffin pan (or pans) with nonstick cooking spray. In Step 4, spoon batter into a muffin pan (or pans). Arrange 24 walnut or pecan pieces on top; press them slightly into the batter. Bake for 16–18 minutes, until set. Remove pan from oven and let cool for 10 minutes. Remove brownie bites from the pan and store in the refrigerator.

RECIPE CONTINUED . . .

1 can (15 oz/425 g) black beans, drained and rinsed (preferably no-salt-added)

2 Tbsp (30 mL) unsweetened cocoa powder

½ cup (125 mL) gluten-free quick-cooking rolled oats (e.g., Bob's Red Mill)

⅓ cup (80 mL) maple syrup or honey

¼ cup (60 mL) canola oil

2 tsp (10 mL) pure vanilla extract

½ tsp (2 mL) baking powder

Pinch of salt

½ cup (125 mL) chocolate chips (sugar-free or semisweet)

½ cup (125 mL) chopped walnuts or pecans (optional)

12 walnut or pecan halves (optional, for garnish)

DR. ED SAYS:

- **Black beans** are part of the legume family. As with most members of this family, they are high in antioxidants, protein, and fiber, and are low in digestible carbs and sugars. Therefore, they have good GI and GL values, resulting in low blood sugar response. They also contain reasonable levels of vitamin E, folate, magnesium, manganese, and zinc.

- **Rolled oats** are a good source of soluble fiber with a low GI if they are not processed too much. Therefore, when possible, choose large-flake cooking oats. The less the processing, the more resistant starch (equivalent to fiber) they will contain, as well as less digestible carbohydrates.

- **Overall,** per serving, we are getting reasonable levels of vitamin E, magnesium, zinc, and folate. Although the brownies are somewhat high in sugar, the beans and oats will help minimize its harmful effects.

> DID YOU KNOW? Generally, the more processed a food, the higher its GI and GL will be. Thus, mashed potatoes (vs baked potatoes), fruit juice (vs raw fruit), and quick-cooking oats (vs large-flake or steel-cut oats), will all have a higher GI and GL.

DOUBLE CHOCOLATE DELIGHTS

PAREVE | GLUTEN-FREE | PASSOVER | FREEZES WELL | MAKES
ABOUT 48 COOKIES

Double your pleasure with this doubly delicious hit of chocolate! These are perfect for Passover or any time of year.

2 large eggs

⅔ cup (160 mL) sugar

1 tsp (5 mL) pure vanilla extract

2 Tbsp (30 mL) unsweetened cocoa powder

3 cups (750 mL) slivered and/or chopped almonds (I like a combination)

¾ cup (185 mL) mini chocolate chips

1. Preheat oven to 350°F (175°C). Line a large cookie sheet (or sheets) with parchment paper (see Norene's Notes).

2. In a large mixing bowl, combine eggs, sugar, and vanilla; mix well. Add cocoa, almonds, and chocolate chips, and stir to combine.

3. Drop in rounded teaspoonfuls onto the prepared cookie sheet(s), making small mounds (these won't spread during baking.)

4. Bake cookies for 15 minutes, until firm. Cool for 15 minutes before removing from pan. Store in a loosely covered container.

67 calories per cookie, 6 g carbohydrates, 5 g sugar, 1 g fiber, 2 g protein, 4 g fat (1 g saturated), 3 mg sodium, 66 mg potassium

NORENE'S NOTES:

- **Position is everything:** If baking two pans of cookies at the same time that don't fit on the same rack, place racks so they divide the oven space evenly into thirds. For even browning, switch (from top to bottom) and rotate pans (from back to front) for the last few minutes of baking.

- **Pan-tastic!** Not enough cookie sheets? While the first batch of cookies is in the oven, place the next batch of dough on a sheet of parchment paper. When the first batch is baked, slide parchment paper (along with the baked cookies still on top) off the pan. Cool pan slightly, then replace with the next batch and bake.

DR. ED SAYS:

- **Chocolate:** Milk chocolate contains about 50% sugar, whereas dark chocolate, with about 70–85% cocoa solids, contains about half that amount. Because of the higher cocoa solids in this recipe, the nutritional density is also higher, including fiber, magnesium, potassium, manganese, zinc, and vitamin B12. Chocolate contains high levels of

RECIPE CONTINUED . . .

gamma tocopherol, a form of vitamin E important to brain health and not readily available in other foods. Therefore, we recommend using dark chocolate with high cocoa solids and, if available, the sugar-free version, which is available from many suppliers.

- **Overall,** this recipe is notable for its use of cocoa powder and chocolate chips and its large quantity of almonds. Each cookie thus provides a good level of important forms of vitamin E, some fiber, protein, and antioxidants. The one drawback of the recipe—its high sugar content—could be improved by using granulated Splenda instead of sugar, and by using sugar-free chocolate chips.

> DID YOU KNOW? Cocoa beans, which originated in Central and South America, were so prized that they were used as currency. Christopher Columbus was the first European to encounter cocoa beans. Originally cocoa beans were used in Europe primarily in chocolate drinks—chocolate candy did not develop until the 19th century.

3-SEED COOKIES

PAREVE | GLUTEN-FREE | FREEZES WELL | MAKES 24–30 COOKIES (DEPENDING ON SIZE)

Addictive! These amazing 3-seed cookies are one of the most popular recipes in my Facebook group, Norene's Kitchen! My friend Rita Gross got the recipe from her friend Elly Shulkin, who got it from her sister, Verna. The add-ins are endless and the cookies taste terrific straight from the freezer. So delicious—bet you can't stop at just one!

1 cup (250 mL) unsalted sunflower seeds

1 cup (250 mL) unsalted pumpkin seeds

½ cup (125 mL) sesame seeds

¼ cup (60 mL) brown sugar, lightly packed

¼ cup (60 mL) dried cranberries or mini chocolate chips

2 egg whites, slightly beaten

Optional add-ins: chopped walnuts, pecans, pistachios, slivered almonds, hemp seeds, raisins, chopped dried apricots

1. Preheat oven to 325°F (160°C). Line a large, rimmed baking sheet with parchment paper.

2. Combine sunflower seeds, pumpkin seeds, sesame seeds, brown sugar, and dried cranberries in a large bowl. Mix together.

3. Pour egg whites overtop and mix until well incorporated.

4. Pack mixture tightly into a mini scoop and release onto the prepared baking sheet. Using light pressure, flatten cookies slightly with a fork.

5. Bake for 20 minutes, until nicely toasted. Remove pan from oven and let cookies cool on the baking sheet for about 10 minutes.

6. Store either on the counter, in the refrigerator, or hide them in the freezer!

76 calories per cookie, 6 g carbohydrates, 2 g fiber, 3 g sugar, 2 g protein, 5 g fat (<1 g saturated), 6 mg sodium, 73 mg potassium

NORENE'S NOTES:

- **"Neat" trick:** My friend Helene Medjuck uses a mini scoop and drops the mixture into muffin tins that have been lined with parchment cupcake liners. This mess-proof method ensures that the cookies will hold together.

- **Eggs-actly?** You may need to add an extra egg white to bind the mixture. Liquid egg whites, the kind that come in a carton, don't bind the mixture as well as when you use real egg whites. Vegans can use aquafaba (see p. 191).

RECIPE CONTINUED . . .

3-SEED COOKIES (continued)

- **Sunflower seeds, pumpkin seeds, sesame seeds:** You can't go wrong with any of these seeds as they are all very low in moisture, which means they are nutrient-dense and mostly made up of protein, good fat, and fiber. This means they have low carbs and sugar, which also results in a low GI and low GL.

- **Cranberries:** Keep in mind that commonly available dried and sweetened cranberries are made up of more than 70% sugar when compared to natural cranberries, which are only about 4% sugar. Consider using no-sugar-added dried cranberries. Check online sources.

- **Overall,** as with most recipes in this section, the sugar levels are on the high side because of the added sugar. However, this is mitigated somewhat by the inclusion of the seeds and cranberries, which contribute significant fiber, folate, vitamin B6, magnesium, and zinc.

> DID YOU KNOW? Glycemic index is only one indicator of the blood sugar impact of a food. A better number is glycemic load, because it is based on the total digestible carbohydrates consumed, which is better correlated with blood sugar response.

BEST OATMEAL COOKIES

PAREVE | FREEZES WELL | MAKES ABOUT 42 COOKIES

These scrumptious cookies are "oat" of this world!

½ cup (125 mL) canola oil

1 large egg (or 2 egg whites)

⅓ cup (80 mL) lightly packed brown sugar

⅓ cup (80 mL) sugar

2 Tbsp (30 mL) water

1 tsp (5 mL) pure vanilla extract

¾ cup (185 mL) whole wheat flour (preferably whole wheat pastry flour)

1½ cups (375 mL) rolled oats (preferably large flake)

¼ cup (60 mL) wheat germ

½ tsp (2 mL) baking soda

1 tsp (5 mL) ground cinnamon

⅛ tsp (0.5 mL) salt

⅓ cup (80 mL) pareve mini semi-sweet chocolate chips

⅓ cup (80 mL) raisins or dried cranberries (optional)

⅓ cup (80 mL) sunflower seeds or chopped almonds, walnuts, or pecans (optional)

1. Preheat oven to 350°F (175°C). Line 2 large, rimmed baking sheets with parchment paper.

2. In a food processor fitted with the steel blade (or in a large bowl and using an electric mixer), beat oil, egg, sugars, water, and vanilla until well blended, about 1 minute. Add flour, rolled oats, wheat germ, baking soda, cinnamon, and salt; mix well. If using a food processor, transfer batter to a large bowl. Stir in chocolate chips, raisins, and seeds or nuts (if using).

3. Drop batter in rounded teaspoonfuls onto the prepared sheets.

4. Bake for 10–12 minutes, until golden. Repeat with the second batch.

63 calories per cookie, 8 g carbohydrates, 4 g sugar, 1 g fiber, 1 g protein, 4 g fat (1 g saturated), 24 mg sodium, 33 mg potassium

NORENE'S NOTES:

- **Wheat germ or wheat bran?** What's the difference? They're separate parts of the same grain—the bran is the outer coating and the wheat germ is the inner part. Wheat germ supplies nutrients such as protein, B vitamins, and vitamin E, whereas wheat bran has more fiber. So, include both in your diet for good health.

DR. ED SAYS:

- **Wheat germ** is a powerhouse of essential brain nutrients. It is an excellent source of vitamins B6 and E and folate, as well as the following minerals: magnesium, potassium, zinc, manganese, and selenium. Its vitamin E content in particular is very high, and just 1 Tbsp (15 mL) provides the recommended daily allowance of 15 mg.

- **Rolled oats** are high in soluble fiber and protein and have a low GI; they also contain good amounts of zinc and selenium. Avoid the quick-cooking or instant varieties, as they have high available carbs and a high GI.

DID YOU KNOW? Wheat germ is only 2.5% of the wheat kernel by weight, but because it is the primary source of nutrients for the new sprout it is highly concentrated in important nutrients.

CRANBERRY OATMEAL FLAX COOKIES

PAREVE | FREEZES WELL | MAKES ABOUT 36 COOKIES

7 Tbsp (105 mL) canola oil

⅓ cup (80 mL) brown sugar, lightly packed

⅓ cup (80 mL) sugar

1 large egg (or 2 egg whites)

1 tsp (5 mL) pure vanilla extract

½ tsp (2 mL) ground cinnamon

½ cup (125 mL) whole wheat pastry flour (or ¼ cup/60 mL whole wheat + ¼ cup/60 mL all-purpose flour)

1 cup (250 mL) rolled oats (preferably large flake)

½ cup (125 mL) ground flaxseed (see Norene's Notes)

½ tsp (2 mL) baking soda

⅓–½ cup (80–125 mL) dried cranberries

½ cup (125 mL) pumpkin seeds

These yummy cookies from Shayla Goldstein of Toronto have become one of my favorites. I've reduced the sugar and added pumpkin seeds and cinnamon. It's a delicious way to incorporate flaxseed into your diet!

1. Preheat oven to 350°F (175°C). Line a large, rimmed baking sheet with parchment paper.

2. In a food processor fitted with the steel blade, combine oil, sugars, egg, vanilla, and cinnamon. Process for 1 minute, until well blended.

3. Add flour, rolled oats, flaxseed, and baking soda; process with quick on/off pulses to combine. Stir in cranberries and pumpkin seeds with a rubber spatula.

4. Drop batter in rounded teaspoonfuls onto the prepared baking sheet, leaving 2 inches (5 cm) between each cookie. Flatten each mound with the tines of a fork.

5. Bake for 10–12 minutes, until golden.

83 calories per cookie, 9 g carbohydrates, 4 g sugar, 1 g fiber, 2 g protein, 5 g fat (1 g saturated), 21 mg sodium, 49 mg potassium

NORENE'S NOTES:

- **Be flax-ible!** Flaxseed increases in volume when ground, so you'll need 6 Tbsp (90 mL) whole flaxseed to get ½ cup (125 mL) ground. Grind flaxseed in a clean coffee grinder or mini processor. While you're at it, why not grind up an extra batch? It keeps for several months in the refrigerator or freezer in a resealable plastic bag or container.

- **Variations:** Use no-sugar-added dried cranberries. Substitute chopped walnuts, pistachios, almonds, or pecans for pumpkin seeds. Add ½ cup (125 mL) mini chocolate chips, if desired.

- **Flaxseed** is a member of the seeds and nuts family and is therefore nutrient-dense. It is particularly known for its high content of soluble fiber, plant Omega-3 fat (alpha-linolenic acid), and the unique antioxidant lignan. Flax contains up to 800 times the lignan content compared to other plant foods. In some studies, lignan has been found to reduce the risk of breast cancer due to its estrogenic properties.

- **Pumpkin seeds** are another very nutritious seed that are rich in important brain nutrients. They do not have the lignan and ALA content of flax, but do have higher vitamin E levels.

> DID YOU KNOW? Flaxseed and its oil are one of the richest sources of plant Omega-3 fat in the form of alpha-linolenic acid (ALA). ALA is a precursor to the formation of the more effective Omega-3 fats EPA and DHA, but it is inefficiently converted to EPA and DHA, especially in older adults. Nevertheless, it has health benefits in its own right. In the eighth century, King Charlemagne required his subjects to consume flaxseeds for their health benefits.

PEANUT BUTTER COOKIES

PAREVE | GLUTEN-FREE | FREEZES WELL | MAKES 26 COOKIES (IF MADE WITH SUGAR) OR 21 COOKIES (IF MADE WITH SWEETENER)

1 cup (250 mL) creamy or crunchy natural peanut butter

¾ cup (185 mL) sugar or granulated Splenda

1 large egg

Three ingredients, three minutes to mix up the batter, and less than three minutes before they're gone! You can make these gluten-free cookies with sugar or Splenda (see Norene's Notes). They are addictive, so practice portion control and save them as an occasional treat.

1. Preheat oven to 325°F (160°C). Line a large, rimmed baking sheet with parchment paper.

2. In a large mixing bowl, combine peanut butter, sugar, and egg; mix well.

3. Drop in rounded teaspoonfuls onto the prepared sheet, leaving 2 inches (5 cm) between each cookie. (If you use Splenda, place a piece of parchment or wax paper on top of the unbaked cookies and press gently to flatten before baking (see Norene's Notes). Uncover cookies before baking them.

4. Bake for 10 minutes, until golden. Remove from oven and let cookies cool on a baking sheet for 10–15 minutes. They will firm up as they cool.

WITH SUGAR: 90 calories per cookie, 8 g carbohydrates, 6 g sugar, 1 g fiber, 2 g protein, 5 g fat (1 g saturated), 3 mg sodium, 3 mg potassium

WITH SPLENDA: 70 calories per cookie, 3 g carbohydrates, 0 g sugar, 1 g fiber, 2 g protein, 5 g fat (1 g saturated), 3 mg sodium, 3 mg potassium

NORENE'S NOTES:

· What's the spread? Cookies made with sugar will spread during baking, whereas cookies made with Splenda will stay in a mound and won't spread unless you flatten them before baking.

· Batter up! You get more batter (and cookies) when using sugar, but less batter (and cookies) with Splenda. That's the way the cookie crumbles!

RECIPE CONTINUED . . .

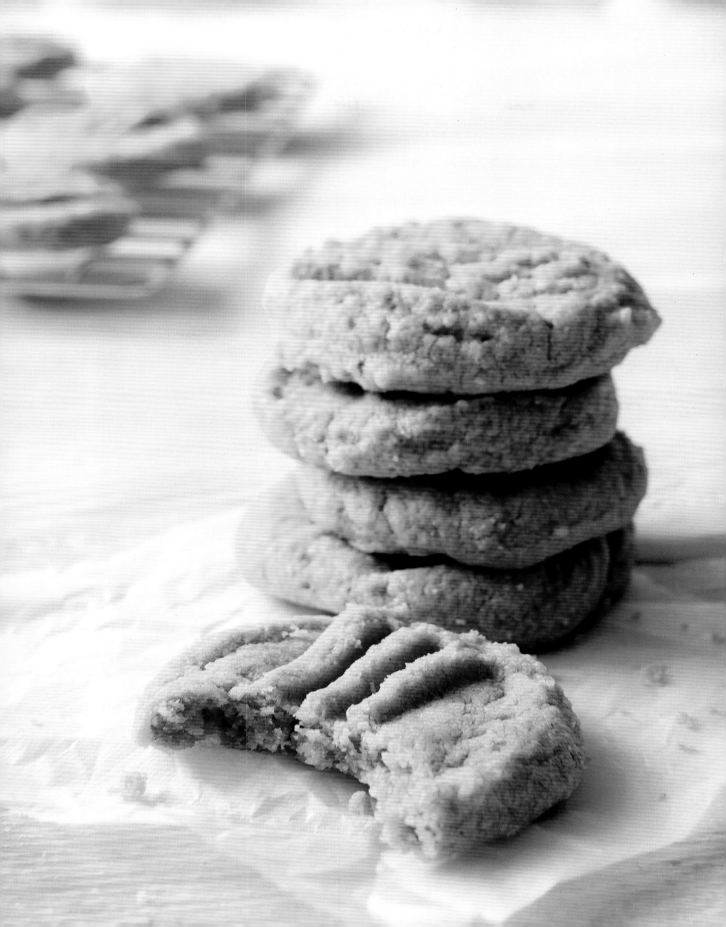

PEANUT BUTTER COOKIES (continued)

DR. ED SAYS:

- **Peanut butter** is mostly good monounsaturated fat, protein, and some fiber. It is relatively low in digestible carbohydrates, and in combination with the high fiber and fat, it has an extremely low GI and GL (7 and 0, respectively). Per 100 g, it is also an excellent source of magnesium, potassium, manganese, and vitamins B6 and E, though each cookie only carries about 5% of these nutrients. Nevertheless, it is a great food for brain health.

DID YOU KNOW? George Washington Carver, a black inventor who lived in the first half of the 20th century, developed over 300 products from peanuts, including soup, bread, cake flour, milk, dye, and cheese.

SUGAR-FREE MERINGUE COOKIES

PAREVE | GLUTEN-FREE | DO NOT FREEZE | MAKES 24 COOKIES

Wendy Baker of New York sent this recipe to me and wrote: "Eureka! At last, a light meringue cookie that works without sugar and still holds up in baking! These are more fragile than meringue cookies made with sugar, so handle them with care." This recipe is a modified version of one she got from a diabetes support newsgroup.

3 egg whites, at room temperature

⅛ tsp (0.5 mL) cream of tartar

1 tsp (5 mL) pure vanilla or almond extract

½ cup (125 mL) granulated Splenda

2 Tbsp (30 mL) grated orange rind

24 semisweet pareve chocolate chips

1. Preheat oven to 350°F (175°C). Line a large, rimmed baking sheet with parchment paper.

2. In a large glass or stainless-steel mixing bowl, using an electric mixer, beat egg whites on medium-high speed until foamy. Add cream of tartar and vanilla and beat until soft peaks form. Reduce speed to low and gradually beat in Splenda. Increase speed to high and continue beating until stiff peaks form. Using a rubber spatula, carefully fold in orange rind.

3. Drop meringue in mounds from a teaspoon onto the prepared sheet. Top each mound with a chocolate chip. Bake for 10 minutes. Turn off the oven with the meringues still inside for 30 minutes to let them dry (no peeking allowed!). Once cooled, store in a loosely covered container so the meringues stay crisp.

7 calories per cookie, 1 g carbohydrates, 0 g sugar, 0 g fiber, <1 g protein, 0 g fat (0 g saturated), 7 mg sodium, 12 mg potassium

NORENE'S NOTES:

- **Bowl them over:** Use either a stainless steel or glass bowl to whip egg whites, as they won't whip well in a plastic bowl. Also, make sure your beaters and bowl are clean and grease-free—even a trace of grease will keep the whites from beating properly. When egg whites are properly beaten, you should be able to turn the bowl upside down without the whites falling out.

- **Freeze with ease:** If you substitute 6 Tbsp (90 mL) sugar for the Splenda then you will be able to freeze these, because meringues made with sugar aren't as fragile.

RECIPE CONTINUED . . .

DR. ED SAYS:

- **Orange rind:** This is a rich source of flavonoid polyphenol antioxidants, especially naringin and hesperidin, which are found in citrus peels. The concentration of antioxidants in orange rinds is higher than that found in lemon or grapefruit rinds. Orange rinds are also excellent sources of fiber and vitamin C, as well as being good sources of B vitamins.

- **Egg whites** are a great source of high-quality protein, but we only get <1 g per cookie since they are used primarily as binding agents in this recipe.

- **Overall,** we do not get a lot of brain nutrients per cookie, but neither do we get deleterious components such as excess calories, sugars, digestible carbs, or saturated fats. We do, on the other hand, get good plant antioxidants from the chocolate chips and orange rind.

DID YOU KNOW? Pesticides tend to concentrate in the peel of the orange as opposed to the fruit, and they can exceed dangerous concentrations, especially in oranges imported from countries that have laxer health control guidelines. It is therefore recommended that one use orange peels from organic oranges and from oranges grown in the USA.

LEMON MERINGUE CLOUDS

PAREVE | GLUTEN-FREE | PASSOVER | FREEZES WELL | MAKES 24 COOKIES

These guilt-free cookies taste a lot like the topping for a lemon meringue pie.

3 egg whites, at room temperature

1 tsp (5 mL) lemon juice (preferably fresh)

6 Tbsp (90 mL) sugar

1 Tbsp (15 mL) grated lemon zest

---

1. Preheat oven to 250°F (120°C). Line a large, rimmed baking sheet with parchment paper.

2. In a large glass or stainless-steel mixing bowl, beat egg whites using an electric mixer on medium-high speed, until foamy. Drizzle in lemon juice and beat until soft peaks form. Gradually beat in sugar, 1 Tbsp (15 mL) at a time. Continue beating until stiff and shiny. Using a rubber spatula, fold in lemon zest.

3. Drop meringue in mounds from a tablespoon onto the prepared sheet.

4. Bake for 1 hour. Turn off the oven, with meringues still inside, for 1 hour longer to let them dry.

5. Once cooled, store in a loosely covered container so the meringues will stay crisp.

15 calories per cookie, 3 g carbohydrates, 3 g sugar, 0 g fiber, <1 g protein, 0 g fat (0 g saturated), 7 mg sodium, 7 mg potassium

NORENE'S NOTES:

- **Egg white wisdom:** Eggs separate best when they're cold, but whip best when they're at room temperature. Make sure no yolks get into the whites or they won't whip properly (see Norene's Notes, p. 565).

DR. ED SAYS:

- **Lemon juice and lemon zest:** These provide vitamin C, fiber, and antioxidants to a limited extent, but the recipe does not contribute much else other than a small amount of good egg protein per cookie. The sugar level per cookie is a bit on the high side at 3 g, so it's best to consume these cookies in moderation.

DID YOU KNOW? Protein and fat tend to bring down the GI of high GI foods, as in this recipe. Therefore, having these cookies with a little cheese will help control blood sugar.

CHOCOLATE ALMOND APRICOT CLUSTERS

PAREVE | GLUTEN-FREE | PASSOVER | FREEZES WELL | MAKES ABOUT 48 CLUSTERS

10 oz (300 g) good-quality dark chocolate (bittersweet or sugar-free; see Norene's Notes)

1 Tbsp (15 mL) vegetable oil

2 cups (500 mL) roasted unsalted slivered almonds

1½ cups (375 mL) cut-up dried apricots (8 oz/235 mL; scissors work best)

These are so good you'll need to pray they last through Passover! Chocolate lifts your spirits when you're feeling tired and overwhelmed with Passover preparations, and these no-bake treats are the perfect "pick-me-up." They also a wonderful and easy gift to bring to a Seder, or to enjoy any time of year. Everyone will cluster around you when you bring these to the table!

1. Break up chocolate into chunks and place in a large, dry microwaveable bowl. Microwave, uncovered, on medium for 2 minutes, then stir. Continue microwaving on medium for 1–2 minutes longer, until barely melted; stir well. Cool slightly, then stir in oil, almonds, and apricots.

2. Drop in teaspoonfuls onto parchment paper–lined baking sheets. Refrigerate for 30–45 minutes, or until firm.

3. Transfer to an airtight container, separating layers with parchment or wax paper. Refrigerate or freeze. Great straight from the freezer—control yourself!

81 calories per cluster, 7 g carbohydrates, 5 g sugar, 1 g fiber, 2 g protein, 6 g fat (2 g saturated), 1 mg sodium, 122 mg potassium

NORENE'S NOTES:

- **Deep dark secrets:** The darker the chocolate, the higher its antioxidant content and the less sugar it contains. Choose the best quality you can get. A 1-oz (30 g) serving of dark chocolate (70% or higher) contains 2–3 g fiber, depending on the brand. Bittersweet and sugar-free chocolate are interchangeable in this recipe, although sugar-free chocolate may not be easy to find during Passover. Check online sources.

- **Chocolate in bloom:** If chocolate is stored above 70°F (21°C), it will "bloom" (get white streaks). Not to worry—the streaks will disappear when the chocolate melts.

- **Melting moments:** Use a bowl that is completely wiped dry, and don't cover it when melting chocolate or the chocolate can "seize" (become solid and grainy). The mixing spoon should also be dry.

<u>**DR. ED SAYS:**</u>

- **Dried apricots** are another fruit with a very high sugar content, at 75% by dry weight. However, they also have a high fiber content, high levels of carotenoid antioxidants, and high potassium, as well as good levels of vitamin B6 and magnesium.

- **Overall,** despite the high sugar and digestible carb levels per cookie, we mitigate this somewhat by the high content of simple and complex antioxidants in the chocolate and apricots, and especially by the vitamin E in the almonds.

> **DID YOU KNOW?** High soluble fiber and fructose levels help reduce the GI of fruits and therefore the blood response. This explains in part why dried apricots have a relatively low GI and GL. Nevertheless, it is advised to eat them in moderation, as is true for most dried fruits.

CHOCOLATE BLUEBERRY BLOBS

PAREVE | GLUTEN-FREE | PASSOVER | DO NOT FREEZE | MAKES
ABOUT 30 PIECES

2 cups (500 mL) fresh
blueberries

8 oz (235 g) good-quality
dark chocolate, broken
up into chunks

These blobs are "berry" easy to make and, as an added bonus, berries will boost your brainpower. Kids and adults alike love these scrumptious, gluten-free treats. What a decadent way to eat your blueberries!

---

1. Line a baking sheet with parchment paper. Rinse blueberries and pat completely dry.

2. Meanwhile, place chocolate into a clean, dry bowl, and place it over a saucepan of simmering water. Melt over medium heat, stirring occasionally. (Alternatively, melt chocolate in a glass bowl in the microwave for 1 minute on medium power and stir well; microwave 30–60 seconds more.)

3. Let chocolate cool to lukewarm before gently mixing in blueberries with a rubber spatula. Continue gently mixing until berries are well coated with chocolate.

4. Drop blobs of the chocolate mixture from a teaspoon onto the prepared baking sheet about 2 inches (5 cm) apart. Refrigerate until firm, about 1 hour. Store in the refrigerator for 1–2 days.

47 calories per piece, 6 g carbohydrates, 1 g fiber, 4 g sugar, 1 g protein, 3 g fat (2 g saturated), 0 mg sodium, 8 mg potassium

NORENE'S NOTES:

- **Variation:** Use a combination of equal parts blueberries and pomegranate arils.

- **Berry important!** Dry blueberries thoroughly before adding them to melted chocolate. If any moisture gets into the chocolate it will seize (get thick and lumpy). Don't use frozen blueberries!

- **Dark secret!** Instead of dark chocolate, substitute 1⅓ cups (310 mL) chocolate chips and 2 tsp (10 mL) canola or grapeseed oil.

DR. ED SAYS:

- **Blueberries:** This recipe has many of the same benefits as Berry-Apple Crisp (p. 537). Blueberries provide very high levels of antioxidants, which are particularly beneficial to cognitive health. The high sugar content is offset by the high fiber content and the overwhelming benefits of the antioxidants.

- **Pomegranate seeds** (see variation in Norene's Notes) are considered an excellent food for the brain. They are low in calories, rich in fiber, and packed with antioxidants.

- **Dark chocolate** is also loaded with antioxidants, and studies have shown it to have cognitive and heart benefits. Chocolate contains high levels of sugar, so sugar-free dark chocolate is a better choice for those watching their sugar intake.

- **Overall,** this is an A+ treat because of the antioxidants in the berries and dark chocolate.

> DID YOU KNOW? Blueberries contain among the highest sugar levels in the berry family and have about three times the blood sugar response as strawberries, blackberries, and raspberries.

CHOCOLATE BARK

DAIRY | GLUTEN-FREE | PASSOVER | FREEZES WELL | MAKES ABOUT
48 PIECES

1 lb (500 g) good-quality
dark chocolate

1½ cups (375 mL) roasted
unsalted whole almonds, divided

2 oz (60 g) white chocolate

Your guests will be barking for more! If you are watching your calories, try to choose smaller chunks, or see Norene's Notes for tips on portion control.

---

1. Break dark chocolate into chunks and place in a large dry microwavable bowl. Microwave uncovered on medium for 2 minutes, then stir. Microwave on medium for 1–2 minutes longer, until barely melted, then stir well. Let cool for 5 minutes. Stir in 1¼ cups (310 mL) nuts.

2. Spread in a thin layer on a parchment-lined baking sheet. Sprinkle with the remaining nuts, pressing them into the chocolate mixture.

3. Melt white chocolate on medium power for 1½–2 minutes and stir well. If necessary, microwave for 30 seconds longer, or until melted.

4. Dip a fork into the melted white chocolate and drizzle over the bark in a zig-zag design.

5. Refrigerate for 30–45 minutes, until hard. Break into small chunks and transfer to an airtight container, separating layers with parchment or wax paper. Store in the refrigerator.

87 calories per piece, 7 g carbohydrates, 4 g sugar, 1 g fiber, 2 g protein, 6 g fat (3 g saturated), 2 mg sodium, 88 mg potassium

NORENE'S NOTES:

- **Instant portion control:** In Step 2, instead of spreading the mixture onto the baking sheet, drop in teaspoonfuls into equal-sized mounds.

- **Allergic to nuts?** Substitute nuts with Passover ready-to-eat cereal, raisins, dried cranberries, or pomegranate arils.

- **Nuts to you:** Instead of whole almonds, use chopped pecans or walnuts.

RECIPE CONTINUED . . .

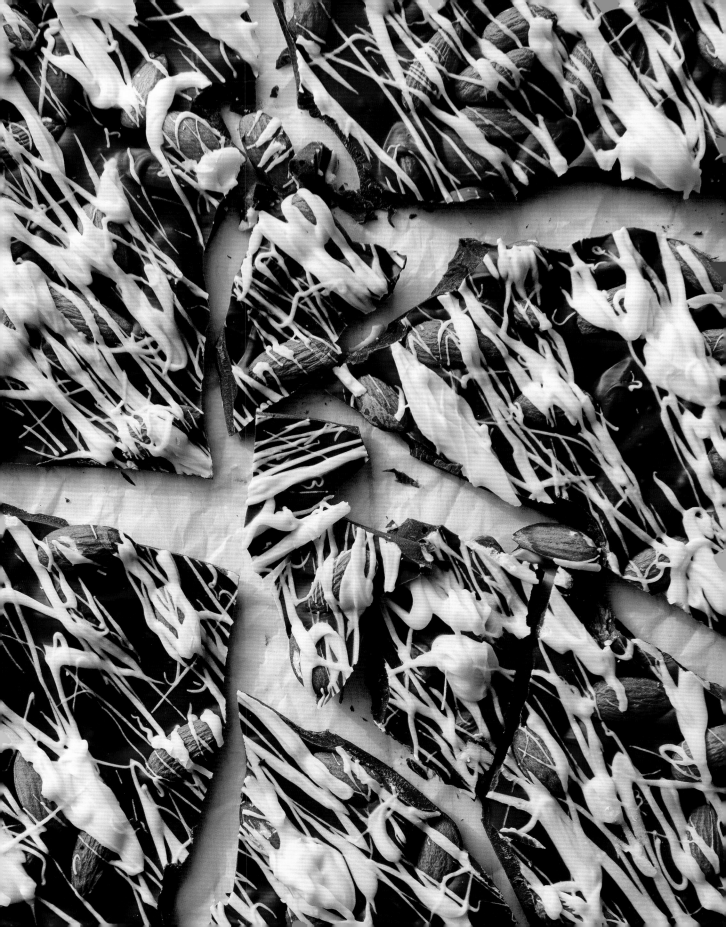

CHOCOLATE BARK (continued)

DR. ED SAYS:

- **Dark chocolate,** which is one of the major ingredients in this recipe, contains more antioxidants than milk chocolate, and is among the foods with the highest antioxidant content. Among its major antioxidants is a group of flavanol antioxidants called catechins which have been linked to healthy brains. Studies with cocoa solids, either as dark chocolate or cocoa powder, have shown increased blood flow to the brain and improved cognition when cocoa powder is consumed on a regular basis. The higher cocoa solids in dark chocolate also contain high fiber, high protein, and high vitamin E in the form of gamma tocopherol, which is important for brain health. Dark chocolate is also an excellent source of magnesium, manganese, zinc, and potassium, and is a good source of vitamin B12 per 100 g. The main drawback with dark chocolate is its high content of saturated fat and high sugar. Sugar-free chocolate will solve the sugar issue, but the saturated fat needs to be controlled by moderate consumption, or by switching to cocoa powder instead of chocolate. If using chocolate, we recommend using one with 70–85% cocoa solids.

- **Overall, t**he combination of 70–85% sugar-free dark chocolate with almonds makes for a great brain dessert.

> **DID YOU KNOW?** Many studies have shown that cocoa solids can reduce risk factors leading to heart disease, and one study over 15 years found that cocoa solids can decrease mortality from heart disease by 50%. This appears to be due to the ability of the cocoa to prevent oxidation of LDL cholesterol, reduce blood pressure, and reduce the risk of diabetes.

CHOCOLATE MYSTERY MOUSSE

PAREVE | GLUTEN-FREE | DO NOT FREEZE | MAKES 4 SERVINGS

Cocoa and tofu make for a delicious pairing, and have more in common than you'd think. Both come from beans (cocoa beans and soybeans), and both are scrumptious in desserts. So, if you can keep a secret, no one will ever guess this luscious dessert has anything to do with tofu, unless, of course, you tell them!

1 pkg (16 oz/500 g) extra-firm or firm silken tofu, well drained

Sweetener equivalent to ¾ cup (185 mL) sugar (e.g., granulated Splenda)

⅔ cup (160 mL) unsweetened cocoa powder

1 tsp (5 mL) pure vanilla or almond extract

Coconut "Whipped Cream" (p. 533) (optional, for garnish)

Grated chocolate (optional, for garnish)

1. In a food processor fitted with the steel blade, process tofu for 1–2 minutes, until very smooth; scrape down the sides of the bowl as needed. Add the remaining ingredients and process until blended, about 20 seconds longer.

2. Transfer mixture into parfait or wine glasses.

3. Garnish with whipped cream and grated chocolate, if desired. Chill for 1–2 hours, or until serving time.

123 calories per serving, 15 g carbohydrates, 2 g sugar, 5 g fiber, 12 g protein, 4 g fat (2 g saturated), 82 mg sodium, 413 mg potassium

NORENE'S NOTES:

- **Doubly delicious:** Some brands of silken tofu come in a 12-oz (340 g) package, but not to worry! Use 2 packages and make 1½ times the recipe.

- **Smooth as silk:** Silken tofu is dairy-free, cholesterol-free, and silky smooth. It provides a wonderful creamy texture that's creamier than cream itself! You can use it instead of whipped cream or whipped topping in desserts.

DR. ED SAYS:

- **Tofu (bean curd):** The difference between firm and extra-firm tofu is that extra-firm tofu has a slightly lower moisture content, with a correspondingly slightly higher nutrient density. Both, however, are a good-quality protein alternative to animal protein. Tofu is also very low in sugar and GI, and has significant quantities of important nutrients such as magnesium, zinc, manganese, and plant Omega-3 fat. The difficulty with tofu and soybeans in general is that they are

RECIPE CONTINUED . . .

CHOCOLATE MYSTERY MOUSSE (continued)

controversial from a health perspective. On the one hand, there is ample evidence showing that they can lower LDL cholesterol, and some data show that they may be useful in preventing cancer, diabetes, and heart disease. On the other hand, studies do exist showing that soy contains antinutrients such as phytates—which combine with minerals, thereby reducing their absorption—and protease inhibitors, which interfere with protein metabolism. Furthermore, in women with a family history of breast cancer, their phytoestrogen content could be a risk factor. Based on all the data, we believe the benefits of soy outweigh the potential health risks when eaten in moderation.

DID YOU KNOW? Tofu is produced in much the same way as cheese from milk: by curdling a water-based extract of soybeans with calcium or other curdling agents. The various methods used in processing tofu account for a large variation in its nutritional profile.

BERRY MANGO SHERBET

DAIRY | GLUTEN-FREE | PASSOVER | FREEZES WELL | MAKES 4
CUPS (1 L)

Keep frozen fruit on hand in your freezer so that you can make this guilt-free dessert in moments. It's "berry" refreshing—great for friends and family!

3 cups (750 mL) frozen strawberries, blueberries, and/or raspberries

1 cup (250 mL) frozen mango chunks

Sweetener equivalent to ¼ cup (60 mL) sugar

1 cup (250 mL) Greek or plain yogurt (skim or 1%)

1. In a food processor fitted with the steel blade, process frozen berries, mango, and sweetener with several quick on/off pulses. Continue processing until the mixture is the texture of snow.

2. Add yogurt and process until very smooth, scraping down the sides of the bowl as needed.

3. Serve immediately in parfait glasses or transfer to a bowl, cover, and freeze.

4. About 30 minutes before serving, remove from freezer and place in the refrigerator to soften. Scoop into parfait or wine glasses and serve.

69 calories per ½-cup (160 mL) serving, 13 g carbohydrates, 8 g sugar, 2 g fiber, 4 g protein, 0 g fat (0 g saturated), 15 mg sodium, 209 mg potassium

NORENE'S NOTES:

- **Mix it up!** Create different flavors by using a total of 4 cups (1 L) frozen mixed fruit.

- **Dessert for one:** To make a small batch, combine 1 cup (250 mL) frozen fruit, sweetener equivalent to 1 Tbsp (15 mL) sugar, and ¼ cup (60 mL) Greek yogurt in a mini prep. Process until puréed.

DR. ED SAYS:

- **Mango** is one of the highest sugar-containing fruits, at 83% by dry weight. Its main nutritional components are vitamins C and B6 and folate. Generally, this fruit should be eaten in moderation.

- **Overall,** this recipe is similar to the recipe for Berry Fool (p. 580) in nutrient quality, except for the high sugar contributed by the mango.

RECIPE CONTINUED . . .

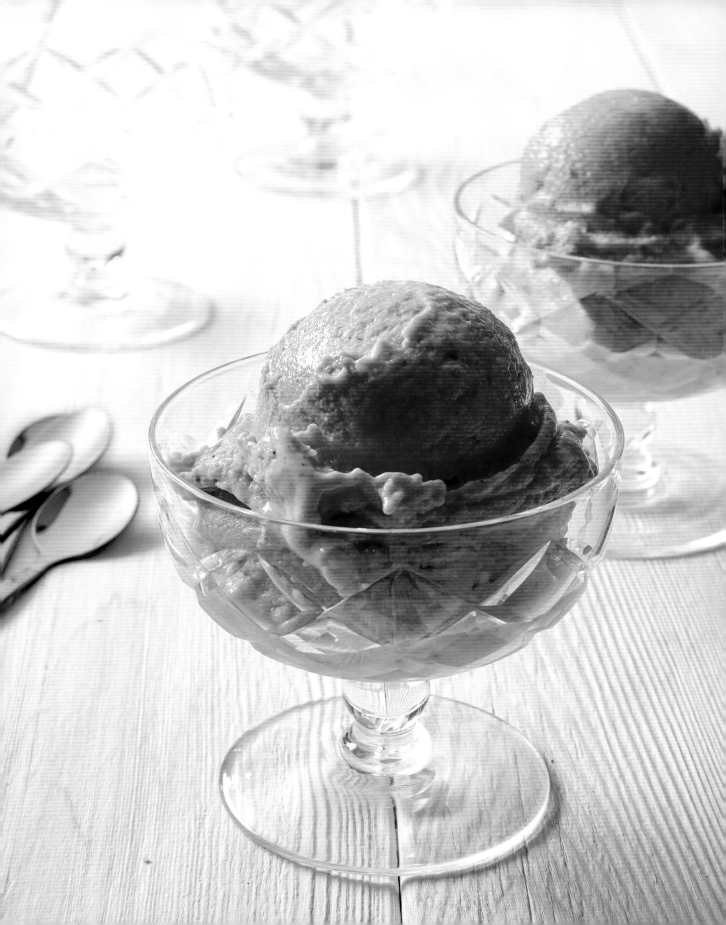

BERRY MANGO SHERBET (continued)

DID YOU KNOW? Mangoes have been used in Southeast Asia for thousands of years and are one of the most cultivated fruits in the region, probably because of their sweet taste. What is interesting about this fruit is that even though it has a very high sugar content and relatively low fiber content, it has a reasonable glycemic index. This is probably due to the fact that a significant part of the sugar content is in the form of fructose, which has a very low blood sugar response. Nevertheless, fructose is not considered healthy.

BERRY FOOL

DAIRY | GLUTEN-FREE | PASSOVER | DO NOT FREEZE | MAKES 4 SERVINGS

3 cups (750 mL) strawberries, raspberries, or blackberries, divided

2 cups (500 mL) plain Greek yogurt (skim or 1%)

Sweetener equivalent to ¼ cup (60 mL) sugar

Although this calcium-packed dessert tastes decadent, you can enjoy it guilt-free—no fooling! Feel free to use any ripe, soft-textured berries, or fruit such as peaches, nectarines, or kiwis.

1. Set aside 1 cup (250 mL) berries. (If using strawberries, thinly slice 1 cup/250 mL and set them aside.)

2. In a food processor fitted with the steel blade, process the remaining berries until puréed, about 15–20 seconds. Add yogurt and sweetener. Process with several quick on/off pulses, just until combined.

3. Pour half the mixture into 4 parfait glasses, then top with half the reserved berries. Repeat with the remaining mixture and berries. Chill for at least 1–2 hours before serving.

107 calories per serving, 14 g carbohydrates, 9 g sugar, 2 g fiber, 12 g protein, 1 g fat (0 g saturated), 42 mg sodium, 324 mg potassium

NORENE'S NOTES:

- **Make-your-own greek yogurt:** Line a fine-mesh strainer with a paper coffee filter, paper towel, or cheesecloth. Place the strainer over a bowl. Spoon 3 cups (750 mL) plain yogurt (skim or 1%, without gelatin or stabilizers) into the lined strainer. Cover and refrigerate for 2-3 hours. You will have 2 cups (500 mL) Greek yogurt plus 1 cup (250 mL) whey. If the strained yogurt is too firm, just stir some of the drained liquid back in. (Use drained whey in muffins, smoothies, and quick breads. It keeps for about 2 weeks in the refrigerator.)

DR. ED SAYS:

- **Greek yogurt** is a good choice for a dessert ingredient. Although it does have some lactose, which is a milk sugar, it does not raise blood sugar significantly and has a low glycemic index and glycemic load. In addition to its high protein content and contribution of vitamin B12, it also contains active probiotics for a healthy gut.

- **Berries:** The choice of berries in this recipe is an excellent one because they have been found to be one of the key ingredients in the Mediterranean, MIND, and Brain Boosting diets that can help reduce the risk of AD/dementia. They also have lower sugar than other fruits, and therefore do not raise blood sugar as much.

- **Overall,** this is a great recipe because of its relatively low blood sugar impact, probiotics, and the inclusion of berries. It's about as good as a dessert can get nutritionally. Each serving also provides vitamins E, B12, and B6 and folate, as well as magnesium and zinc.

> **DID YOU KNOW?** A significant part of our immune system resides in the gut, and the type of bacteria that reside there can affect inflammatory response. Inflammation, in turn, is thought to be a risk factor for cognitive decline, and probiotics may help in controlling this inflammatory response.

MAPLE BALSAMIC STRAWBERRIES

PAREVE | PASSOVER | DO NOT FREEZE | MAKES 4½ CUPS (1.12 L)

4 cups (1 L) sliced strawberries

1–2 Tbsp (15–30 mL) balsamic vinegar

1–2 Tbsp (15–30 mL) maple syrup

This is a beautiful blend of flavors. Berry good!

1. Combine strawberries with balsamic vinegar and maple syrup in a medium bowl and mix gently.

2. Cover and refrigerate for at least 1 hour before serving (the longer they marinate, the better they taste). Serve chilled in stemmed wine glasses.

42 calories per ¾-cup (185 mL) serving, 10 g carbohydrates, 7 g sugar, 2 g fiber, 1 g protein, 0 g fat (0 g saturated), 2 mg sodium, 157 mg potassium

NORENE'S NOTES:

- **A different twist!** Add a grinding or two of black pepper to add a kick!

- **Passover variation:** Use a brand of maple syrup that has been certified for Passover. Alternatively, substitute honey or a sugar substitute for maple syrup.

DR. ED SAYS:

- **Strawberries** are the major ingredient in this recipe. Strawberries were studied in research showing the effects of berries on AD/dementia, so this recipe is great for the Mediterranean, MIND, or Brain Boosting diets.

- **Overall,** this recipe is great because it fits in well with diet plans shown to reduce the risk of AD/dementia and reduce cognitive decline. It contains high amounts of vitamin C, fiber, and antioxidants. The sugar level per serving is somewhat high, but its impact is reduced by the fiber, acidity, and fructose content, which have a low glycemic response. Using a commercially available sugar-free syrup will help significantly reduce the sugar content.

DID YOU KNOW? The top four fruits for total antioxidant capacity are all berries. Strawberries are just below cranberries, blackberries, and raspberries on the list, and vitamin C is an important contributor to these antioxidant levels.

Acknowledgments and Dedication by Norene Gilletz

We are so proud of our book, *The Brain Boosting Diet: Feed Your Memory*! Our gratitude and appreciation go out to the incredible team of people who generously contributed their knowledge, time, and treasured recipes that we modified as needed to fit into a brain-healthy lifestyle.

Dr. Edward Wein, my co-author, was my teacher and guide in selecting the ingredients that starred in the recipes for this book. He taught me the science behind the recipes, and I taught him that no matter how healthy a recipe is, it has to taste good or no one will eat it!

Thanks to Sharon Fitzhenry, our publisher, for seeing the potential in this book and the importance of its message. Patrick Geraghty, we appreciate your fastidious editing of our massive manuscript. To the Whitecap team for their professional expertise, guidance, and patience—we gave you a lot to digest, literally. Nick Rundall, former publisher at Whitecap, provided guidance and encouragement during the initial stages.

Stephanie Von Hirschberg, our publishing consultant, once again stepped up to the plate and provided her wisdom and support.

Sharona Abramovitch, RD, provided us with the nutritional analyses for the recipes in this book. Her numbers kept us on track, making sure we kept the flavor while keeping carbs and added sugars within reason.

A huge "thank you" goes to Renée Owieczka-Colton for sharing her time, energy, and commitment for this important project. Her organizational skills raised it to new heights. She was dedicated, fastidious, and passionate, helping with everything from recipe testing to keeping me focused and on track. Her fingers on the keyboard were often ahead of my brain as we worked together in synchronicity.

Shirley Millett has run my office efficiently for 20+ years. She proofread recipes, offered helpful suggestions, and her eagle eye caught many tiny errors or inconsistencies that we had missed.

Marilyn Glick recipe-tested over the miles and was always honest when a recipe didn't measure up to my guiding principal: "Food that's good for you should taste good."

Abe Wornovitzky, our photographer, provided his artistic eye and creative talent to bring food to life through the magic of his camera.

Special thanks to our families and friends for their encouragement and support behind the scenes.

To my children, Jodi and Paul Sprackman, Steven and Cheryl Gilletz, Doug and Ariane Gilletz, and my grandchildren, Lauren, Camille, Max, Sam, and

Zak—your phone calls, visits, and messages were always a breath of fresh air. To my sister Rhonda Matias and her family, thanks for your love and support. My devoted dog, Maizie, who was my chief taster and always preferred "people food" to dog food.

To my fabulous friends: Elaine Kaplan, who was there when this journey began, and who helped shape the book proposal. Helene Medjuck, Tolsa Greenberg, and Cindy Beer provided continued encouragement and a listening ear. From grocery shopping to sharing special celebrations and everything in between, they're my sisters from other mothers! Thanks to Shim and Vivian Felsen for introducing me to Ed and Anita Wein. Cheryl and Len Goldberg included me in their Friday night dinners when I was too tired to cook. The recipes in this book were inspired by you, my loyal readers, friends, and fans, including the 8600+ members of my Facebook group, Norene's Kitchen! and my dedicated admins, especially Carol Press and Lisa Neuman, who watched over my virtual kitchen while I was writing this book. Thank you one and all for your continued support during my 50+ year culinary career.

This book is dedicated to my late parents, Max and Belle Rykiss, especially my mother, who was my first cooking teacher and has always been my culinary inspiration. She taught me that homemade is always best!

Acknowledgments and Dedication by Dr. Ed Wein

Norene has done a wonderful job of acknowledging the great team that was involved with this book and I am in wholehearted agreement with what she has said. She is the first person I wish to acknowledge because she introduced me to the magic world of recipe creation and taught me that, although health may be number one, taste is an important number two. There are, however, some other behind-the-scenes participants who have contributed significantly to the completion of this book.

First, I would like to thank my wife, friend, and companion, Anita, who is a voracious reader and understands grammar, vocabulary, and syntax much better than I ever will. She helped bring me down to earth and made the science part of the book much more readable.

Secondly, I would like to thank my friend and associate, Paul Bendheim, MD, Clinical Professor of Neurology at the University of Arizona, who kindly shared with me his extensive knowledge of Alzheimer's disease and dementia, and with whom I have had many fascinating discussions on the role of nutrition in maintaining memory and cognition.

I would like to thank Dr. Paul for graciously agreeing to write the foreword to this book and for many helpful and relevant suggestions in his review of our writing.

I also want to recognize the role of family and friends who supported me in the long haul of completing the book. My caring sons Kevin and David, my sister Linda, my sister-in-law Mindy, and my friends, Vivian and Shim Felsen, who introduced me to Norene.

Finally, I would like to thank my grandchildren, Eden, Dalia, and Noa, who are always a joy to be with, and who keep me young at heart.

I would like to dedicate the book to my parents, Karl and Minnie, who were responsible for instilling in me the value of education and never ceased impressing me with its importance, especially when I was distracted by other life experiences.

APPENDIX 1

Seafood is the major source of the best Omega-3 fatty acids for the brain, EPA and DHA. However, EPA and DHA are not uniformly distributed in fish species. Generally speaking, the more fat a fish contains and the darker the flesh, the higher the Omega-3 content of EPA and DHA. Thus, fish such as herring, sardines, salmon, and mackerel will have higher concentrations of EPA and DHA than less-fatty fish such as cod, sole, or pollock. Below, we have summarized the content of EPA and DHA in various fish species. Recommended intake by government authorities varies in a range from 250 to 1000 mg per day, though for cognitive maintenance we recommend at least 1000 mg per day. The highest concentrations of EPA and DHA in terms of grams per serving are in caviar (5.6 g), cooked fish roe (2.6 g), herring (1.8 g), anchovies canned in oil (1.8 g), and cooked, farmed Atlantic salmon (1.8 g) and American shad (2 g).

Table A1. Omega-3 content in selected seafood.

EPA+DHA per 90-g Serving	Fish Species
>1000 mg	Caviar (red and black)
	Fish roe
	American shad
	Herring (Atlantic)
	Salmon
	Anchovy
	Mackerel (Pacific, jack, and Atlantic)
	Tuna (bluefin)
	Whitefish

(CONTINUED NEXT PAGE)

Table A1. Omega-3 content in selected seafood. (CONTINUED)

EPA+DHA per 90-g Serving	Fish Species
500–1000 mg	Sardines (Atlantic, canned)
	Trout (rainbow)
	Tuna (canned in water)
	Swordfish
	Shark
	Mussels
	Sea bass and striped bass
	Bluefish
<500 mg	Crustaceans
	Turbot
	Carp
	Catfish
	Cod
	Haddock
	Halibut
	Tuna (skipjack and light, canned)

Source: health.gov/dietaryguidelines/dga2005/report/HTML/table_g2_adda2.htm: Go to this site for more detailed list.

APPENDIX 2

There is some variation between the US and Canada on what constitutes a serving size, but these tend to be minimal. Where different, Canadian values are shown in brackets.

Table A2. Serving size calculator.

Food Type	Example of Serving Size	Size of
Grains	1 slice bread	Hand
	1 oz (30 g) dry cereal	Fist
	½ cup (125 mL) cooked rice, pasta, or cereal	Small baseball or half fist
Vegetables	1 cup (250 mL) raw leafy vegetables	Small fist
	½ cup (125 mL) cut-up raw or cooked vegetables	Half fist
	½ cup (125 mL) vegetable juice	Half fist
Fruit	1 medium fruit	Small baseball or half fist
	¼ cup (60 mL) dried fruit	Cupped Hand
	½ cup (125 mL) fresh, frozen, or canned fruit	Half fist
Dairy	1 cup (250 mL) milk	Fist
	1 cup (250 mL) yogurt	Fist
	1½ oz (45 g) cheese	Six stacked dice or two thumbs

(CONTINUED NEXT PAGE)

Table A2. Serving size calculator. (CONTINUED)

Food Type	Example of Serving Size	Size of
Lean meats, poultry, and seafood	3 oz (90 g) cooked meat	Computer mouse or palm of hand
	3 oz (90 g) grilled fish (CAN: 2½ oz/75 g)	About the size of a check book or palm of hand
	3 oz (90 g) cooked meat	Computer mouse or palm of hand
Fats and oils	1 tsp (5 mL) soft margarine	Thumb tip
	1 Tbsp (15 mL) mayonnaise	Thumb
	1 tsp (5 mL) vegetable oil	Thumb tip
	1 Tbsp (15 mL) regular salad dressing	Thumb
Nuts, seeds, and legumes	⅓ cup (80 mL) or 1½ oz (45 g) nuts (CAN: ¼ cup/60 mL)	One-third of a fist (cupped hand)
	2 Tbsp (30 mL) peanut butter	Two thumbs
	2 Tbsp (30 mL) or ½ oz (15 g) seeds	Two thumbs
	½ cup (125 mL) dry beans or ¾ cup (185 mL) peas	Half fist (Fist)
Sweets and added sugars*	1 Tbsp (15 mL) sugar	Thumb
	1 Tbsp (15 mL) jelly or jam	Thumb
	½ cup (125 mL) sorbet or ices	Half fist

Source: American Heart Association and EatRight Ontario
*Limit baked goods, candies, and salty snack portions to as small as you can.

APPENDIX 3

Table A3.1. Imperial/metric pan equivalents.

Pan*	Metric Measure	Capacity
8- × 8- × 2-inch (square) pan	20 × 20 × 5 cm	2 L (8 cups)
9- × 9- × 2-inch (square) pan	23 × 23 × 5 cm	2.5 L (10 cups)
9- × 5- × 3-inch loaf pan	23 × 13 × 6 cm	2 L (8 cups)
10- × 3½-inch fluted tube/Bundt pan	25 × 9 cm	3 L (12 cups)
10- × 4-inch tube pan	25 × 10 cm	4 L (16 cups)
8- × 2-inch round layer pan	20 × 5 cm	1.5 L (6 cups)
9- × 2-inch round layer pan	23 × 5 cm	2 L (8 cups)
7- × 11- × 2-inch glass baking dish	18 × 28 × 5 cm	2 L (8 cups)
9- × 13- × 2-inch glass baking dish	22 × 33 × 5 cm	3.5 L (15 cups)
9-inch pie plate	23 cm	1 L (4 cups)
10- × 15- × 1-inch cookie sheet	25 × 38 × 2.5 cm	2.5 L (10 cups)
9-inch springform pan	23 cm	2.5 L (10 cups)
10-inch springform pan	25 cm	3 L (12 cups)
5-quart casserole dish	47 × 32 cm	5.7 L (23 cups)

*Note that to prevent sticking, you should use a nonstick spray made of canola oil to spray pans lightly. When baking in glass or dark baking pans, reduce temperatures by 25°F (10°C).

Table A3.2. Imperial/metric measurement equivalents.

Inches	Cm
⅛ inch	0.3 cm
¼ inch	0.6 cm
½ inch	1.2 cm
1 inch	2.5 cm
4 inches	10 cm
6 inches	15 cm
12 inches	30 cm

Table A3.3. Imperial/metric temperature conversions.

°F	°C	Comment
0°F	–18°C	Freezer temperature
32°F	0°C	Water freezes
40°F	4°C	Refrigerator temperature
68°F	20°C	Room temperature
105–115°F	41–46°C	Water temperature to proof yeast
212°F	100°C	Water boils

To convert from °F to °C: (# of °F minus 32) divided by 1.8 = # of °C.
To convert from °C to °F: (# of °C multiplied by 1.8) plus 32 = # of °F.

Table A3.4. Oven temperatures.

°F	°C
250°F	120°C
275°F	135°C
300°F	150°C
325°F	160°C
350°F	175°C
375°F	190°C
400°F	200°C
425°F	220°C
450°F	230°C
475°F	240°C
500°F	260°C

MEASUREMENTS FOR VOLUME AND WEIGHT

Quick Conversions (approx.)

TO OUNCES: Drop the last digit from the number of milliliters (mL) or grams (g) and divide by 3. For example, 156 mL is about 5 oz (15 divided by 3 equals 5).

TO MILLILITERS OR GRAMS: Multiply the number of ounces by 30. For example, 1 ounce is about 30 mL or grams.

Table A3.5. Approximate imperial/metric equivalents (volume).

Imperial	Metric
¼ tsp	1 mL
½ tsp	2 mL
1 tsp	5 mL
1 Tbsp	15 mL
2 Tbsp	25 mL
¼ cup	50 mL
⅓ cup	80 mL
½ cup	125 mL
¾ cup	185 mL
1 cup	250 mL
4 cups	1 L

Table A3.6. Approximate imperial/metric equivalents (weight).

Imperial	Metric
1 oz	30 g (actual is 28.4 g)
2 oz	60 g
3 oz	85 g
3½ oz	100 g
½ lb	250 g (actual is 227 g)
¾ lb	375 g
1 lb	500 g (actual is 454 g)
2 generous lb	1 kg

Table A3.7. Packaging equivalents (common can/bottle sizes).

Imperial	Metric
3 oz	85 g
5½ oz	156 g
7½ oz	213 g
8 oz	227 g
8.8 oz	250 g
10 oz	284 g
12 oz	340 g
14 oz	398 g
16 oz	454 g
17.6 oz	500 g
19 oz	540 g
28 oz	796 g
35.2 oz	1 kg
48 oz	1.36 kg

Table A3.8. Equivalents for ingredients.

Weight (Metric)	Volume	Weight (Imperial)
Butter, Margarine		
115 g	½ cup	¼ lb
250 g	1 generous cup	½ lb
Cheeses, Hard		
125 g	1 cup grated	¼ lb/4 oz
227–250 g	2 cups grated	½ lb/8 oz
Cheeses, Soft (Cottage/Ricotta/Cream Cheese)		
125 g	½ cup	¼ lb/4 oz
227–235 g	1 cup	½ lb/8 oz
454–500 g	2 cups	1 lb/16 oz
Chocolate, Chocolate Chips, Cocoa		
30 g	¼ cup grated chocolate	1 oz (1 square)
175 g	1 cup chocolate chips	6 oz
110 g	1 cup cocoa	3¾ oz
Cream, Milk, Sour Cream, Yogurt		
227–250 mL/g	1 cup	8 oz
454–500 mL/g	2 cups	16 oz
1 L	About 4 cups	35.2 oz
Dried Fruits, Nuts		
150 g	1 cup dates, raisins	5¼ oz
115 g	1 cup chopped walnuts	4 oz
110 g	1 cup ground almonds	3¾ oz

(CONTINUED NEXT PAGE)

Table A3.8. Equivalents for ingredients. (CONTINUED)

Weight (Metric)	Volume		Weight (Imperial)
Fish/Meat/Poultry, Fruits/Vegetables (Fresh)			
227–250 g	½ lb		
454–500 g	1 lb		
1 kg	2.2 lb		
1.5 kg	3½ lb (an average chicken)		
5 kg	11 lb (an average turkey)		
Fruits and Vegetables (Frozen)			
300 g	10-oz pkg		
454–500 g	16-oz pkg (1 lb)		
1 kg	2.2 lb		
Flour, Cornstarch, Crumbs, Cereal			
145 g	1 cup all-purpose flour		5 oz
125 g	1 cup cornstarch		4½ oz
110 g	1 cup cookie crumbs		3¾ oz
125 g	1 cup dried bread crumbs		4½ oz
90 g	1 cup oats		3¼ oz
Pasta, Grains, Dried Beans			
200 g	1 cup split peas, lentils, rice		
235 g	8-oz pkg		
375 g	12-oz pkg		
454–500 g	16-oz pkg (1 lb)		
1 kg	2.2 lb		
Sugar, Honey			
200 g	1 cup sugar		7¾ oz
170 g	1 cup packed brown sugar		6 oz
150 g	1 cup icing sugar		5 oz
340 g	1 cup honey		12 oz

NUTRITION FACTS TABLES

Nutrition Facts labeling is extremely useful in helping you decide which foods to choose and how much of each to eat. US and Canadian Nutrition Facts tables are in the process of changing, and both the current and upcoming labels are presented in this appendix. New labels for both countries will be enforced in 2021.

Figure A1. US Nutrition Facts table examples.*

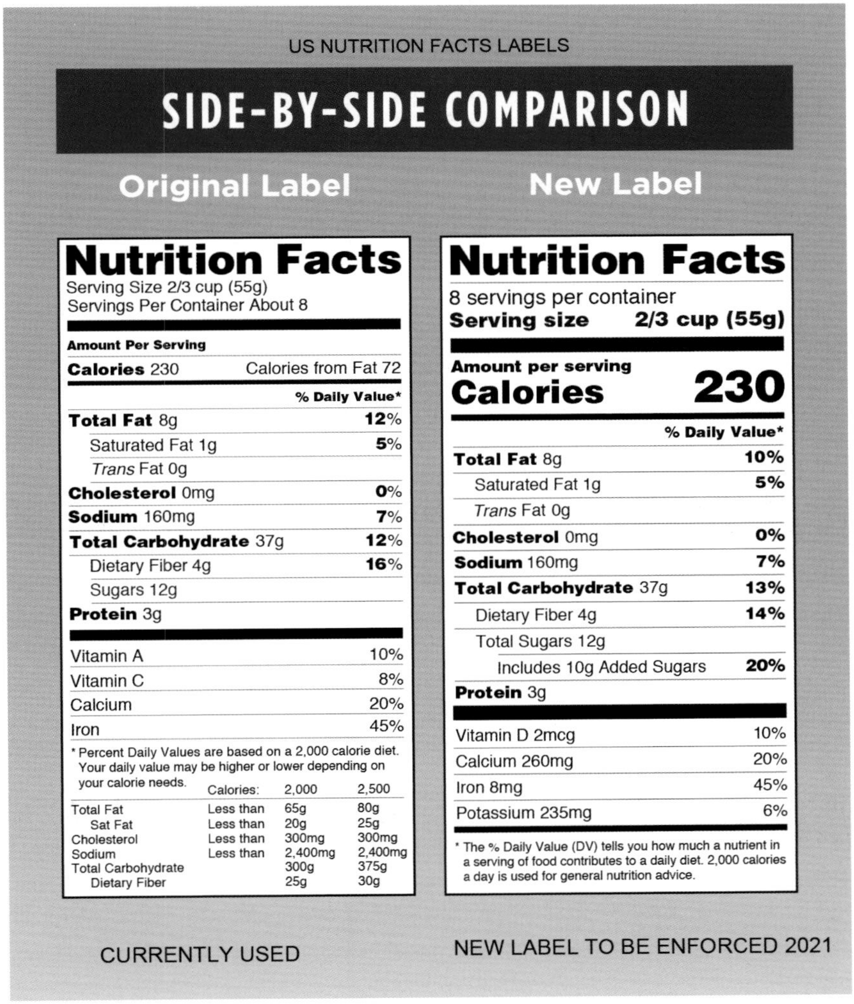

Source: FDA.

* Canadian Nutrition Facts table is available on p. 42.

The new table will have more information available, which will enable you to make wiser food choices:

- Total and added sugars will be listed instead of just total sugars. Shoot for a maximum of 6 g total sugar per 100 g of food, and choose foods that have the lowest added sugar.
- Actual quantities of contained nutrients will be listed, so you don't have to make calculations from the daily values. Potassium levels per serving should be at least 1–1½ times the sodium levels.
- Subtract the dietary fiber number from the total carbohydrates to get an estimate of the amount of digestible carbs you are consuming.
- Keep in mind the calories per serving you are consuming so that you can control your portion size.
- Keep in mind the saturated fat content per serving so you can control your intake and ensure it does not exceed the daily value.

INDEX

NOTE : Recipes have been indicated with an (R) – e.g., Florentine Cupcakes (R), 150-51